DIAGNOSING DESIRE

ABNORMATIVITIES: QUEER/GENDER/EMBODIMENT
Scott Herring, Series Editor

Diagnosing Desire

Biopolitics and Femininity into
the Twenty-First Century

Alyson K. Spurgas

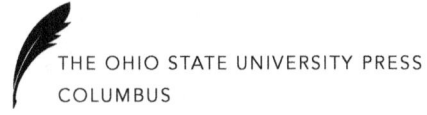
THE OHIO STATE UNIVERSITY PRESS
COLUMBUS

Copyright © 2020 by The Ohio State University.
All rights reserved.

Library of Congress Cataloging-in-Publication Data
Names: Spurgas, Alyson K., 1981– author.
Title: Diagnosing desire : biopolitics and femininity into the twenty-first century / Alyson K. Spurgas.
Other titles: Abnormativities: queer/gender/embodiment.
Description: Columbus : The Ohio State University Press, [2020] | Series: Abnormativities: queer/gender/embodiment | Includes bibliographical references and index. | Summary: "Examines how low female desire is produced, embedded, and lived within neoliberal capitalism. Rethinks 'femininity' by investigating sex research that measures the disconnect between subjective and genital female arousal, contemporary psychiatric diagnoses for low female desire, and new models for understanding women's sexual response"—Provided by publisher.
Identifiers: LCCN 2020022197 | ISBN 9780814214510 (cloth) | ISBN 0814214517 (cloth) | ISBN 9780814280751 (ebook) | ISBN 0814280757 (ebook)
Subjects: LCSH: Sexual desire disorders. | Women—Sexual behavior. | Femininity. | Sex therapy.
Classification: LCC HQ29 .S68 2020 | DDC 306.7082—dc23
LC record available at https://lccn.loc.gov/2020022197

Cover design by Regina Starace
Text design by Juliet Williams
Type set in Adobe Minion Pro

CONTENTS

Acknowledgments   vii

INTRODUCTION	Diagnosing Gender through Desire: How You Know You're in Bed with a Woman	1
CHAPTER 1	Sexual Difference and Femininity in Sex Therapy and Sex Research: Examples from the Nineteenth, Twentieth, and Twenty-First Centuries	29
CHAPTER 2	Interest, Arousal, and Motivation in Contemporary Sexology: The Feminization of Responsive Desire	63
CHAPTER 3	Women-with-Low-Desire: Navigating and Negotiating Sexual Difference Socialization	107
CHAPTER 4	Embodied Invisible Labor, Sexual Carework: The Cultural Logic and Affective Valorization of Responsive Female Desire	148
CHAPTER 5	Reclaiming Receptivity: Parasexual Pleasure in the Face of Compulsory and Feminized Trauma	184
CONCLUSION	The Freedom to Fall Apart: Feminine Fracturing and the Affective Production of Gendered Populations	221

Appendix	235
References	239
Index	263

ACKNOWLEDGMENTS

This book was conceived during my (first) time living in Brooklyn, from 2006 to 2014, and it owes much to the trials and tribulations of those deeply important years of my life. Symone, who has now passed on, was with me for the majority of this project, and her interspecies love got me through the best and worst times. And Kim Bernstein—thank you for knowing me better than anyone.

At the City University of New York, Victoria Pitts-Taylor, Patricia Ticineto Clough, and Barbara Katz Rothman were fundamental in guiding this work and provided excellent feedback on the earliest drafts. Thanks also to Deb Tolman and Michelle Fine for their time and intellectual insight. Members of the NeuroCultures Seminar and the Mellon Committee for Interdisciplinary Science Studies also helped contour this project, and I'd like to thank Jason Tougaw, Rachel Liebert, and Kim Cunningham, in particular. I made some of the best friends ever while at CUNY and I'm honored to have Amanda Matles, Patrick Sweeney, Emma Francis Snyder, Shay Thompson, Ali Lara, SAJ Jones, Chris Sula, John Andrews, Zoë Meleo-Erwin, Kate Jenkins, Sandra Trappen, Marnie Brady, Valerie Francisco-Menchavez, Dominique Nisperos, Jesse Goldstein, David Spataro, Steve McFarland, John Boy, Justin Myers, Colin Ashley, Josh Scannell, Jesse Schwartz, Jeremy Rayner, John Gergely, and Natalie Havlin—among too many others to name—as comrades, collaborators, and intellectual interlocutors. I love you all forever, and especially C. Ray Borck, who has really been there since the beginning of all of this.

Upon moving to St. Louis and Southern Illinois University (SIUE), I was lucky enough to be connected to Cynthia Barounis before I even got to the Midwest (thank you Linda Nicholson via Patricia Clough for that life-changing introduction!). Cynthia is a seriously amazing friend and one of the most intellectually generous people I've ever known. Thank you, Cynthia, for helping me develop so many of the ideas in this book.

I am thankful for conversations at Washington University I had in St. Louis in late 2014, and specifically to Linda Nicholson for the opportunity to engage, and to Amber Musser for insightful feedback. My colleagues and students at SIUE were of the utmost support during that time in my life, and I'd like to thank the awesome faculty in the Sociology Department, including Flo Maätita, Kiana Cox, Sandra Weissinger, Connie Frey Spurlock, Dave Kauzlarich, Linda Markowitz, Mark Hedley, Liz Stygar, Megan Arnett, and Marv Finkelstein. Folks in Philosophy and Women's Studies at SIUE have also been wonderful friends and interlocutors—Alison Reiheld, Saba Fatima, and Richard Fry stand out as some of the people I relied on most to help me think through these ideas. Debbie Nelson, Abbie Hall, and Hayden Treadway are amazingly brilliant and I'm so lucky to have had you all as students and now as friends.

Also in St. Louis, this project benefited immensely from the super-smart and deeply ethical sensibilities of Stephen Inman and Baylee, both of whom will always have a big piece of my heart and whose imprints on this project are huge. Allison Kirschbaum, Sarah Lacy, Jenny Johnson, Jae Shepherd, and Les Stitt have been incredible sources of support, sustenance, and radical connection.

When I started at Trinity College and moved back to Brooklyn/Hartford in 2017, I found myself surrounded by amazing folks in both New York and Connecticut. Thanks to Laurel Mei-Singh for excellent feedback in our mini-writing group that fall, and thanks to other writing group friends and interlocutors at Trinity for encouraging me to further flesh out the race and class analyses in the conclusion—including Shunyuan Zhang, Karen Buenavista Hanna, Julie Gamble, and Gabriella Soto. Thanks especially to Justin Fifield for being a great friend and collaborator and for reading so much of my work over the last few years. The final stages of this project benefitted immensely from the support of my colleagues in Sociology and Women's, Gender, and Sexuality Studies at Trinity—so a big thanks to Johnny Eric Williams, Steve Valocchi, Xiangming Chen, Tanetta Anderson, Dan Douglas, Diana Paulin, Janet Bauer, Zayde Antrim, Kifah Hanna, and Rob Corber. My students, teaching assistants, and advisees at Trinity have inspired me immensely—including Tiana Starks, Sam McCarthy, Lindsay Pressman, Caitlin Southwick, Victoria Guardino, Gwen Sadie, Rocio Fernandez Gutierrez, Keji Oladinni, Lucemy

Perez, Simran Subramaniam, Anne Valbrune, Felicia McDevitt, Jyles Romer, Jederick Estrella, Jason Farrell, Eddie Hayes, Giovanni Jones, Zorawar Singh, Alex Gnassi, and Jake McBride, among many others. I am grateful to Stefanie Chambers, Isaac Kamola, Serena Laws, Emily Cummins, Kari Theurer, Josh King, and Mark Stater for their steadfast support and invaluable friendship since I arrived at Trinity.

Thanks to Taylor & Francis for publishing my article, "Interest, Arousal, and Shifting Diagnoses of Female Sexual Dysfunction, or: How Women Learn about Desire," in *Studies in Gender and Sexuality* in 2013, now revised as chapter 2 of this book. And many thanks to Scott Herring and Tara Cyphers at The Ohio State University Press for their faith in this project.

Many other folks from all walks of my life have helped me through this process. My parents, Bob and Ellen Slagle, and my sister, Robyn Showanes, have always come through for me, and my niblings—Tenley, Elsa, and Teddy—inspire me every single day. Ari Meyer Brostoff is an amazing editor, co-conspirator, and friend and I am indebted to their sharp political insight, extensive intellectual and theoretical vocabulary, and uncanny ability to always help me say what I always wanted to say. Thanks to Lisa Jean Moore and Monica Casper for sharing thoughts on an earlier draft of this manuscript, in addition to several anonymous reviewers of various articles, chapters, and other pieces of this project. Other folks who have offered generous feedback and support through different stages of this process, and with whom I am deeply grateful to be in dialogue, include Christine Labuski, Alain Giami, Georgiann Davis, Livi Faro, Robin West, Katherine Rowland, Holly Laws, Jenny Vilchez, Bhakti Shringarpure, K. J. Cerankowski, Theodora Danylevich, Alyson Patsavas, Robert McRuer, Morgan Holmes, Katie Gentile, Peggy Kleinplatz, and the late Muriel Dimen. None of this would have been possible without Kelly Roberts, who has seen me through this project and life and is a true best friend, and Christian Rutledge, who is the best partner I could have ever hoped to love and fight alongside. Thank you, Christian, for reading every word of this book so many times in all its different permutations and for talking me through it when I was in every single possible mood at once.

And, finally: Thanks to everyone who spoke with me in the interviews for this book. All the folks I interviewed about sex, desire, and power were so open, generous, and detailed with their time and stories; I hope I did you all justice with the final analysis. And to the clinicians, therapists, researchers, and activists I interviewed and whose work I have been closely following for years now: Even though we don't agree on everything, I am awed by your own strength and spirit and I am proud to be in conversation with such smart and powerful women.

INTRODUCTION

Diagnosing Gender through Desire
How You Know You're in Bed with a Woman

In 2009, popular writer Daniel Bergner published two articles on the complexities of female sexuality and desire in the *New York Times Magazine*. The first, published in January 2009, was titled "What Do Women Want?" and the second, published later that year, in November, "Women Who Want to Want." It was in these two popular pieces, over a decade ago now, that the seeds of this book were sown. Twenty-first-century women were apparently stricken with low desire, and their sexuality, their femininity, was a frontier to be explored. Bergner's articles described the new pioneers—the explorers were young, smart, ambitious, and energetic; they called themselves feminists. These new scientists were there to help women figure out what the problem was, why they weren't in the mood. It was upon reading these articles that I realized that what I now refer to as the "new" science of female sexuality was blossoming, and that it was going to be—already was—very big.

In the second of his two articles, Bergner points to both the ambiguous nature of female sexuality and to the ambiguously feminist nature of the driving force behind this new science: "More than by any other sexual problem—the elusiveness of orgasm, say, or pain during sex—women feel plagued by low desire." Many low-desiring women, however, *want to want*. He describes how, in her efforts to help these women, the Canadian sex researcher and clinician he interviews in the article, Lori Brotto, deals "in the domain of the mind, or in the mind's relationship to the body, not in a problem with the body itself." Bergner suggests that the ultimate therapeutic goal for clinicians like Brotto, then, might be to help women repair this estranged mind/body connection by suturing (physical) sensation and (subjective) sexual self-image, and cultivate their own desire, even in the face of what he calls "women's complex sexual beings." Questions of women's sexual complexity, responsiveness or receptivity, and how their minds and bodies line up (or, more often in these accounts, do not) seemed to be at the heart of this new science and its accompanying sexual response models and treatment protocols for low female desire. But how had it come to be that at the beginning of the twenty-first century, self-identified feminist sex researchers described women's sexuality as reactive, receptive, and responsive? Did these researchers believe, as these popular articles implied, that women's sexuality operated according to a completely different logic than men's sexuality? Why were women's sexual problems, no longer the result of hysteria or frigidity, still so confounding to scientists? And if, as these popular articles posited, women were so sexually complex, in many cases lacking an urgent sense of lust yet also demonstrating strong physiological arousal and a fluid responsiveness and receptivity—how did they get to be that way? Furthermore, how was the problem of women's low desire to be solved?

A few aspects of Bergner's articles, and others like it, jumped out at me. One was that the new science of female sexuality described desire from what we might call a behaviorist perspective. In this way of thinking about sex, human beings are almost robot-like organisms with instincts and drives. The desire for sex, in this framework, is sometimes understood as inextricable from the drive to reproduce, as one might expect given behaviorism's frequent pairing with evolutionary psychology. Even more to the point, though, the behaviorist perspective reduces desire to a cost-benefit analysis of what the organism is willing to seek out for sex—or more often, for women, what the organism will be receptive to. The idea is that, like Pavlov's dog, we learn (or are trained) to find certain stimuli desirable, weighing internal and external criteria to make rational, incentive-motivated, and reward-seeking decisions about whether or not to engage in sex. Particularly in the first decade of the twenty-first century, this cost-benefit analysis was often portrayed as being more complex for women than for men, in part because the related evolutionary psychology discourse views women as beholden to a maternal drive that complicates their sexuality and orients it toward finding a good mate. I came to identify behaviorism and evolutionary psychology as the twin foundations of several contemporary sexual response models that I will describe in this book. I also came to see that, in these models, desire, per se, wasn't part of the sexual equation. And this seemed to be especially true for women.

This absence of desire in the new science of female sexuality was jarring for me. For Freud, Lacan, all of the many queer, feminist, and postcolonial scholars that followed (and critiqued) them, desire was about aims, objects, fantasies, fetishes, power, and trauma. Desire was sexy, it was hot, sometimes it was ugly, shameful, and unspeakable, but it was never fully capturable or controllable; there was a *je ne sais quoi* that was indeed constitutive of it. It was sometimes differentiated along the lines of gender in these theories, but rarely reduced to evolutionary adaptations or machinelike rationality. For post-Freudian psychoanalytic thinkers like Laplanche (1976), there may be a mechanics or hydraulics to desire, a libidinal economy, but there was still a *wiliness* to it that couldn't be trained away—or conjured up—by any proverbial Skinner Box (the behaviorist black box trope of cognitive psychology and operant conditioning designed by founding father B. F. Skinner [1938]). If anything, as Jagose (2013) has pointed out regarding behaviorism and sexuality, whatever it is that cognitive conditioning models have tried to *do* to human sexuality, from the sensate focus techniques of Masters and Johnson in the 1960s to the erotic conversion therapy (including "orgasmic reconditioning") used on gay men in the same era, these models cannot account for desire's vicissitudes. There is always an excess, a part of desire that cannot be fully redirected, even if behaviors themselves can be changed. This is in part because, unlike most other human behaviors, *fantasy* is constitutive of sexuality in a way that suggests that desire—that fundamentally intersubjective and unrequited wanting or longing—is never reducible to behavior or motivation and can never be approximated or fully delimited.

Beyond the lack of attention to desire, another thing stood out to me about these popular articles and other discussions of the new science of female sexuality, including the research studies that I began to voraciously read. Many of these studies were deeply invested in making comparisons between the objective arousal of the body, as measured by a subject's physiological sexual response (determined by attaching machines to her genitals), and her subjective experience of arousal—the desire she experiences in her mind, abstracted into quantitative and behaviorist terms. These two measurements were increasingly taken in laboratories, and the gap between them was made to say a lot of things about gender (long story short: women have a much bigger gap). This seemingly new trend, what I have come to call *the work of the gap*, was all over the place in the scientific research and its popular interpretations. I learned that experiments that used arousal-measuring instruments were called volumetric studies, and that the use of these machines was called plethysmography (the machine for people with penises was sometimes called a penile strain gauge). In his first 2009 *New York Times Magazine* piece, for instance, Bergner describes the work of the Canadian experimental sex researcher Meredith Chivers. Chivers uses plethysmography to measure her subjects' physical arousal, then compares the results to the numbers these subjects record on an "arousometer," a tool for registering how turned on they feel. In many of these volumetric studies, cisgender men and cisgender women[1] are compared in terms of this gap.

The studies work something like this: A person sits down in a LaZBoy recliner, alone in a lab, and inserts a probe into their vagina (in more recent studies, measuring devices may also be attached to the labia or clitoris) or attaches one to their penis. They watch different films or other stimuli, maybe listen to an audio recording. Some films are considered neutral (like a documentary on lei-making in Hawai'i—true story), while some feature sexual content. The sexual stimuli include a variety of scenes and situations—men having sex with women, women having sex with women, men having sex with men, a naked man alone walking on a beach, a woman working out. Sometimes there are rape scenes. Sometimes there are animals having sex, like bonobos, overdubbed with loud ape sex noises. Across these studies, the common finding has been that cis men—both gay and straight—tend to have physiological and subjective experiences of arousal that line up with each other. They are "concordant." Cis women, on the other hand, particularly those attracted to cis men, tend to be physically aroused by everything, or at least any "relevant sexual stimuli," even when they report low levels of subjective desire via the arousometer. They are "discordant." In other words, women who are attracted to men have the biggest gap.

This was the cutting-edge research of the twenty-first century. I had spent many years in graduate school reading Freud, Foucault, Fanon, Butler, and many other bad guys, girls, and genderqueers of critical race and queer theory, cultural studies, psychoanalysis, and poststructuralist feminism, but I was way more shocked by the new science of female sexuality than I was reading about hysteria, wish fulfillment, and the repressive hypothesis. In the January 2009 article, Chivers tells Bergner that she hopes one day to develop a "scientifically supported model to explain female sexual response." Bergner writes:

---

1. In some cases, such as in a study conducted by Lawrence, Latty, Chivers, & Bailey (2005), the subjects are also transgender women, who are referred to as "male-to-female transsexuals" and are said to "display male-typical [sic] category-specific sexual arousal" (p. 135). The potentially violent cisnormativity and heternormativity inherent in the methodology of studies like this—particularly those conducted in the first decade of the twenty-first century—is a theme I will interrogate throughout this book. See chapter 2 especially for more on the construction of "category-specificity" in terms of genital sexual response.

When she peers into the giant forest, Chivers told me, she considers the possibility that along with what she called a "rudderless" system of reflexive physiological arousal, women's system of desire, the cognitive domain of lust, is more receptive than aggressive. "One of the things I think about," she said, "is the dyad formed by men and women. Certainly women are very sexual and have the capacity to be even more sexual than men, but one possibility is that instead of it being a go-out-there-and-get-it kind of sexuality, it's more of a reactive process. If you have this dyad, and one part is pumped full of testosterone, is more interested in risk taking, is probably more aggressive, you've got a very strong motivational force. It wouldn't make sense to have another similar force. You need something complementary. And I've often thought that there is something really powerful for women's sexuality about being desired. That receptivity element."

I read these words and saw the history of sexology flash before my eyes. I was immediately struck by how this idea of female reactivity, responsiveness, receptivity, that had been supposedly abandoned with all the other misogyny of the premodern sciences (including psychoanalysis, abandoned much to my dismay) had somehow been maintained in the twenty-first century. How were words like these being uttered by a feminist scientist in 2009? Why was this being discussed in the *New York Times Magazine*? What would the impact be? Then I read the comments. Of course, many people lauded the *Times* for publishing such an article. Others said this research diminished the variation across women's sexualities. And plenty said that the "gap" of female discordance identified in this research indicates that women are lying about what turns them on, or that they don't know the truth of their own desire. For instance, commenter "George" from Irvine says: "Undamaged, quality women want real men. They want the strength, protection, leadership, stability and commitment of a man who isn't afraid to express his masculinity. A man who understands that women are driven by their emotions, not necessarily by logic and reason, as the article well points out. When men understand this, they can have their way with women." Similarly, "David" from Boston tells us: "So, the conclusion among leading (female) sexologists is: Women are selfish narcissists who don't know what they really want, except that, underneath it all, what they really want is to be ravished against a wall in a dark alley by a stranger. Well! Any man could have already told you that!"

Beyond the retrograde nature of the scientists' words and the way they were being taken up by everyday misogynists, another thing that caught my attention in these articles was the focus on new ways for women to enhance their desire, including through sex therapy techniques that utilize cognitive behavioral methods and mindfulness. Although at the end of the first decade of the twenty-first century, plenty of antimedicalization feminists were focused on critiquing pharmaceutical interventions like Addyi for women, in the wake of the supreme success of Viagra for men (see the work of the New View Campaign[2] for the quintessential example of this anti–Big Pharma movement), I was more interested in what other sexual enhancement techniques were being developed and deployed. This was in keeping with my interest in the work of French theorist Michel Foucault and his notion of biopolitics (1978, 2000, 2003)—or the ways that our lives are governed, in late neoliberal capitalism, through technologies that don't so much discipline us as *make us live* in certain ways. Bergner underscores some of these new techniques and associated research in his second 2009 *Times* article. For instance, according to Bergner, while Brotto's "patients' genitals commonly pulse with blood in response to erotic images or their partners' sexual touch, their minds are so detached—distracted by work or children or worries about the way they look unclothed, or fixated on fears that their libidos are dead—as to be oblivious to their bodies' excitement, their bodies' messages." Mindfulness, by combining an attention to bodily sensations with the "power of positive thinking," allows women to cultivate a subjective sense of sexual arousal or "trains patients to immerse themselves in physical sensation"—that is, it trains them to work to bridge the mind/body gap. Through Bergner's interviews with Brotto and another Canadian sex researcher, Rosemary Basson, readers also learn about women's tendency toward "responsive" or "receptive" desire, and the formulation of a new "trigger-based" sexual response model. For women, Basson reports, "the start of plenty—and maybe the great majority—of sexual encounters is defined not by heat but by slight warmth or flat neutrality." This was the new "arousal-first" sexual response model for women, based on reactivity, receptivity, and *bridging the gap*: I will refer to it from now on as the *circular sexual response cycle*, as it is described in the literature. "Basson's lesson for women, which has been distilled by sex therapists into three words, 'desire follows arousal,' is a real rearrangement of expectation and a reweighting of sexual theory," Bergner wrote. But was it really so new? The idea that women lack free-flowing desire and require sexual activation (by men) seemed pretty old to me. Indeed, it appeared in some of the earliest sexological texts, including in those by Wilhelm Stekel, Havelock Ellis, and Richard von Krafft-Ebing.

The final thing that stood out to me as I read these articles over a decade ago was the way they discussed diagnoses for sexual dysfunctions, including low desire. In the second of his 2009 articles in the *Times,* Bergner raises questions surrounding the next incarnation of the *Diagnostic and Statistical*

---

2. Website: http://www.newviewcampaign.org/

Manual of Mental Disorders, or *DSM,* the psychiatric bible since the 1950s that infamously once included an entry for homosexuality. The volume was scheduled to be updated and rereleased in 2013. What would the new low desire diagnosis look like, Bergner asked, given all of this new research into female sexuality? The existing unisex diagnosis of hypoactive sexual desire disorder, or HSDD—defined in the *DSM-IV* as "persistently or recurrently deficient (or absent) sexual fantasies and desire for sexual activity"—struck him as "simplistic," or at least as insufficiently complex to apply to women. Bergner wouldn't know it for certain yet, but similar concerns would eventually lead to the development of a new female-specific diagnosis for low-desiring women— female sexual interest/arousal disorder, or FSIAD. And so it was, that in an attempt to depathologize women's responsive desire, the *DSM-5* (2013) sexual and gender identity disorders work group included a new criterion for women only (three out of six criteria are required for an FSIAD diagnosis): "does not initiate/is not <u>receptive</u> *to a partner's initiations.*" The scientific research and clinical treatments described in Bergner's articles and in other popular accounts, and later the revised low female desire diagnosis itself, in concert indicate that women should not be diagnosed with a disorder just because they lack fantasies or a strong initiating sexual urge (they aren't men, after all?). These discourses instead suggest that if more women knew about their own *responsive* desire, then maybe they wouldn't feel like their desire was *low.* And here, I began to see, is where all the pieces fit together.

Throughout the rest of this book, I will refer to the broad paradigm connecting these strands as the *feminized responsive desire framework.* This paradigm, which became ubiquitous at the turn of the twenty-first century and which has left its imprint through today, consists of all the themes I just outlined: the absence of desire from behaviorist models of sexuality; plethysmographic research suggesting a commonplace discordance between objective and subjective experiences of female arousal; a theory of circular sexual response for women in which desire is said to be triggered by receptive arousal, and new *DSM* diagnostic criteria for low desire in women codifying that theory; and finally, new modes of treatment for women's discordant desire/arousal system, including mindfulness practices intended to work on the gap by bringing the undesiring mind into line with the aroused body. Something didn't sit well with me about this entire framework, and this book is an attempt to explain, analyze, and theorize what that reaction was and where it came from.[3] It is only in a moment in which liberal feminism has

---

3. Since the publication of the *DSM-5* in 2013, several of the experts involved in this original line of research have stated that responsive desire may be common in men, too, and more research has since been conducted on men in this vein. I am aware of the quickly shifting

been mainstreamed, right alongside evolutionary psychology, that this model of female sexual response could make it into the media spotlight and be read as feminist. And it was only at the turn of the twenty-first century, with no critical or activist response, that this type of reductionist, hetero-/cisnormative, and anti-intersectional thinking about female sexuality could become common parlance across the Global North, and particularly in the North American context.

While the new science of female sexuality and the feminized responsive desire framework are certainly meant to be feminist, and in fact came into being as a response to what was understood to be a restrictive male-oriented model of desire (Tiefer, 1991, 1995, 1996), I question the feminism of this new paradigm on a variety of bases. My concerns include the way that "women" are (re)produced as a population here; how this population is read as white, wealthy or middle-class, straight, and cisgender; how widespread gendered, raced, and classed trauma too often goes unaccounted for in this framing; and how this feminized population is positioned to be managed through new techniques framed as "safe" simply because they don't involve psychopharmaceutical drugs or hormones. I argue that this framework must be interrogated as it plays into tropes about white cisgender heterofemininity, and particularly because it will invariably affect a lot of other people who don't fall into this category. I write from a crip-queer-femme perspective, and want to attend to the ways in which these discourses pathologize queer femmes and nonbinary and gender-nonconforming folks, including femmes of color and trans women. A further gap that I will explore in this book is why trauma—including banal, everyday, and insidious forms of trauma including but also beyond childhood sexual abuse—has been largely unaccounted for when considering the differences between men's and women's desire. My analysis suggests that this is a direct result of a shift away from psychoanalytic/psychodynamic thinking in mainstream psychology. But what is also important to consider is how women—cis and trans, across racial backgrounds, of different embodiments and other disparate statuses—understand their own desire, or lack thereof. My

---

terrain of sexual science and recognize that much has changed even in the last five years, but in this book, I want to emphasize how these reductive ideas about women's desire have been taken up broadly in the mainstream since the turn of the twenty-first century through today. One problem is how quickly media latch on to scientific explanations for gender differences in sexuality; however, over the course of the last two decades, the scientists themselves have also made broad, sweeping claims in both media interviews *and* in their expert publications, even when their findings are actually just hypotheses in an ever-shifting world of scientific knowledge (see DeJesus et al., 2019 for empirical evidence [!] on problems with scientific overgeneralizing). Thus, I argue that even as they move their research agendas forward in the spirit of feminist inquiry and ethics, these experts must first reckon with their own recent pasts.

main quest was to seek information from these folks themselves about how well this feminized responsive desire framework applies to them. And I found out that for a lot of them, it doesn't work so well. Certainly, some of these folks *do* feel receptive and responsive, but those experiences are often related to trauma, and with how the people we call women are socialized; they are not neutral or natural. So, let me be clear: My project here is not to make the case that men's and women's sexualities, or that masculine and feminine desires, are exactly the same. Instead, I argue, along with the new scientists of female sexuality, the pioneers and explorers of this frontier, that many women are absolutely different from many men. But in this book, I consider and honor how they've come to be that way, rather than simply describing them as such.

To this end, I want to explain how I use the term *femininity* in this book, and why I chose to use *she/her* pronouns in most cases throughout the text. I did this for a couple of reasons, and my decision-making here was an incredibly fraught and difficult process. First, for reasons that I will explore throughout this book, it was primarily cis women who responded to participate, and all participants used *she/her* pronouns at the time of the interviews; however, these interviews represent only a snapshot in time in terms of participants' gendered subjectivities. I strongly suspect that in the case of at least a few folks, their pronouns have changed, but conducting follow-up interviews about participants' gender identities to confirm this is the province of a future study. Indeed, how trans women, nonbinary, two-spirit, agender, genderqueer, and gender-nonconforming individuals uniquely experience these heteropatriarchal medical and scientific norms regarding femininity should be explored further and in greater depth. How some trans men have potentially experienced coercive medicalized norms for responsive femininity pre-transition is imperative to study, as well, particularly insofar as these men have a unique perspective to offer on the gendering of desire and sexual expectations. Second, and relatedly, I talk about *women* and *femininity* throughout this book because those are the terms used—and taken for granted—in much of the medical and scientific literature that I engage with and critique, and it is this research that I argue produces these very categories (categories that individuals, in the case of this study assigned-female-at-birth, or AFAB, individuals, are then forced to navigate—and in some cases reject but are often still haunted by). I hope that readers will understand the delicacy of choosing language to use for a project such as this one, dwell with me in this conceptually difficult space, and read my use of the terms *women* and *feminine* throughout the text as somewhat tongue-in-cheek—yet also uttered with a certain sobriety and solemnity. The truth is that I know these categories could never be so monolithic, and that they are coproduced with race, class, nationality, and so many other categories of difference. This is precisely why I wage the critique that I wage in this book—the "femininity" that clinical and experimental researchers too frequently imagine belongs to a white, cisgender, middle-class or wealthy, normatively able-bodied woman in the Global North. But this femininity is then deployed as timeless and universal—even evolutionarily ordained.

In this vein, I am not describing femininity as an *identity* in this book; instead, I describe it as a *process*—one that is embodied and experiential but not essential, one that in its hegemonic or dominant formulation may be experienced as coercive, and one that is most specifically connected, in my analysis, to the traumatizing effects of receptivity as a clinical protocol, as a technoscientific framework, and as a lived—but extremely mercurial and unstable—materialization of sexual difference. Here, women-with-low-desire, sexuality, and contemporary sexology are co-constituted; there is no natural category of "woman" here to be recuperated. Femininity is then a material-discursive socialization process, enacted in part through medicine and science, and it is the project of this book to connect that process to its promulgation via contemporary sexological discourse and that discourse's popular framings. My formulations here of femininity-as-process have much in common with other contemporary sociotechnical investigations of gender, including with the pharmacopornographic or techno-chemical dimensions of gender in the work of Preciado (2013), the biopolitics of gender in the post–John Money era as analyzed by Repo (2016), and the production of gender via scientific and medical categories, particularly as they pertain to discourses around hormones and to treatment of intersex, as described by Jordan-Young (2011) and Jordan-Young and Karkazis (2019). Other important recent interlocutors include Labuski (2014, 2015, 2017), who considers how vulvodynia and its treatment inform experiences of race, gender, and (a)sexuality, and Ward (2015), who examines straight white men's sexual behaviors outside of the deterministic logics of biology and identity but instead as part of a culturally delimited process that is bound up with misogyny and white supremacy.

Ideas about women's responsive sexuality and fluidity are found in myriad popular cultural domains today. And it is the pervasiveness and popularity of "expert" discourses on receptive femininity that are precisely why many of the AFAB folks I interviewed—most of whom identify as women but some of whom also reinvent or reject femininity—still have to navigate and grapple with these ideas about women (and what it means to be one) throughout their lives. So, although all the participants in this study describe interacting with femininizing discourses, technologies, and protocols, they absolutely occupy a diversity of spaces in relation to femininity and feminine or femme identity. This is in no small part due to the fact that they come from a diversity of racial, ethnic, cultural, religious, and other backgrounds in addition to being of diverse sexualities; a fact that emphasizes the need to implement an intersectional feminist framework and to consider the racialized Eurocentric and white supremacist origins of sexual difference, which I address below.

Race, Femininity, and the Whiteness of Sexual Difference

Very little work has looked at the phenomenon of low desire through an intersectional (Collins, 1990; Crenshaw, 1991) lens, so desire issues have either been framed as universal for women *or* the impression has been given that concerns about desire are specifically problems encountered by white women (my data suggest otherwise). Following the recent work of Snorton (2017) and Schuller (2018), I seek to highlight the racialized terrain of sexual difference production—for this project, within contemporary discussions of female sexual dysfunction and women's low and/or responsive desire. Schuller (2018), for instance, argues that discourses of sexual difference are not only related to racial difference narratives, but that sex difference is a *function* of racial difference—that is, without the evolutionary logic embedded within racist scientific discourses of the nineteenth century and before (including, for Schuller, impressibility and sentimentalism—white people are more "receptive in a good [evolved] way," according to these logics), there would be no civilizing project in which *male* and *female* as distinct types emerged.

The idea encapsulated in early racist scientific narratives is that as the "races" became more evolved and civilized—moving up the "great chain of being"—masculine and feminine types became more distinct. The white European male was produced as anatomically, behaviorally, and psychically distinct from the white European female; in some sense, the passive, receptive nature of the white European female became the constitutive ground for white European male rationality and objectivity, while white femininity became produced as something in need of protection (in most cases from the figure of the Black male rapist). Of course, the other constitutive ground here has always been Black femininity—conceived initially as not very differentiated from Black masculinity (i.e., "Black gender" or "flesh" for Spillers, 1987), and then as hypersexual, exotic, and tempting to white men (Collins, 2004; Hammonds, 1994, 1999).

Black feminist scholars have opened up critical investigations of the ways in which notions of sexual difference have always rested upon regimes of racial difference—to the point where neither can be examined alone. Spillers (1987) argued that the treatment of Black bodies under slavery produced them as ungendered flesh—that bodies that were enslaved and produced as Black were not gender differentiated or subject to the same regimes of sexual difference as white bodies, and further that sexual differentiation was part and parcel of narratives of racial evolution and civilization. Hartman (1997) extended this argument and examined the ways that Black womanhood (or the figurative lack thereof) was codified under regimes of slavery in the US and thus illuminated "the contingency of woman as a category" (p. 101). In *Scenes of Subjection,* Hartman (1997) examines sexual injury as it relates to conceptualizations of femininity, addressing how Black women were legally figured as "unrapeable" and thus as not really "women" at all, stating:

> By interrogating gender within the purview of "offenses to existence" and examining female subject-formation at the site of sexual violence, I am not positing that forced sex constitutes *the* meaning of gender but that the erasure or disavowal of sexual violence engendered black femaleness as a condition of unredressed injury, which only intensified the bonds of captivity and the deadening objection of chattel status. (p. 101)

Hartman's discussion of the relationship between sexual injury and femininity has special import for the current project—particularly in that my project investigates the widespread popular deployment of expert discourses of purportedly "unmarked" feminine receptivity and responsiveness, discourses that have their origin in colonialist science, but that are now disseminated broadly and sometimes taken up by—or forced upon—women of diverse backgrounds.

Scholars who critically interrogate philosophies and histories of science have also added much to this conversation about racialized femininity. McWhorter (2004, 2009) makes a case for the co-constitution of biopolitical regimes of racial and sexual difference, and Somerville (1994, 2000) has described the ways in which the designation of the "homosexual" has always been a racially freighted category. Somerville (1994) illuminates how the pathologization of the purported anatomical idiosyncrasies of lesbian bodies (large labia and other genital anomalies) were bound up with racialized descriptions of the supposedly abnormal bodies of Black women (the so-called hottentot apron, or enlarged labia, also analyzed by Fausto-Sterling, 1994). Markowitz (2001) extended the conversation by looking specifically at how ideas about female pelvic size were used in conceptualizing racist frameworks of sexual difference. In both early comparative anatomy and sexology, including in the work of Havelock Ellis, white women were figured as having larger pelvises than Black women—a trait that was said to have evolved because white women needed to have more pelvic space in order to give birth to white babies (who were figured as having larger skulls according to the logics of craniology and phrenology!). At the same time, Black women, who in these early discourses were regularly framed as having larger and more voluptuous lower bodies than white women, were said to look this way due to "steatopygia"—a physical anomaly that included large buttocks, which gave the (compensatory and deceptive) *appearance* of a larger pelvis without actually having that "evolved" trait (Markowitz, 2001).

Snorton (2017) has recently revisited these themes, as he analyzes how the formation of white femininity quite literally relied on medical experimentation conducted on Black women by early gynecologists such as J. Marion Sims. Snorton argues that the regular occurrence of vesicovaginal fistula (VVF) in Black women slaves was a product of the circumstances of living on the "medical plantation" of chattel slavery, but was simultaneously blamed on the lack of expertise of Black midwives and/or posited as a product of the biologically inferior and categorically "unfeminine" bodily constitution of the Black woman. Snorton (2017) sums up this paradox, and the imbrication of racial difference and sexual difference, stating: "The founding of the field of American gynecology thus raises a number of questions, including how race constructs biology, and whether sex is possible without flesh" (p. 20). Importantly, these differences in discursive production and material treatment of real live (Black) bodies is not just a thing of the past—Black women today experience disproportionately poor treatment in terms of gynecological care and sexual and reproductive outcomes, including in maternal and infant mortality rates (Casper & Moore, 2009; D. C. Owens, 2017; Washington, 2006).

All of these scholars illuminate the whiteness of sexual difference discourses as these are produced under colonialist medicine and via scientific racism. Whiteness is similarly the foundation of the feminized responsive desire framework I analyze in this book. If sexual difference is, in fact, a function of race (and I argue, along with the scholars cited above, that it is), then there can be no feminine receptivity without race—or, more specifically, without the privileging of whiteness. White feminine receptivity has always been produced against Black feminine hypersexuality as its counterpart. Further, white women have traditionally been *framed* as more sexually receptive, but women of color have traditionally been *expected to actually be* more receptive to sex. In this study, I do not extensively examine the Black hypersexuality against which white receptivity is framed, but rather illustrate the dominant white discourses and the insidiousness of their reach, as I critique a particular moment in contemporary popular psychology that is very much white (i.e., the publication of the *DSM-5* and its related discursive formations). While these discourses about women's sexuality are racialized as white or are left "unmarked," my findings importantly suggest that women across racial identities experience low desire and are forced to navigate this white framework of receptive femininity.

In spite of a plethora of excellent intersectional research from critical scholars, contemporary scientific narratives of sexuality and gender continue to reify binary conceptions of sexual difference, specifically since the modern Darwinian synthesis in which male and female were firmly cast as distinct and complementary types, with all of their binary trappings, and since the X chromosome was formally posited as the "female" chromosome (Richardson, 2012). Beginning with this neo-Darwinian shift and through to today, (discursively unraced) women are broadly understood as being more sexually receptive, responsive, and reactive than (discursively unraced) men—and this is in part due to how ubiquitous experiences associated with white feminine sexuality have become. Part of what I will engage with in this book is how the idea that women *as a whole* are sexually "receptive" became popularized and how it has come to affect diverse individuals. How did sex difference as binary become such a truism in popular culture in the Global North, and how is this idea perpetuated through expert knowledge? What are the contemporary technologies that produce binary sex difference? And why is it that so many women today do, in fact, end up experiencing their desire as low or lacking?

Diagnosably Low Female Sexual Desire: A Brief Clinical History

Although the contemporary iteration of feminized responsive desire is my focus in this book, the main sexual complaint that women tend to present with clinically is "low desire."[4] Indeed, sexology, sex therapy, and sexual medicine shifted to a responsive model of female desire in part because of the prevalence of this complaint. Beginning in roughly the 1970s, antimedicalization feminists began to argue that a male model of spontaneous desire had been applied to women, and that women were therefore pathologized (or pathologized themselves) when in fact their desire was simply different from men's:

---

4. Although there is little to no epidemiological data on racial or class demographics of the women who seek medical help for low desire, due to the very structure of what it means to "present clinically," particularly in the US, where health insurance is a commodity, we can assume that most of these presenting women are white, cisgender, and middle-class or wealthy. However, due to the way that expert discourses travel in the popular sphere, many other women may *self*-diagnose as low in desire and self-treat. That is precisely what this book is about.

potentially weaker, more receptive or responsive, often following arousal and needing to be triggered. However, as "low desire" has been registered as women's key complaint and as the notion of women's responsive desire only entered mainstream medical discourse in its newest guise around the turn of the twenty-first century, I will elucidate a brief history of low female desire here.

Many sexual disorders are accounted for in the American Psychiatric Association's *Diagnostic and Statistical Manual of Mental Disorders,* but none included the language of desire until 1980. That year, two new disorders—inhibited sexual desire (ISD) and sexual aversion—were introduced into the *DSM-III,* both emphasizing desire disorders as dyadic; in other words, they were said to afflict the (implicitly heterosexual) couple rather than just one partner, and were brought to bear in the context of sex therapy treatment. In the *DSM-III-R,* published in 1987, ISD was divided into two categories: hypoactive sexual desire disorder (HSDD) and sexual aversion disorder (SAD), and when the *DSM-IV* was introduced in 1994, these diagnoses remained the same. Up until the publication of the *DSM-5* in 2013, both men and women could be diagnosed with hypoactive desire, although women have consistently been diagnosed much more frequently than men. In the *DSM-IV-TR* (text revision), HSDD was defined as "persistently or recurrently deficient (or absent) sexual fantasies and desire for sexual activity." The 1999 National Health and Social Life Survey (NHSLS) reported that around 32 percent of women between the ages of eighteen and thirty-nine were afflicted with low desire (as compared to about 14 percent of men in the same age range). A nationally representative study conducted in 2008 suggested that 26.7 percent of premenopausal women and 52.4 percent of naturally menopausal women fit the criteria for diagnosis with HSDD (West et al., 2008), and another study suggested that up to 40 percent of women lack interest in sex (K. R. Mitchell et al., 2013).

Even within the terms of these studies, these numbers should be qualified. The number of low-desiring women reported by the NHSLS study has been critiqued as inflated, including by the main researcher on the study. Meanwhile, these percentages are often dramatically reduced when potential diagnosees must also be "troubled" or "distressed" by their lack of sexual desire in order to receive a diagnosis, a criterion that is built into the new *DSM-5* diagnosis (i.e., women who are not distressed by their low desire should not receive the diagnosis, as some may identify as asexual instead). According to most contemporary estimates, the number of women who lack sexual motivation and who are concomitantly troubled by this experience hovers at around 12 percent (Shifren, Monz, Russo, Segreti, & Johannes, 2008). Regardless of the details of these studies, the prevalence of low female desire remains a cultural trope, and statistics continue to be cited as proof of the pervasiveness of the phenomenon. Although recent estimates do not indicate an increase in the actual number of women afflicted with diagnosably low desire over the last few decades, widespread attention to women's desire problems in clinical literature, a proliferation of recent reports in the popular media (for examples, see Bergner, 2009a, 2009b, 2013a; Elton, 2010; Gottlieb, 2014; Schreiber, 2012), and an increase in reports of women who lack interest in sex as demonstrated in both clinical settings and on national surveys gives the impression that low desire in women is on the rise, at least in the Global North. Further, as pointed out by Charest and Kleinplatz (2018), there has been a shift from an emphasis on sexual problems as dyadic to the increased pathologization of individuals with sexual complaints—and in the case of low desire, this is most often individual women.

Hence, in most clinical and popular discourses today, it is widely accepted that men and women have very different sexual problems (Basson et al., 2001; Basson, Brotto, Laan, Redmond, & Utian, 2005; Brotto, 2010a; Leiblum & Rosen, 1988; Tiefer, 1991, 1995). Low sexual desire appears not only to occur more regularly in women, it is *expected* to be a more common experience for women. Here, it is important to recognize that many women do in fact experience themselves as low or lacking in desire, and this experience now cuts across race and class lines, among other categories of difference. The questions I seek to answer in this book do not challenge the reality or validity of this highly gendered sexual experience of low desire, but instead, its etiology and assumptions: *Why* are women more likely to be afflicted with this problem? Do we assume this gendered experience is natural, biological, hardwired? What does that assumption look like, or how does it manifest, and with what consequences, in our contemporary climate? Unlike much feminist analysis in the medical sociology and social psychology traditions, which tends to argue that sexuality is socially constructed, and that heteronormative gender expectations influence us to pathologize women's low desire when it is actually just "normal variation"—or, more recently, that women's desire may not be disordered but simply "responsive" and "receptive"—I want to consider how these ideas about receptivity, responsiveness, and even "normal variation" themselves become gendered, and how this framing influences men's and women's lived experiences of desire and their sexual expression more broadly. I want to think about how gender differences in desire are carved out in the world, in all their specificities, and with what effects, including for women who come to identify as either deficient or disordered, or as normal—but receptive and responsive. Is there a way to understand low desire as disorder, yet simultaneously to question and complicate its supposed neurobiological or essential origins? Is there a way to look beyond both social constructionism and biological determinism when it comes to sexual difference? Relatedly, is there a way to think beyond disability, debility, and disorder as objective, medical, and measurable, yet to simultaneously foreground their material and embodied existence? And is it possible to endeavor a deep critique of the racialized and gendered nature of scientific and medical discourses while at the same time acknowledging that some women are disturbed by their lack of desire and want treatment for it?

Theoretical and Methodological Framework

Before beginning my analysis, I posed a number of research questions: How do contemporary and historical scientific, medical, and therapeutic discourses define sexual desire? How do these discourses (and the experts themselves) frame sexual difference? Do they identify gender differences in desire, arousal, and sexual behavior? If so, how do they interpret and explain these differences? Are masculine and feminine desire framed differently across sexual medicine, sex therapy, and clinical psychology paradigms over the last two centuries? Is anything consistent across these paradigms? And finally, how do women themselves understand the machinations of their own desire, or lack thereof?

Because I wanted to focus on the low desire diagnoses in the new *DSM-5* and related feminized responsive desire framework, I interviewed women identifying as low or lacking in sexual desire, including those who have either sought medical or alternative therapeutic treatments or who have considered seeking treatment. However, I chose to include within my study interviews with women who had *not* undergone medical treatment or received a diagnosis, for a few reasons. It is actually quite difficult to acquire a low-desire diagnosis from a psychiatric practitioner due to obstacles within the US health care system, internalized shame about female sexuality, and a variety of other factors (additionally, this population is also very difficult to reach due to medical gatekeeping). But I was also actively interested in speaking not only with women who have received official diagnoses and medical treatment for low desire but also with *potential* consumers of medicine—or of alternative therapies such as mindfulness, yoga, tantra, and feminine energy "healing" workshops—intended to remedy low desire. In other words, I was interested in how not only the low desire diagnosis itself but also the broader feminized responsive desire framework I outlined at the beginning of this introduction affects a broad population of women. This study deals with medicalization and healthism (to be defined below), but it is *not* a medical ethnography. I am more interested in how the logic of feminine receptivity impacts women broadly than in the experience of patients who have been diagnosed with a specific disease state or disorder. Or, rather, I am interested in the increasing blurriness of these categories—the diagnosed and the undiagnosed—particularly as self-medicalization becomes more and more prevalent due to the impact of the internet and social media.

The sociological study and critique of medicalization—what Conrad (1992) referred to as "a process by which non-medical problems become defined and treated as medical problems, usually in terms of illnesses and disorders" (p. 209)—has been an important subfield within sociology since the 1960s, borne out of the symbolic interactionist and sociology of knowledge traditions. Early theorists of medicalization included Szasz (1960), who wrote about the historical invention of mental illness; Zola (1972), who argued that medicine has become an institution of social control; and Conrad (1975), who argued that hyperkinesis or attention deficit disorder (ADD) in children, among other disorders, were iatrogenically produced.[5] These sociologists examined how disorders are socially constructed via powerful medical discourses, and how they then affect individuals and the "biosocial" communities who take them up, contest them, or navigate them in a variety of other ways (Rabinow, 1996). More recent scholars in this area have focused on biomedicalization (Clarke, Shim, Mamo, Fosket, & Fishman, 2003) and healthism or healthicization (Crawford, 1980). These terms reflect a shift in which the dominant status of medical professions has diminished under neoliberal capitalism, and increasingly, individuals are targeted by corporations; they may self-diagnose and self-treat (via online protocols); and alternative, functional, holistic, and "Eastern" medicine and extramedical protocols have become more popular, both within so-called Western medical arenas and also outside of the clinic.

The medicalization of sexuality—and specifically the project of making sexual difference a focal point of psychiatric interest and intervention—has a long history in the Global North, particularly in the Anglo-American context. Many feminist scholars have suggested that medicine and science, including psychology and psychiatry, should be deemed irresponsible not only for their

---

5. Goffman, with his work on institutionalization (1961) and stigmatization (1978), and Foucault, with his genealogical analyses of madness (1965), the productive power of expert discourse (1972), the development of the clinic and the clinical gaze (1973), and disciplinary regimentation within surveilling institutions (1977), are also associated with the sociological critique of medicalization. For this project, I am more interested in Foucault's later work on governmentality, regimes of sexuality, and the biopolitical production and management of populations, as I elaborate below.

social control techniques in general, but for their social control of women as deviant others in particular (Birke & Hubbard, 1995; Boyle, 1993; Harding, 1986; Hubbard, 1990; Irvine, 2002, 2005). Feminists of the 1960s and 1970s analyzed the legacy of psychoanalysis in this regard, and much of the pathologization of women's minds and bodies has been attributed to Freud's drive model of sex, and the concept of penis envy. These scholars further argued that the "feminine neuroses"—female masochism, hysteria, frigidity, and even eating disorders today—were socially constructed as ways to pathologize femininity or, alternatively, that they were the tangible and devastating material results of the suffocating societal control of women. For other scholars, these illness experiences may also be read as radical forms of feminist refusal or resistance to patriarchal modes of being (Bordo, 1993; Ehrenreich & English, 1978).

Today, disability studies scholars such as Garland-Thomson (2002) and Kafer (2013), and feminist psychiatric disability and madness studies scholars such as Donaldson (2002), Johnson (2010, 2013, 2015), and Mollow (2014) in a crip theoretical frame (McRuer, 2006) offer a way of understanding gendered and racialized illnesses as being simultaneously real and legitimate (rather than just "socially constructed"), yet still emergent as social products and not simply forms of refusal. Some feminist and sexuality studies scholars have also taken up critiques of sexism and misogyny in sexual dysfunction discourses and in the areas of women's sexual, reproductive, and mental health more broadly (Angel, 2010, 2012; Cacchioni, 2015; Labuski, 2015; Moore & Clarke, 1995; Tiefer, 1995). Additionally, asexuality studies scholars have highlighted regimes of compulsory sexuality (Barounis, 2014, 2015, 2019; Flore, 2014, 2016, 2018; Gupta, 2011, 2015, 2017; Kim, 2014; Milks & Cerankowski, 2014; Przybylo, 2013, 2014), and feminist science studies scholars have unpacked categories of diagnosis, including in regard to intersex embodiment, exposing the heteronormative rhetoric that operates under the guise of scientific objectivity (Fausto-Sterling, 1992, 1994, 2000; Jordan-Young, 2011; Jordan-Young & Karkazis, 2019; Karkazis, 2008). As mentioned above, many scholars in this vein have importantly highlighted the whiteness of these regimes and of racialized sexual difference more broadly (Hartman, 1997; Markowitz, 2001; McWhorter, 2004, 2009; Schuller, 2018; Snorton, 2017; Somerville, 1994, 2000; Spillers, 1987). I offer an analysis of low desire in women that is in conversation with all of this scholarship.

Recent sociological critiques of the medicalization of sexuality, including prolific critiques of the social construction of female sexual dysfunction and low desire, have primarily taken an antimedicalization, antipharmaceuticalization or anti-"Big Pharma," anti-"disease-mongering" stance (Jutel, 2010;

Moynihan, 2005; Tiefer, 1995, 1996, 2006). By contrast, I focus on the ways in which sexual difference is carved out through clinical discourses, how gendered ways of being are thus prescribed within these domains, and ultimately, how discursive regimes for active masculinity and receptive femininity become circuitously attached to bodies and lived out socially. In the present study, I address these crucial—and too often neglected—components of the current context within which "female sexual dysfunction" (FSD) and low female desire are constructed, debated, and, by some critics, denounced as wholly fictitious. I do not think non-asexual women's low desire is fictitious or purely "socially constructed," but nor do I think it is simply "normal variation," in the most generous reading, or essential to female sexual constitution, in the most reductive reading (it is worth noting that both "normal variation" and "female essence" here operate within the logic of a reductive biological frame). Instead, I want to turn the gaze back upon the very feminist-identified clinicians and scientists who study and work on women's desire, and show how they are complicit with the production of receptive femininity as something to be regulated, controlled, and optimized. Women-with-low-desire here is produced as a category, as a population to be managed, and the members of this population are in many cases produced and managed by self-identified feminist researchers and clinicians themselves.

In this vein, my research questions further lend themselves to a theoretical exploration proceeding from a biopolitical framework. Beginning with the work of Foucault in the late 1970s, there has been much attention to the dynamics of identity and population production, embodiment, and other forms of corporeal politics in late neoliberal capitalism (Clough, 2007, 2018; Cooper, 2008; Cooper & Waldby, 2014; Mbembe, 2003, 2019; Murphy, 2012, 2017; Puar, 2007, 2011, 2017; N. Rose, 2001, 2007; Weheliye, 2014). Scholars following and critiquing Foucault began to explore these questions within a biopolitical and affective framework beginning in the late 1980s. The primary common claim is that neoliberal discourses under late global capitalism—which are attuned to and productive of race, gender, sexuality, nationality, (dis)ability, and other categories of citizenship and governance—manipulate, surveil, and affectively control bodies and populations, increasingly through consensual rather than disciplinary means. Some of these control mechanisms operate through the domains of medicine, science, and psychiatry—and their popular instantiations that are now accessible through new media, digital formats, and self-help techniques—and they regulate and manage the health, illness, capacity, debility, life, and death of various populations and the body politic at large. This management is increasingly performed in the name of "self-improvement" and individual "health" to the benefit of certain groups at the expense of certain others (all of whom are raced, gendered, sexualized, and nationalized). All of these investments are part of a larger neoliberal project of submitting social life—including family configurations, sexual relations, and other embodied aspects of this sociality—to market logic. My project, as it examines the lived experience of racialized and gendered medical and scientific discourses—including those that extend beyond the clinic—and their effects on women's bodies and psyches, and insofar as it focuses on the management, regulation, and production of certain iterations of feminine desire, is firmly situated within this biopolitical framework.

In order to investigate how individuals live out low or responsive female desire discourses, I employed a mixed methodological qualitative approach. I utilized three different sociological research methods, including critical discourse analysis of peer-reviewed scientific and sexual medicine journal articles, a limited amount of analytic observation[6] at medical clinics and sexual enhancement workshops, and in-depth interviews with thirty-seven individuals. Most of these interviews were with cisgender women who identified as currently lacking in sexual desire or who have experienced problematic low desire at some point in their lives. I also conducted a small number of interviews with a variety of practitioners who do "desire work," including clinical psychologists, sex therapists, yogic/tantric practitioners, sexual enhancement workshop leaders, and antimedicalization activists. By analyzing emergent themes through in-depth qualitative data-analysis techniques, I was able to excavate the parallels and tensions between "expert" discourses on low female desire and the experiences of low-desiring women themselves.

How do women think about low desire, receptivity, responsiveness, complexity, and sexual flexibility? How do they experience their sexualities and genders? How do they characterize their current and past sex lives? What turns them on or off? How could their sexual partners help them increase their desire and give them more pleasure? Why do women themselves think their desire is low, or has been throughout their lives at different times and with different partners? In order to shed light on these questions, among others, I conducted in-depth, one-on-one, semistructured, qualitative interviews with thirty low-desiring women. These interviews ranged from thirty to 210 minutes in length, but most were between one and three hours long. Most participants contacted me on the basis of experiencing low desire currently or because they had experienced troublingly low desire at some point in

---

6. I use the term *analytic observation* rather than *participant observation*, as I was not actually a participant in any of these spaces. Rather, I conducted interviews in medical and alternative therapeutic spaces and was able to observe certain dynamics in these "clinics" during the interviewing process.

their lives; two had participated in medical treatment programs that utilized behavioral, therapeutic, and pharmaceutical interventions to treat sexual pain and concomitant low desire. They ranged in age from twenty-one to fifty-six years, but most were between the ages of twenty-five and thirty-seven, and all except for one were premenopausal. These women were of diverse racial and ethnic backgrounds, with about one-third of the sample identifying as women of color. They grew up with a multitude of cultural, community, and religious backgrounds. Most were born in the US, and almost all had at least a college education (or were currently attending college). They were of diverse sexualities (most were straight or bisexual; some identified as queer) and lifestyles (some were married or in long-term partnerships, some were single, some were polyamorous or in open relationships, and only a few were pregnant or had children), but all of the women I interviewed who identified as low-desiring (or who had previously experienced distressingly low desire) had been sexually involved with cisgender men at some point in their lives. One participant identified as being on an asexual/pansexual spectrum, and one identified as genderqueer/nonconforming. A participant also interviewed me, using the same interview schedule I had used with all of the low-desiring women I interviewed. See the appendix (Table 1 and Table 2) for full participant and expert demographic information. All of the names used for participants in this study are pseudonyms. The names in Table 1 (low-desiring participants) were chosen by the participants themselves. I selected the names in Table 2 (the experts; although some of the experts agreed to use their real names, not all did, so in order to be consistent, I gave them all pseudonyms. All of the experts are white).

Most of the participants responded to a flyer I posted in a variety of spaces around Brooklyn, Queens, and Manhattan in New York City—including in college health centers and other university settings, coffee shops and restaurants, grocery stores, yoga and dance studios, and other public places with bulletin boards for posting events and activities. The flyer was also disseminated to initial participants to email to their friends and post on their Facebook and other social media pages, so many of the later participants were recruited via snowball sample (Berg & Lune, 2011; Miles, Huberman, & Saldaña, 2013). I also posted the recruitment flyer on my personal blog, Facebook, and Twitter pages and made it shareable so others could post it. This type of convenience sampling is appropriate given the sensitive nature of the interview topics, and is useful for making exploratory grounded theoretical observations that are not generalizable to any larger population.[7] My sample could be said to be

---

7. Most of the interviews were conducted at my apartment, at the participants' apartments, or in a public space such as a café or park (in all cases, the participants chose where they preferred to be interviewed—and a handful of interviews were conducted via Skype or

somewhat disparate, but I argue that this makes sense and is in keeping with the scientific literature, as what it means to be a "low-desiring" woman is confusing and ill-defined, and the medical discourse itself is confusing and ill-defined. There is no consensus in experimental or clinical psychology or sexual medicine or sex therapy on what "desire" even is, or what "low desire" indicates, and the new female sexual interest/arousal disorder diagnosis attests to this, as I will explain in chapter 2.

In the remaining six interviews, which were conducted with clinicians, therapists, activists, and yogic/alternative health practitioners, emergent themes included these experts' thoughts on feminine receptivity, innate or neurological differences between men and women, evolutionary sexual adaptations, and gender differences in mind/body disconnects or alignments (i.e., arousal/desire "concordance" versus "discordance"). I also examined how practitioners dealt with the same themes that emerged from the low-desiring women's interviews. Different practitioners grappled with these themes differently, and they had diverse ideas about the most appropriate and effective treatments for low female desire. I utilize these expert interviews sporadically throughout the remainder of this book, primarily to frame the textual analysis and low-desiring participants' interview data.

Chapter Overview

In the first half of *Diagnosing Desire,* I examine historical and contemporary formulations of both clinical and popular discourses about femininity, sexuality, and gendered sexual response; in the second half of the book, I turn more closely to the interviews and the themes that emerged from them.

In chapter 1, I examine how femininity, women's sexuality, and female desire have been framed in sex therapy, sex research, and specifically as part of conceptualizations of human sexual response, from the nineteenth century through to today. I pay special attention to how notions of feminine responsiveness and receptivity have been maintained through different sexual response models, from early psychoanalytic configurations to more behavioristic accounts to evolutionary psychology formulations of sexual difference. Although paradigms through which sexuality is interpreted have shifted immensely (and much has been lost in the movement from trauma-based psychoanalytic/psychodynamic theories to the more reductive evolutionary

---

FaceTime) between 2012 and 2014. I did not compensate any of the interviewees monetarily, although I did offer to buy them coffee or tea if we were at a café, and if they came to my apartment to conduct the interview, I cooked dinner for them and/or provided food and beverages.

psychology and behavioristic models), the idea that men and women operate on different sexual planes of existence has remained constant.

In chapter 2, I pick up with contemporary behavioristic and evolutionary models and focus on the trajectory of the new science of female sexuality as it relates to these models, and specifically on the development of the circular sexual response cycle as part of the feminized responsive desire framework. I show how these models for thinking about women's sexual response began to take hold over the last twenty-five or so years, and came fully into the popular spotlight during the first decade of the twenty-first century, and I consider how the notions of sexual "interest," "arousal," and "motivation" have come to replace the language of (female) "desire" and have simultaneously come to dominate in individualized sex therapy, sexual medicine, and contemporary sexology. I further show how this feminized responsive desire framework—along with experimental psychology research on women's subjective/genital discordance—culminated in the newly gendered FSIAD diagnosis in the 2013 edition of the *Diagnostic and Statistical Manual of Mental Disorders* (*DSM-5*). The feminization of responsive desire is not only an issue for those who are diagnosed with FSIAD, however—because of the far reach of ideas about feminine sexual receptivity via popular media, many women have internalized these notions, and will self-diagnose and seek treatment, including through mindfulness-based sex therapy, or MBST, one of the most popular methods of treatment today. I analyze this entire framework as it relates to themes about women's sexuality that have emerged in evolutionary psychology, and consider treatments—including mindfulness to enhance desire—through a biopolitical lens. Members of the population women-with-low-desire are produced as such through sexual medicine and treatment protocols and come to regulate themselves accordingly. This self-surveillance rehearses antiquated narratives about (white) feminine receptivity and has dire negative consequences for women's sexual agency—which is paradoxical, in that the framework and treatments are designed to "empower" women.

Through the qualitative analysis of interview data, several primary themes emerged as specifically affecting women who identify as low in sexual desire, and they are the topics of the remaining chapters. In chapter 3, I examine concepts associated with the FSIAD diagnosis, such as "interest," "arousal," "motivation," and "receptivity," and consider how well they apply (or do not apply) to the women I interviewed. I also examine how second-wave feminism, specifically cultural feminist strains within the "psychology of women," and even ideas about women that have emerged from antimedicalization activism, have been imported into the feminized responsive desire framework. Today, this model of women's sexual response is offered as "feminist"—however, I argue that it can only be interpreted as such if women's empowerment is defined narrowly within a white liberal feminist framework. I argue that more in-depth, intersectional feminist goals are undercut by the racialized, cisnormative, and heterornomative contours of the feminized responsive desire framework itself. The primary theme that emerges from my interview data here is the notion of *sexual difference socialization,* or the experience of one's sexuality (and femininity) through pervasive scientific, therapeutic, and popular discourses that prescribe gender differences in sexual desire and behavior. Here, I consider how the category women-with-low-desire is not only produced discursively via sexual medicine but also how members of this population are socialized into being, through gendered sexual expectations that are part and parcel of contemporary sexology and its associated scripts.

In chapter 4, I consider embodied invisible labor in the form of sexualized social reproduction, or what I call *sexual carework.* This theme from my interview data does not only concern the ways women are expected to sexually service men under heteropatriachy (although it does concern that). I also focus on how the medical and scientific discourses I analyze in the first part of the book support notions of feminized sexual carework, which has particular import for women-with-low-desire, and even more specifically for women of color in this category. Further, I consider how, under regimes of compulsory gendered (hetero)sexuality, sexual carework becomes a mandate for *self-*care—for the good of the hetero/cis relationship, the bourgeois family, the nation/state, and sometimes the woman's "own health"; here, alternative therapies, including mindfulness, become tools of *self-care as self-regulation,* and femininity becomes a duty. Feminized sexual carework is thus a biopolitical mandate, and feminine carers are a population to be invested in and who are expected to invest in themselves in order to *self-appreciate* (in the sense of accruing value, or making oneself more valuable).

In chapter 5, I analyze the interviews and consider how and why some low-desiring women are drawn to submission in bondage and discipline/ dominance and submission/sadism and machochism or BDSM practice, and concomitantly interrogate the problem of the missing discourse of trauma within the feminized responsive desire framework. In this vein, I consider the fraught nature and importance of sexual intentionality—including the necessity of actively negotiating sexual taboos and attempting to build sexual trust (particularly for women who have sex with men)—in the face of many low-desiring women's frequent experiences with and histories of feminized trauma as a result of gendered and sexual violence. Here, I further expose the violence inherent in the feminized mandate to sexual receptivity, including as it is deployed via the FSIAD diagnosis and mindfulness-based sex therapy and related discourses. I show, however, that receptivity can be and is reclaimed by women, including through mindful and intentional submission, for instance via BDSM. This intentional and queer reclamation of receptivity via submission throws into stark relief the (ironically) more self-disciplinary mandate of enhancing one's own responsive desire via biopolitical techniques such as mindfulness, and thus what I refer to as *parasexual* pleasure is able to be experienced even in the face of compulsory and feminized trauma. Here, I add to ongoing conversations about asexuality, demisexuality, and other non-normative versions of erotic life.

I bring all of these themes together in the conclusion of *Diagnosing Desire* and consider a different model of care and parasexual agency through the lenses of crip theory, critical feminist disability studies, and feminist madness studies. Here, I think through the implications of the biopolitical analysis of femininity that has been laid out in the book; if the responsive feminine are produced as a population, then there may be an experience of vitality to be found in "falling apart" or "fracturing" together—rather than self-surveilling and constantly seeking to individually enhance under white supremacist, ableist, cisheteropatriarchal capitalism. There is revolutionary potential in falling apart in the face of trauma and low desire, with others, in radical community, rather than using biopolitical techniques in order to simply "get by."

•

I want to acknowledge a few final things before I go any further. First, while I will argue throughout this book that contemporary discourses of femininity are framed as universal or are racially "unmarked," but that they ultimately recapitulate ideas about white women's sexuality (founded in early scientific discourses of racialized sexual difference), the one-on-one interviews for this this book did not focus on race in an in-depth way. I reflexively acknowledge the limitations of this book in this vein; while I did speak with several women of color for this project, we did not extensively discuss the many ways that race, racism, and white supremacy undoubtedly impact their experiences of their own sexuality and desire. To some extent, this was a limitation of my interview schedule and the substance of the overarching research question that brought these participants to speak with me in the first place (the connection between gender and low desire), but my own whiteness surely influenced how I chose to analyze the interviews and what themes I ultimately centered in the final analysis. There is a strong connection between my own work here and research that suggests how (sexualized/gendered) trauma and (sexualized/gendered) carework are disproportionately experienced and enacted by poor women, women of color, and folks of other marginalized statuses, and I highlight that research throughout the text with a nod to the limits of my own project. I take seriously Nash's (2019) critiques of the burden thrust upon feminist scholars of color to do intersectional work and Puar's (2017) critiques of the ways in which (white) new materialist feminist scholars specifically have too often ignored an intersectional frame. I hope that my research here on the whiteness of the contemporary medical and scientific milieu of sexual difference production and regulation can open the door for more in-depth analyses of racialization and unmarked whiteness as it travels in this milieu (and it is white scholars, including me, who should endeavor to perform these analyses).

A few final points I'd like to acknowledge include the time scale of this research, the pervasiveness of what may appear to be a narrow discourse, and the complexity of the experts I analyze. The science that I have been studying moves fast, and narratives and hypotheses offered in experimental and clinical psychology publications have changed quickly since I began this project. Thus, this book focuses primarily on a very specific time period: the first ten to fifteen years of the twenty-first century, when women's (receptive) desire increasingly came into the spotlight, and the discursive space of "feminism" was increasingly occupied by mainstream sexual medicine practitioners, researchers, and sex therapists. This book, then, is also a critique of white liberal feminism as it has been taken up in mainstream psychology.

In this vein, one of my goals is to inspire an interdisciplinary dialogue. Many popular mainstream psychologists are still primarily working with the categories of "males" and "females," are only recently beginning to examine the social construction of gender, and assume universal sex categories without analyzing their founding within colonialism and white supremacy. By contrast, scholars in critical race and sexuality studies, disability studies, queer and feminist theory, and queer of color and crip of color critique have moved well beyond social constructionist arguments and forefront white supremacy as undergirding all of our medical and scientific categories. I hope this book can promote useful and practicable discussions among these scientific researchers and cultural theorists, so that our most cutting-edge science and medicine can be informed by our most cutting-edge theories of gender, sexuality, race, and embodiment. These discussions will be imperative in improving both clinical/therapeutic treatments for marginalized populations, and the scientific research upon which those treatments are based.

Finally, it must be noted that this project has been difficult in part because of the complexity of the medical figures and experts who have become the primary characters in this story. While I critique the way their various research projects, treatment protocols, and activist endeavors have come together to form the feminized responsive desire framework that I see as ultimately detrimental and retrograde, I also recognize that these women are progressive and innovative scholars in their fields and have done much to shift the terrain of mainstream psychology and sexology. They have moved sex therapy and research forward in many invaluable ways, and my intervention here is meant in the spirit of feminist dialogue and critical engagement with those projects. We are all steeped in our own disciplines and have to navigate the constraints therein, and I hope that my argument and analysis in this book will provoke a necessary conversation.

CHAPTER 1

Sexual Difference and Femininity in Sex Therapy and Sex Research

Examples from the Nineteenth, Twentieth, and Twenty-First Centuries

In 1931, toward the end of his career, Sigmund Freud published an essay titled "Female Sexuality" wherein he lays out his case for sexual difference in development—women are naturally more "bisexual" than men (here, he means more prone to taking up both "male" and "female" gender orientations and associated sexual behaviors), they are more sexually receptive, and, when properly developed, they are sexually passive (albeit active in terms of a maternal instinct). Proper female adulthood is signified by a shift in libidinal energies from the clitoris to the vagina. All of this is "natural"—just a part of human psychosexual development, given by body parts and their obvious uses. By the time this essay was published, psychoanalysis, Freud's much lauded and reviled theory of human psychology, had been in clinical practice for more than two decades in the US and Europe. In addition to psychoanalytic sessions, variations of psychoanalysis were used to treat a broad swath of related and sometimes indistinguishable feminine neuroses, including hysteria and frigidity, in quasi-gynecological settings (Ehrenreich & English, 1978)—in this way, psychoanalysis was clearly an important moment in the trajectory of the development of sex therapy in the Global North. Beginning in the second half of the twentieth century, psychoanalytic theorizations and protocols would fall out of vogue, at least among practicing psychologists, psychiatrists, and sex therapists, in favor of biopsychiatric, neurobiological, evolutionary psychological, and cognitive behavioral frameworks.

One might have hoped that such universalizing and essentializing theories of human sexual development would have been abandoned along with these irresponsible uses of psychoanalysis (how much Freud condoned these usages himself is debated to this day). But, almost eighty years later, prominent experimental sexologists, theorizing sex differences in response to pornographic videos shown in a laboratory to subjects whose penises and vaginas are hooked up to machines that gauge their physiological sexual arousal, make conjectures about gender differences in sexual response that sound remarkably similar to those for which Freud was so villainized. For instance, in an archetypal article in the preeminent scientific journal *Archives of Sexual Behavior,* some of the most renowned sex researchers of the twenty-first century describe differences in male and female arousal, positing that women may experience less mental/physiological alignment or "concordance" than men do (that is, women's minds and bodies often do not agree about what turns them on) for evolutionary reasons: "Another possible explanation for the sex difference in concordance is that men and women are designed differently in terms of their physiological and psychological sexual response systems" (Suschinsky, Lalumière, & Chivers, 2009, p. 571). In support of this theory of evolved sexual difference, the researchers cite sociobiology and evolutionary psychology forerunner Donald Symons, who argues for the importance of mate choice in guiding ancestral women's interest in sexual activity—which could really be boiled down to interest in motherhood (for women, "quality over quantity" is the general rule, which evolutionary psychologists claim is an adaptation inherited by women today; according to this theory, even though women tend to be physically aroused by many things, including bonobos having sex or other entities/acts that do not align with their stated sexual preferences, they often are either subjectively unaware of their objective arousal or choose not to "follow" it in order to make better mate choices, although this is not conscious). The researchers extend this evolutionary psychology argument about evolved adaptations—in this case, automatic, rapid, and easy physiological arousal in women—to the hypothetical pervasiveness of rape in prehistoric environments:

> Reflexive vaginal responding may have been beneficial because vaginal vasocongestion results in lubrication of the genital tract, reducing the likelihood of injury and subsequent infection resulting from vaginal penetration. Ancestral women who did not reflexively lubricate and who experienced unwanted sex would have been more likely to experience injuries or infections that could have rendered them reproductively sterile or resulted in their deaths after sustaining injury during genital penetration. (p. 571)

Alongside describing what has since come to be known as "the preparation hypothesis" for hardwired reflexive female genital response,[1] these researchers cite the work of psychologist Roy Baumeister, who argues that women's sexuality is naturally more "erotically plastic" and influenced by nurture, culture, and the external environment than is men's sexuality, which is inherently more "in-born," goal-oriented, and biologically driven. So, over the span of almost a full century, similar guiding themes regarding feminine complexity, receptivity, and responsiveness are maintained, even though the theoretical frames doing the guiding are, on their face, very different. This observed continuity raises several questions: What are the consequences of these universalizing theories of sexual difference on treatments for low desire and sexual dysfunction in the twenty-first century? Beyond dysfunction, how do these ideas impact how we perceive "healthy" sexuality, desire, and gendered sexual behavior? And finally, even when contemporary experimental sexological research produces evidence-based theories and hypotheses, does that mean they are sound or worth investing in? How are these hypotheses implemented, how are resulting theories utilized, and what ideologies are inextricable from even the most replicable and reliable scientific evidence?

This book analyzes the science and medicine of low female desire, and the related contemporary notion of "female sexual dysfunction." That history cannot be discussed without critically analyzing the corollary notion of feminine sexual receptivity—and specifically that receptivity within the framework of institutionalized heterosexuality, or what social theorists call *heteronormativity* (Fischer, 2013; Ingraham, 2008; Pascoe, 2011; Wade; 2017; Warner, 1991). In each of the sex therapy and research paradigms I examine, the story remains the same: Female sexuality is murkier, more complex, more flexible, fluid, or subject to the influence of "nurture" or the external environment, and thus it is more receptive or responsive than male sexuality. A variety of histories, including pre-sexological and premodern medical histories, could be places to begin this story. In the interest of time and space, and because in the popular imagination of contemporary psychology, psychoanalysis is often considered to be synonymous with misogyny, I begin with Freud.

---

1. At the time of this writing, the empirical status of the preparation hypothesis regarding cis women's reflexive genital response as evolutionary adaptation still has great import and much support, and continues to be a topic of debate in the experimental community. For instance, in their in-depth review of studies on related topics since the 1990s, Lalumière, Sawatsky, Dawson, & Suschinksy (2020) ultimately conclude that "the evidence presented in [their] article suggests that there is a coordinated perceptual, cognitive, emotional, physiological, and neural system that facilitates an automatic sexual response to sexual stimuli [in cis women]—a coordinated system that may serve protective functions" (n. pag.).

Just as peculiar female sexuality has consistently posed a problem for sexology, sex therapy, sexual medicine, and psychoanalysis, these medical frames and associated technologies have been vexing for feminists. The history of psychoanalysis in this regard is particularly noteworthy; whereas many feminist thinkers have taken up psychoanalytic perspectives on gender, from Lacanian to object-relations traditions, others have abandoned psychoanalytic theory completely and argue that it is inherently sexist, particularly as psychology has moved toward what are claimed to be less "theoretical" or "political" frameworks in the last several decades. In light of this split among feminists, it is useful to consider what Freud actually said about female sexuality, how these notions have been taken up in practice beyond his writings and possibly without his consent, and what these ideas have in common with contemporary conceptions of sexual difference. This is imperative also as many contemporary practicing psychologists, sex therapists, and clinicians (feminist-identified or not) have disregarded Freud while simultaneously maintaining some of the worst—and most misogynistic—aspects of his theories of psychosexual development. That is, in an effort to be apolitical and atheoretical (i.e., to distance themselves from psychoanalysis) many contemporary psychologists have embraced evolutionary and behaviorist models of human sexuality, giving up a focus on trauma and even socialization, and, paradoxically, they have maintained notions of essential feminine responsiveness and receptivity in the process.

Here, I critique early psychoanalytic theories of gender and sexual development, while also acknowledging the utility of psychoanalysis as a therapeutic framework for understanding trauma—including gendered and sexual trauma—and for understanding the impact of early experiences on our psychic lives. Freudian psychoanalysis has become a stand-in—to the point of caricature—for all that is misogynistic about modern psychology, a point that Angel (2010, 2012, 2013) has elaborated at length. Even in light of warranted critiques of Freud's writings on femininity, not to mention his lack of attention to difference across race, class, and culture, there are many aspects of psychoanalytic therapy that are useful and should be carried forward, including psychoanalytic insight into causes of sexual problems, acknowledgment of the unconscious and the notion that human behaviors are often guided by things that are not directly within our awareness, and acknowledging prior trauma as a cause of pathology, in addition to processing this trauma as a part of treatment. While vulgar psychoanalytic theorizations (read: narrowly Oedipal explanations) are often the focus when Freud is discussed in contemporary mainstream psychology, or misogynistic work with "hysterical" women is described when discussing psychoanalytic treatment, there is much more to both psychoanalytic theory and associated therapeutic treatments. An important positive aspect of psychoanalytic work is its use of narrative techniques for uncovering the deeper roots and explanations for understanding sexual desire or lack thereof. Also valuable is the psychoanalytic attribution of dysfunction to experiences of trauma, which has been lost in the present behaviorist focus on immediate symptoms and brief treatments. And finally, contemporary psychoanalytic conceptions are quite nuanced in their renderings of brain-body connectivity (E. A. Wilson, 2015); *distributive ontologies* or *neurological intimacies* are more intersubjective, affective, and trauma-informed psychoanalytic explications than the ones we might be used to, and they allow us to consider the connections between psychoanalysis and neuroscience, or to think of "the body in conversation with itself" (E. A. Wilson, 2004, p. 98)—and in conversation with its environment and other bodies therein.

Throughout the rest of this chapter, I analyze the production of femininity and sexual difference as these have been configured in some of the key sex therapy paradigms in the nineteenth, twentieth, and twenty-first centuries, focusing on the major figures that institutionalized these protocols: Freud and psychoanalysis, Masters and Johnson and the physiological or behaviorist approach, Helen Singer Kaplan and the further instantiation of behavioristic sex therapy (but with a renewed acknowledgment of desire), and those who implement contemporary individualistic sex therapy techniques, which often utilize psychopharmacology, cognitive behavior therapy, and increasingly, mindfulness as treatments for low desire—and who tend to theorize about sexuality and gender from the perspective of evolutionary psychology (if they theorize at all).[2] Even when a clear theorization for gender differences is lacking in cognitive research today, evolutionary psychology is often in the backdrop ("we became different as cavepeople"), and gets cavalierly thrown in as an explanation—if not by the researchers themselves, then by those who interpret the research (whether that is other researchers and "experts" or popular writers and journalists).

For each therapeutic model described below, I ask a series of questions: Is it the couple or the individual with sexual problems that is treated? What kind of treatment is deemed most appropriate (e.g., psychodynamic, behavioral, or pharmaceutical methods, or some combination of these)? Is treatment conceived of as necessarily different for men and for women? A thorough exami-

---

2. I do not attend to a deeper history of eighteenth- and nineteenth-century sexology here; ideas about femininity as "inverted" masculinity and the "one-sex" model of human sexuality are fundamental to understanding these contemporary modes, however, and more extensive analyses can be found in Laqueur (1992).

nation of the legacy of these regimes and treatment protocols for desire and behavior abnormalities and sexual dysfunctions is warranted in light of the themes that emerged from my interview data; the low-desiring women who participated in my qualitative study had much to say about how this history and associated notions of femininity and female desire have made it into their psyches, bodies, and bedrooms.

Freud and Deficient Womanhood: "The Little Creature without a Penis"

Even though these ideas could be traced to well before this time period, passive femininity and "receptive" versus "frigid" female desire were popularized and given broad cultural sway along with the psychoanalytic turn of the late nineteenth and early twentieth centuries. In the US and Europe, Sigmund Freud's influence on pre–sex therapeutic treatment of women's sexual problems was profound, and this was mostly clearly linked to his writings on the two (active or "masculine" and passive or "feminine") phases of female sexual development, the female-specific instantiation of the Oedipus and castration complexes, and the primarily feminine pathologies, including frigidity, hysteria, and other feminine neuroses. Freud was a complicated figure. He is also known for his seduction theory, for instance, the proper interpretation of which has been debated by feminists for decades. Depending on which stance you take, this theory either tells us that young women have been largely traumatized by very real sexual violence at the hands of their male elders (see Kleinplatz, 2018 for a discussion of this interpretation) or that at the core of feminine sexuality is the fantasy of incest, the notion that young women masochistically wish to be violated by men, including their fathers and other adult male family members or adult men in their lives (see Ahbel-Rappe, 2006 for a full discussion of both perspectives). Here, I will focus specifically on Freud's later work on female psychosexual development, specifically his 1931 essay on this topic, as it is this thread that appears to have had the greatest effect on popular ideas about female sexuality within contemporary psychology, about Freud and psychoanalysis more generally, and about Freudian or psychoanalytic theories of sex and gender.

Although Freud believed that both men and women were driven by the singular force of the libido, he argued that the libido's modes of sexual gratification could be either active or passive. Proper human sexual development resulted in very different libidinal formations for men and women, corresponding to active and passive impulses—that is, masculinity and femininity, or dimorphic yet complementary gender formations and corresponding healthy behaviors and desires, along with potential dysfunctions or neuroses. According to Freud, human development at its earliest stages is not sexually differentiated; in the pre-Oedipus phase, both boys and girls are attached to the mother, yet also project sadistic impulses onto her, as she is a frustrating denier of masturbation and loathsome disseminator of a variety of other prohibitions. This pre-Oedipal phase of attachment to the mother is significantly longer and more complex in girls, though; once "the little creature without a penis" (Freud, 1931/1952, p. 259) discovers the truth of her castration—her lack of a penis and subsequent horrifying realization that she will never acquire one—she quickly comes to blame her mother for this lack, which then results in a lifetime of ambivalent and often hostile feelings toward loved ones (i.e., the feminine neuroses). For Freud, the sexuality of the young child is ambivalent, as it lacks an object and thus an aim. But this ambivalence is more pronounced, profound, and formative for female children than it is for males due to the "biological reality" of penis envy—the feminine manifestation of the castration complex, which is characterized by a lifelong sense of "organic inferiority" (Freud, 1931/1952, p. 259)—and the fact that surmounting or breaking down the Oedipus complex is simply less important to the development of proper and healthy femininity than to its masculine equivalent. As a result, adult women are less apt to adequately overcome the childish love of their fathers and find an appropriate replacement object than men are to overcome the immature love of their mothers, and thus, women are always less sexually developed and appropriately goal-oriented than are men. In Freud's formulation, women's one true and authentic desire is motherhood, which should be understood as very different than the sexual desire and concomitant individuated selfhood that defines the distinct ego that healthy men develop.

Freud (1931/1952) writes, "We have long realized that in women the development of sexuality is complicated by the task of renouncing that genital zone which was originally the principal one, namely the clitoris, in favor of a new zone—the vagina. But there is a second change which appears to us no less characteristic and important for feminine development: the original mother-object has to be exchanged for the father" (p. 252). Although Freud acknowledged that the linkage of these two "tasks" was elusive, in this statement he set forth a project in which the biological body, gendered behavior, and sexual or object orientation become fused. It was not the first time in medicine or science that this fusing had been articulated, and it certainly would not be the last. What is important and notable about Freud's formulation is how he links a zone of the body itself (the vagina) to an essential kind of energy: feminine passivity, responsiveness, or receptivity. Later in the essay, Freud discusses the two phases of women's sexual development, "the first of which is of a masculine character [and is thus active, and guided by the clitoris], whilst only the second is specifically feminine [it is oriented around the vagina]" (p. 255). He goes on to state:

> Thus in female development there is a process of transition from the one phase to the other, to which there is nothing analogous in males. A further complication arises from the fact that the clitoris, with its masculine character, continues to function in later female sexual life in a very variable manner, which we certainly do not as yet fully understand. Of course, we do not know what are the biological roots of these specific characteristics of the woman, and we are still less able to assign to them *any teleological purpose.* (pp. 255–256; italics added)

This excerpt is crucial to analyze, as it pertains to two specific points that relate to contemporary conceptions of femininity and the treatment of female sexual dysfunction. First, Freud's discussion of proper gendered sexual development and how it is correlated with teleological, evolutionary reproduction in a (cishetero)normative sense has been a running theme through different medico-scientific paradigms throughout the twentieth and twenty-first centuries, and it has made a distinct, forceful, and contentious comeback in the last forty years with the advent of sociobiology, evolutionary psychology, and gender- and sexual orientation–focused experimental psychological research that compares subjective and objective sexual arousal. The second crucial point is that here we see the first full instantiation of the enduring scientific notion that women's sexuality is inherently more complex and enigmatic than men's, and that, as a corollary, adult women are more likely to retain their originary polymorphous perversity, or the bisexuality that is present in all children early on. For Freud, women's sexual development *ought* to result in "definitive femininity" via the passage from clitoral aggression to vaginal passivity correlated with desire for the father or the paternal man who replaces him. In fact, though, femininity is inherently more circuitous, fraught, and less likely to be effectively and completely achieved in the woman than masculinity is to be achieved in the man. Put simply, when it comes to female sexual development, there are more chances for things to go wrong. According to Freud, women are innately prone to feel conflict between, on the one hand, their drive to be masculine (a holdover from the active phallic state during which they first come to experience the forbidden *activity* of the clitoris), and, on the other hand, an essential inferior *passive* feminine state (and thus relegation to a life of receptivity, penis envy, and subsequently, of proper, vaginally focused, "true" femininity). The irony here is that even though women's sexuality is conceived as more complex and complicated than men's sexuality, due to its multiple steps to normative achievement, this complexity does not ultimately indicate that it is more evolved. Instead, male sexuality is equated with proper sublimation, internalization of the paternal function, development of the superego, and ultimately citizenship within "civilized society" (Freud, 1931/1952, p. 256), whereas female sexuality is always inherently closer to the ambivalent, immature, and objectless sexuality of the infant, associated with an inability to fully emerge from the Oedipus complex into adulthood. This fraught, complex, complicated, and less teleological or less evolved sexual state has been maintained as the essential characteristic of female sexuality in scientific discourses from the heyday of psychoanalysis through to more contemporary conceptions of sexuality within the realm of experimental research informed by evolutionary psychology, the consequences of which I will elaborate in chapter 2.

What would eventually become an affinity between Freudian notions of the feminine and more recent neuro-evolutionary conceptions is also foreshadowed at the end of the essay, when Freud states:

> Subsequently, biological factors deflect them [libidinal forces in children] from their original aims and conduct even active and *in every sense masculine* strivings into feminine channels. Since we cannot dismiss the notion that sexual excitation is derived from the operation of certain chemical substances, it would at first seem natural to expect that someday biochemistry will reveal two distinct substances, the presence of which produces male and female sexual excitation respectively. But this hope is surely no less naïve than that other one which has happily been abandoned nowadays, namely, that it would be possible to isolate under the microscope the different causative factors of hysteria, obsessional neurosis, melancholia, etc. (p. 268; italics added)

In our current biomedical and technoscientific landscape, it seems that we have returned to this exact "abandoned" project. Testosterone and estrogen have become stand-ins for masculinity and femininity in popular renditions of scientific discourse (Jordan-Young & Karkazis, 2019; Oudshoorn, 1994), and different levels of hormones such as oxytocin combined with how brightly various parts of the brain light up on a PET scan or fMRI become correlated with gender differences in arousal and desire patterns and with both sexual orientation and loving/nurturing behaviors. Thus, the above passage arguably demonstrates that the normative project of blueprinting proper sexual development as inherently gendered, binary, and rooted in a hetero-reproduction-oriented and teleological biology might have been laid out in particularly clear terms in the early twentieth century by pioneering psychoanalysts (the Freud we love to hate!), but it is a project that has been maintained to this day, under myriad and diverse biomedical guises. Feminists have elaborated and critiqued patriarchal societal structures, institutions, and social, sexual, and reproductive relations as these structures are supported by medical and scientific discourses about sexually differentiated hormones, biology, and gendered sexual natures (for examples, see Fausto-Sterling, 1992, 2000; C. Fine, 2010; Jordan-Young, 2011; Jordan-Young & Karkazis, 2019), and in subsequent chapters, I analyze what some low-desiring women have to say about how these notions have made their way into their experiences of their own sexualities, desires, romantic and familial relationships, and current and past sex lives.

Whatever stance one takes on psychoanalysis, we arguably still feel the effects today of the later Freud's writings on femininity, although the scientific paradigm for excavating sexual truths has clearly shifted away from psychoanalysis to cognitive psychology, neuroscience, behavioral biology, and genetics in the past few decades. More recent conceptions of the sexual nature of women, rooted in evolutionary psychology and neurocognitive paradigms, promulgate very similar themes to those first articulated within early psychoanalytic configurations—including the notions that women are more sexually receptive or responsive than are men; more flexible and fluid; more driven toward monogamy and romantic intimacy or attachment (although this is currently being challenged in some scientific and popular discourse); more reserved or conservative when it comes to their in-the-moment sexual desire (which is described as being at odds with their longer-term and more defining desire to secure a high-quality male mate to father their children and to protect them); and, according to some researchers, more likely to be aroused by submissive or masochistic sexual acts and dynamics. The diametric correlate of all of these characterizations of femininity is, of course, the purported activity, linearity, and spontaneity of male sexuality—that is, a high and free-flowing sex drive, naturalized *as masculinity*. What is perhaps most interesting about what Freud introduces in his 1931 essay is thus the notion that masculinity and femininity literally consist of different biological substrates, or that they operate on different planes. It is this theme that would in some ways be challenged by Masters and Johnson and the behavioristic models of sex therapy beginning in the 1950s, but would ultimately never fully go away. And it is this theme that would eventually make a huge comeback with the evolutionary psychology and sociobiology of the 1970s, '80s, and '90s, and, as I will show, that would ultimately be conscripted to do the dirty work of compulsory heterosexuality in the guise of liberal feminism in the 1990s and early 2000s by a variety of evolutionary sexologists and clinicians who would, to varying degrees, take up the notion that male desire is biological or natural, whereas female desire is cultural or influenced by the infamous "nurture."

Masters and Johnson: The Human Sexual Response Cycle and the Focus on Behavior

In the 1950s and 1960s in the US, research on sexuality began to take a distinctly experimental, cognitive-rational, and behavioristic turn, focusing on the physiology of the body and sexual response in clinical laboratory settings.[3] This type of scientific inquiry is exemplified in the work of William Masters and Virginia Johnson—who are now widely recognized as the founders of modern-day sex therapy. Following the program of gathering data on human sexuality that Alfred Kinsey began in the '50s, Masters and Johnson began their own study, which culminated in their first publication in 1966—the now-classic *Human Sexual Response*. Whereas Kinsey conducted interviews with people regarding their sexual behaviors, thus assessing certain demographic trends (for instance, regarding fluidity in sexual orientation) in the US population, Masters and Johnson conducted research on real human subjects performing sexual acts in their St. Louis–based clinic. They understood their research to be explicitly more scientific than psychoanalysis was, as their work was founded upon clinical observations of masturbation and sexual intercourse. Masters and Johnson believed that their work was thus more objective than the "theoretical" ponderings of the Freudian method, and that it was more neutral and non-ideological, as it equally assessed male and female sexual response in the controlled space of the laboratory.

The most enduring aspect of Masters and Johnson's research program was the development of the four-stage human sexual response cycle (HSRC), consisting of excitement, plateau, orgasm, and resolution. In addition to developing the gender-neutral HSRC (note the absence of desire as a part of this model), their research shed much light on many neglected aspects of sexual-

---

3. It is worth noting that Freud and other psychoanalysts in the early twentieth century also understood their methods to be experimental, scientific, objective, and medically sound in the hypothetico-deductive tradition—but since psychoanalysis began losing its clout and authority within the medical profession in the second half of the twentieth century, the endeavor has been popularly framed as outside of the realm of testable, empirical, scientific analysis. This has been the case in spite of scientific evidence suggesting that psychoanalytically informed therapeutic treatments are, in fact, highly effective (for an example, see Shedler, 2010).

ity, including the extensive capacity for orgasm in women and the unique qualities of the human clitoris. Thus, Masters and Johnson ultimately did much to challenge the scientific ideas of their day about the sexually different responses of men and women to sexual stimuli, including the notion of innate feminine receptivity and vaginal passivity. Even so, their research program has since been roundly critiqued on the grounds of its lack of generalizability (it was conducted in an artificial laboratory setting on a mostly white, educated, middle- to upper-class, heterosexual sample; "homosexuals" were included only to formulate initial hypotheses and ultimately to make conjectures about deviant sexuality); its consequent heteronormativity (not only were members of the sample largely straight, the research agenda assumed that normal sexuality was reproductively oriented and thus focused primarily on penile-vaginal intercourse); and due to the fact that the conclusions of the study rendered sexuality a mechanical, linear, and goal-oriented process (it primarily focused on orgasm as the key to function, and its lack to dysfunction).[4] On this last point, a more recent critique is also that Masters and Johnson's research agenda was ultimately a means to pathologize purportedly abnormal or inadequate sexual response—this is clear in that their second major text was titled *Human Sexual Inadequacy* and explored "deficient" sexual responses (i.e., those that deviated from the linear, orgasm orientation of the HSRC). Thus, Masters and Johnson's research paved the way to an entire field of nonpsychoanalytic medicine devoted to treating the sexually dysfunctional or incompetent—or those figured as such in light of so-called healthy, penetration-driven, orgasmic response.

Regardless of these legitimate critiques, in their time, Masters and Johnson undeniably heralded a revolutionary movement in sexology. These researchers made a few moves, all rooted in the premises of science and medicine, that are noteworthy and remarkable, in spite of their undeniably heteronormative and, in some senses, conservative agenda. The ambivalence here is palpable. First and foremost, they argued that sex was a natural function of the human species and nothing to be ashamed of, neither for men nor for women.[5] They studied the similarities in male and female sexuality, or "the parallels in reactive potential between the two sexes" (Masters & Johnson,

---

4. Leonore Tiefer lays out these critiques of the linearity and universality of the HSRC clearly in much of her own work, including *Sex Is Not a Natural Act and Other Essays*, published in 1995.

5. This formulation of sex as "natural" would ultimately be critiqued by sexuality studies scholars, feminist theorists, queer theorists, and contemporary asexuality studies scholars. Although these critiques are warranted, and indeed, this book proceeds from this critique of "compulsory sexuality," Masters and Johnson arguably helped to destigmatize sex during a cultural moment in which it was, in fact, stigmatized—due, at least in part, to the conservatism of the 1950s in the US and in the aftermath of a cultural vilification of psychoanalysis (which

1966, p. 273) rather than assuming that women are less orgasmic, active, or interested in sex than men—a highly provocative move at the time. Masters and Johnson also called attention to the cultural neglect and simultaneous restriction of female sexuality, as discussed above, for instance by gathering scientific data on certain women's multiorgasmic capacities—from both clitoral and vaginal stimulation—and they directly challenged the notion of a distinct difference between the clitoral and vaginal orgasm, and the notion that the (clitoral and vaginal) structures themselves are separate. They even wrote of a "double standard" applied to men's and women's "sexual value systems" in which men have consistently been encouraged to develop their own sexualities, as they are afforded the opportunity to explore their sexual urges and engage in sex without reprobation. Unfortunately, and somewhat paradoxically, for all they did to challenge Freudian assumptions about "natural" feminine receptivity, shedding light on women's agentic participation in sex, the fact that they conducted their research so disproportionately on cis men and cis women engaged in penile-vaginal penetrative intercourse and assumed that this configuration was the evolutionarily proper and natural way to have sex (not to mention that they assumed that the heterosexual population they studied were the only people who were having "healthy" or "normal" sex) significantly compromised the revolutionary potential of Masters and Johnson's project. Perhaps their ambivalence around sexuality, gender, and biological versus sociocultural influences on sexual response is best summed up in the following quote from *Human Sexual Inadequacy* (1970): "Sociocultural influence more often than not places woman in a position in which she must adapt, sublimate, inhibit or even distort her natural capacity to function sexually in order to fulfill her genetically assigned role. Herein lies a major source of woman's sexual dysfunction" (p. 218). Here, it is clear that Masters and Johnson acknowledged the toxic effects of cultural repression on women's sexuality, but they simultaneously believed that women's sexuality should be "liberated" primarily so that women can fulfill their naturally ordained reproductive duties—to procreate and mother. This theme of sexual liberation as a means toward a heteronormative and gender-reductive end would occur again and again over the next several decades in sex therapy discourse, through to today. It can be seen in evolutionary sexology in the twenty-first century, including in research and treatment enacted under a white liberal feminist protocol.

In another notable and less fraught contribution, Masters and Johnson studied couples having sex in addition to individuals masturbating, and thus

---

had come, perhaps unjustly, to be associated with a certain stigmatization and pathologization of sexuality).

provided a stepping stone toward the inception of the robust field of sex therapy that would develop over the next several decades and that would make sexual relationships (rather than individuals) the focus of treatment—including, eventually, treatment for low desire. This focus on couples was important, as it represented a turn from the sexology that had been in vogue before the modern medical period, and also a movement away from the individualized focus of early psychoanalysis. Their treatment protocol ultimately lost some of its ubiquity closer to the turn of the twenty-first century, with the advent of psychopharmaceuticals, biopsychiatry, cognitive behavioral methods, mindfulness modalities, and gender-specific group therapies. As Kleinplatz (2018) and Kleinplatz, Rosen, Charest, and Spurgas (2020) have noted, the field of sex therapy has splintered over the course of the second half of the twentieth century into the twenty-first, which occurred alongside a rise in specialist sexual medicine, and which subsequently resulted in communication breakdowns among these different specialists. This communication breakdown has posed particular problems for the treatment of low desire, as the etiology of desire problems is characteristically difficult to identify—especially post–Masters and Johnson through to today, a time during which the "organic" versus "psychogenic" causes of sexual dysfunctions continue to be contested (i.e., some specialists focus on biological factors, whereas other sexual medicine practitioners and therapists emphasize subjective and psychogenic elements in a—still often highly medicalized—"biopsychosocial" model).

Alongside their focus on couples, Masters and Johnson also developed short-term behavioral treatments, including "systematic desensitization" and "sensate focus" techniques, which are still used with individuals and couples today. Desensitization, related to the concept of *extinction,* emerged from the behaviorist tendency developed within classical conditioning or a cognitive learning model of psychology—the notion that in order for a pathology to be remedied, the patient must be exposed to the aversive experience until it is no longer offensive, or rather until it is extinguished (in nonsexual behaviorist psychological arenas this may include overcoming a phobia by being exposed to a thing one is afraid of until the fear subsides—a form of behavioral learning or training). As applied in sex therapy, it meant doing whatever the patient was either unable or unwilling to engage in sexually—until they were able to tolerate the act or change their response. For example, in regard to the treatment of vaginismus, the patient might be instructed to insert dilators of increasing sizes into her vagina over and over again until she was able to relax her pelvic muscles enough to engage in intercourse (see Kleinplatz, 2018 for a discussion of this "bridging" technique as it emerged from Masters and Johnson's work and influenced the sex therapy of Helen Singer Kaplan). Once the patient was able to be penetrated successfully during heterosexual intercourse, the treatment was considered successful. Desensitization-related techniques continue to be used in sex therapy today; dilators are still a popular method of treating genito-pelvic pain/penetration disorder (GPPPD) and vulvodynia, and contemporary mindfulness and cognitive behavioral techniques have much in common with this classical conditioning extinction-oriented frame. In recent years, classical and operant conditioning techniques have also been used to study potential methods of extinguishing "aversive" sexual behaviors and desires in male and female patients in laboratories, where subjects are conditioned via positive and negative stimuli—including a sharp pain to the wrist as a negative stimulus (for an example, see Brom, Laan, Everaerd, Spinhoven, & Both, 2015).

Sensate focus, perhaps Masters and Johnson's most important technical contribution to the field of sex therapy, was originally used with sexually dysfunctional couples to allow them to move past their own performance anxiety and focus on exploring one another's bodies. For Masters and Johnson, the touching was oriented more toward the person doing the touching than the person being touched, at least in its initial stages. It was a way for a person with anxiety around sex to break their own anxiety cycle and stop focusing so much on their own performance—for instance, a person who is prone to "spectatoring," or imagining how they look in the moment, watching themself as a third party, with a judgmental attitude, might be treated with sensate focus to bring them "back into the moment." Weiner and Avery-Clark (2014) have recently argued that sensate focus has been misinterpreted by sex therapists broadly and used in a way that is not true to Masters and Johnson's original framework. This protocol, according to Weiner and Avery-Clark, is not about pleasing the partner and instead is about allowing oneself to focus on (voluntary) sensations, thus overcoming the (involuntary) dysfunctional response. It is more about being in tune with one's own body and experience than with one's partner's body and experience (and it is not really about either partner's sexual pleasure, per se). These sex therapists also made the case for the compatibility of sensate focus with depth psychology—as an attempt to think of sex therapy in a more long-term vein, much differently than the way it was originally used at the Masters and Johnson Institute, which was very much within a short-term and behavioristic framework.[6]

---

6. Although they developed the now-standard short and intensive treatment protocol for sexual dysfunctions, a protocol that focused on the immediate causes of sexual problems (over deeper, "remote" psychological issues), Masters and Johnson also noted that the vast majority of sexual concerns (in both men and women) were psychogenic or psychosomatic in nature. This stands in stark contrast to the way that sexual dysfunctions came to be framed in the following decades, through to today.

Although sensate focus was initially developed for use with couples (and before desire was included in the behaviorist models of sexual response), it was later taken up in programs targeted to individual women with low desire, as a way for these women to get "back in touch" with their own bodies, desires, and sensations—for instance, in the treatment protocol of Heiman, LoPiccolo, and LoPiccolo described in their 1976 book *Becoming Orgasmic*. A version of this technique is also used in the self-directed mindfulness protocols of the twenty-first century as well (see Brotto, 2018 for an example), in which women cultivate their desire by sensually focusing on their own aroused bodies, autonomic sensations, or an external object, such as a raisin, in order to let distracting thoughts pass so they can be present, or "in the moment," and thus available for sex. It is clear that in many ways the behaviorist technique of sensate focus is a precursor to mindfulness in sex therapy, as both emphasize reducing distractions, and are thus in some sense part of the brief-but-intensive treatment approach to sexual problems—and, importantly, both are also understood as alternatives to the long-term, narrative-based protocol of depth psychologies and psychoanalysis. But why is it that behaviorism and psychoanalysis have come to be framed as mutually exclusive when it comes to sex therapy, and to psychological interventions more broadly? In what type of sociopolitical environment do therapists prescribe methods to reduce distractions and be more in the moment, and why do people feel so distracted in their daily lives to begin with, including in their sex lives? Why are these methods so widely utilized, and why do they have such broad appeal? Which populations are most heavily targeted as in need of these treatments, and what assumptions are made about the individuals under these protocols today? In short, why are *women* so sexually distracted (or assumed to be)? Why are women (particularly white, middle- or upper-class, cis women) those who are most often prescribed treatments to help them get back "into the present moment?" Is this treatment modality and its theoretical orientation to desire spreading to other folks as well? Does the treatment come first, or the need for it? And finally, how are these treatments feminized (applied to folks who are *not* women or femmes but who are still treated in accordance with the feminized logic of ameliorating distractibility while simultaneously cultivating desire)? These are the questions I will seek to answer in the rest of this book. They are important to address, as sex therapy has a long history of functioning as a mechanism of social control—a project that continues in the present day, under a new biopolitical protocol, and under the sign of feminism.

Masters and Johnson's desensitization and sensate focus work with couples was taken up in the subsequent research and sex therapy paradigm of Helen Singer Kaplan, who arguably did plenty of pathologizing of "deviant" sexualities herself, but who also maintained a relational focus on the problems of couples rather than putting all of the blame for sexual problems on individuals and their purportedly autonomous issues—as is the case more often today. Kaplan was also unique for her consideration of both "remote" and "immediate" psychosomatic causes of sexual dysfunction and for her consideration of the intricacies of desire—which she paid attention to rather than maintaining the mechanical, cognitive, and behaviorist focus attributed to Masters and Johnson, or by focusing only on deep psychic pathologies, as Freud is remembered for doing.

Helen Singer Kaplan: Behavioristic Sex Therapy and the (Re)Introduction of Desire

Whereas Freud's formulation of female sexuality was specifically concerned with women's desire as it was oriented toward or deviated from feminine passivity, and Masters and Johnson were primarily concerned with the rote physiology of sexual arousal and assumed a sexually differentiated reproductive drive that inspired it (even as their HSRC was gender-neutral), Austrian American behaviorist sex therapist Helen Singer Kaplan's work on sexual disorders and her particular brand of sex therapy techniques in the 1970s brought desire—and its absence in both the sexual medicine of the day and in many of her sex therapy clients, especially women—back into the clinical spotlight. Building on the work of Masters and Johnson, Kaplan abandoned the Freudian focus on "immature" (clitoral) versus "mature" (vaginal) female sexuality, and instead looked at the larger mechanics and determinants of women's arousal patterns. In her classic text, *The New Sex Therapy* (1974), Kaplan states that in formulating her therapeutic project, she strove to bring together knowledge from the diverse theoretical realms of traditional psychoanalysis and psychodynamic therapy, behaviorism and behavioral therapy, psychosomatic medicine, and group therapies. In the preface to the original 1974 volume, she asserts that "modern medical treatment owes its power to the adoption of a *rational* model of intervention" (p. 1; italics added). For Kaplan, this focus on rationality, inherited from Masters and Johnson, meant that effective therapeutic treatment of any sort must move beyond the "grand speculations" of Freud and empirical treatment based on "trial and error and untested or unsubstantiated hypothesis" (p. 1) to focus instead on specific behaviors and acts and whether or not they elicit desired responses. Thus, the "new sex therapy" would utilize the confirmed anatomical knowledge of sexual arousal, response, and basic reproductive and genital anatomy offered in the work of Masters and Johnson, combined with a goal-oriented, practical, and behavior or "sexual task"-oriented (hence her use of the term *rational*) approach to the treatment of dysfunction—including low desire and arousal, which she referred to, as she observed these primarily in her female patients, as "frigidity." For Kaplan, the goal was a higher frequency of pleasurable sexual experiences for any given sexually suffering couple. But what might be considered pleasurable? And on which partner's terms was pleasure to be measured for the (cisgender, heterosexual, usually married) couples that Kaplan treated? These were questions left largely unanswered by Kaplan and her followers, in spite of their insistence on a shared responsibility of the couple—by both partners seeking therapy—to increase sexual pleasure through sensate focus and other exercises designed to reconfigure and enhance their portfolio of "sexual transactions."

There was much about this trend in sex therapy that was, in fact, new—and very exciting. Kaplan's triphasic focus (developed in her 1979 book *Disorders of Sexual Desire*) on dysfunctions of desire, excitement/arousal, and orgasm in both men and women paradoxically meant that, perhaps for the first time in the history of Western sex therapy, women were acknowledged as having the capacity for sexual desire to begin with. In the wake of Masters and Johnson's conclusion that clitoral and vaginal orgasms were actually always both, that there was really only one kind of female orgasm that incorporated the stimulation of both clitoral and vaginal structures, it seemed that women's sexuality was finally about to be taken seriously in the clinic (and hopefully, by extension, in the bedroom), that women's sexual needs were finally going to be attended to—instead of being neglected in lieu of a focus on attention to male pleasure, as they had been up to that point within clinical and therapeutic spaces. In many ways, Kaplan's model was evidence of a new look at sexuality as dynamic and relational, as involving multiple organizing factors in its constitution, expression, and aim, and of dysfunction or disorder as involving many etiologic factors as well. Despite examining the multicausal etiology of sexual problems, though, Kaplan's theoretical orientation was fraught and ambivalent, and ultimately did not adequately challenge the notion of women's sexuality as more responsive, receptive, and emotionally driven than men's sexuality. In fact, she added new research to bolster and extend these notions, even as she reconfigured the importance of sexual desire in the linear process of arousal, adding it as the important first step to Masters and Johnson's four-stage human sexual response cycle, and even as she examined contextual factors that might influence women's (and men's) desire.

The notions of desire and sexual response were gender-differentiated in Kaplan's theory; men's desire was conceptualized as more attached to the physiological pursuit of sexual pleasure (which was conceived in biological terms as easier for men to achieve) and rooted in an evolutionary drive to procreate, whereas women's desire continued to be understood as "more variable than the male's, presumably because it is far more susceptible to psychological and cultural determinants" (Kaplan, 1974, p. 33). This notion of the complex nature of woman's desire, which is more receptive to the vicissitudes of her environment, was in keeping with Masters and Johnson's analysis, and would remain a running theme in sexology and sex therapy through to today. However, even more so than Masters and Johnson, Kaplan gives airtime to the cultural pressures to which women are sexually subjected. She briefly elucidates some of these potentially influential psychological and cultural determinants in a section on female sexual dysfunction, a move that could certainly be considered progressive at the time:

> Multiple factors can impair the development of sexual autonomy in women. In the past we have looked only to psychoanalysis for our answers and have paid insufficient attention to the destructive effects of a culture which places women in a subservient and dependent role. . . . [U]nconscious conflicts about sexuality, fear, shame, and guilt due to a restrictive upbringing, conflicts about the female role and about independence and dependency, about activity and passivity, fear of men, fear of losing control, fear of rejection and abandonment, a hostile and rivalrous marital relationship, and severe psychopathology can all be instrumental in producing any or all of the female sexual dysfunctions. (p. 359)

It is clear from this passage that Kaplan has truly considered the social factors that might influence women's sexuality, and sexuality in general. Unfortunately, these musings do not influence her approach to sex therapy, an approach that (consistent with Masters and Johnson's approach) tends to focus on the amelioration of what she calls "immediate" causes of sexual dysfunctions over a deeper examination of the "remote" causes ("remote" causes here mean psychoanalytic causes, not social factors). Although Kaplan recognizes that social factors influence sexuality, she gives this little attention in her 544-page tome, continuously juggling the descriptive "empirical" work of Masters and Johnson with the Oedipally focused "theoretical" psychoanalysis of Freud, but ultimately coming down on the side of a behavioristic and rationalistic approach to sex therapy. Again, psychoanalytically informed investigations of desire (and trauma) are relegated to the Oedipal. Kaplan sees utilizing psychoanalytic and even psychodynamic frames as inherently requiring the exploration of incestuous seduction wishes, infantile transference, penis envy, and castration anxiety, and thus as being too time-consuming and cumbersome (in addition to being increasingly passé to a psychology that was increasingly seeking to redefine itself as "atheoretical" and "apolitical"). In a particularly revealing discussion of Freud, in which she praises him for his discovery of the "dark continent of The Unconscious" and subsequent revelation that most sexual conflict is beyond conscious awareness, Kaplan (1974) states: "In retrospect, his greatest error was that he ignored all other potential sources of sexual conflict except early incestuous wishes of the child toward his parents" (p. 138). Statements such as these demonstrate how psychoanalysis came to be reduced to the Oedipus complex for post-Freudian psychologists and thus relegated to an antiquated past, while behaviorism and associated cognitive behavioral treatments were increasingly seen as the way of the future. This tendency continues to this day in twenty-first-century psychology, wherein sex therapy (insofar as it still exists as a field) and related treatment schemas for enhancing desire do not engage with narrative-based interpretations or protocols, and "immediate" causes of dysfunction and their quick and measurable alleviation remain the focus.

Helen Singer Kaplan's (1974) notion of "bypassing" may be the clearest example of how, even as she acknowledged cultural constraints on women's sexuality, she ultimately centered brief, rationalistic, behavioral treatment for sexual problems in her new sex therapy model—with potentially deleterious effects for women's sex lives. Regarding the importance of rapidly resolving "here and now" conflicts that impede sexual performance, she states: "Symptom relief can be obtained by modifying the immediate products of conflict without necessarily eliminating the conflict itself.... [A]lthough we give recognition to the deeper source of conflict, sex therapy does *not* ordinarily deal with this deeper structure unless this proves to be specifically necessary ... [and] in the majority of sexually dysfunctional patients, basic conflicts can be bypassed and defenses built up to allow the patient to function well sexually" (pp. 150–151). Kaplan explicitly makes the case that so-called remote causes of sexual dysfunction, including traumatic sexual violence, which could result in low desire or "frigidity," are some of the main issues that sex therapists will need to be prepared to help their patients bypass. Bypassing trauma sounds a lot like using cognitive behavioral therapy (CBT) or mindfulness to avoid distractions that prevent one from engaging in sexual activity;[7] the therapeutic point here is that bypassing versus processing trauma are two very different ways of thinking about how to manage traumatic experiences that may have

---

7. I thank Peggy Kleinplatz for our discussions of the connection between bypassing and mindfulness in sex therapy.

contributed to sexual problems. In this light, it seems obvious that bypassing, CBT, and mindfulness could potentially have unintended negative effects, including in perpetuating cycles of coercion—particularly for women (who were and are more likely to be encouraged to use these techniques).

It might be argued that, as a clinical psychologist and sex therapist, Kaplan could not have been expected to integrate feminist and sociopolitical analyses into her treatment protocols. But I want to argue, along with Kleinplatz (2011, 2018), among others, that it is imperative that sex therapists consider the diverse etiologies of sexual troubles, including the ways these troubles can traumatically arise both from personal experience and relational history, as well as from structural and cultural influences—in addition to the unique ways in which sexual concerns may be manifested by women and gender-diverse individuals, and particularly folks of color in these groups, in light of their disproportionate experiences of trauma—when designing treatments. It is for precisely this reason that sociological, critical, and intersectional feminist analyses of sexuality and gender must be integrated into clinical and therapeutic treatment programs. Clinicians must take responsibility for the powerful assumptions they make—and expertly disseminate—about the bases of sexual difference and behavioral sexual relations between men and women.

In *The New Sex Therapy*, even in light of what seems at times like a revolutionary attention to sociocultural determinants of desire (or its lack), and an attention to both immediate and remote causes of dysfunction, Kaplan also actively naturalizes women as more emotionally complex, finding in the emerging field of neurology evidence for the feminine drive to love, and thus promulgating the notion that romance is a purported necessity for female pleasure. Although in 1974, Kaplan was not yet writing explicitly about sexually disparate desire patterns in women and men, she appears to assume this differentiation in her discussion of the emotionally charged sexual "flashbacks" that some of her female patients report (and she makes it clear that she has only witnessed this phenomenon in women):

> Sometimes the day after they [women] have engaged in a particularly arousing sexual act with an especially loved and desired partner, they experience profoundly pleasurable "flashbacks." These are triggered by memories of the erotic experience and are accompanied by intense erotic sensations and feelings of euphoria and love. (p. 44)

In this passage, we see the early formulations of a neurological linking of sex and love, for women, specifically. This theme of the importance of romantic attachment and sentimentality for women will be reiterated throughout the latter half of the twentieth century to the present day in medical and scientific research on sexuality, and will become a prerequisite—an assumed variable—within later studies of female desire, which is generally configured as distinct from "pleasure-seeking" and "goal-oriented" male sexuality within clinical experiments, quantitative survey research, qualitative social psychology research, and eventually in neuroimaging studies. Although Kaplan does not explicitly define desire disorders as part of the landscape of potential sexual pathology until 1977, her discussion of women's sentimental sexual feelings, emotional erotic life, and romantic "flashbacks" lays the foundation for the first reinstantiation of the concept of desire—and its corresponding gendered pathos—in the post-Freudian psychiatric and therapeutic milieu of the day.

In articulating the importance of the relationship, partner, and other external factors on the health of the body itself, Kaplan demonstrates her belief that relational context, erotic environment, or what she calls the "sexual system" of the relationship, can affect biology—in a type of feedback loop of embodied imprinting or psychic learning. Like many other clinicians during this time (including Masters and Johnson, more than is often acknowledged in popular representations of their work), Kaplan was very attentive to the effects of psychosomatic problems on sexual response and experience, and also to how these produced "specific learned inhibitions" or "aversive conditioning" (Kaplan, 1974, p. 63). Her elucidation of how chronic stress, depression, fear of failure and other performance anxiety issues, and even guilt and "threat of injury" can influence hormonal constitutions and the functioning of the hypothalamic-pituitary axis (HPA) comes just shy of acknowledging the physical effects of trauma on the brain and neurocircuitry—and of acknowledging the sociopolitical reasons these might affect men and women differently, beyond assumed a priori biological differences in sex drive. But ultimately, even in her brief discussion of "traumatic early sexual experience," Kaplan evades a full engagement with the social, cultural, and political traumas that influence women's sexualities, bodies, and senses of desire, constituting them—in specific ways, to different degrees, and in some cases—as distinct from men's. She instead distinguishes between the trauma of an "immediate obstacle" to successful sex, such as premature ejaculatory tendencies that result in subsequent performance anxiety (here, she focuses on men's trauma), and the "gross trauma" of being the victim of incest, pederasty, or childhood rape. She states that the "destructive potential" of these gross traumas is "obvious" (p. 176). Across her clinical writing, gender differences in exposure to these different types of traumas are left largely unexplored—or at least rarely considered in her theoretical formulations or technical protocol.

So, the feedback loops she takes into account only go so far (or deep), and Kaplan generally does not take an in-depth approach to trauma in her later conceptualization and treatment of "inhibited sexual desire" (ISD). Unfortunately, the casual and cavalier nature of these comments about trauma would come to set the tone for the next several decades of research on and treatment of sexual dysfunction. In the following chapter, I demonstrate the import of this legacy on today's sexual medicine, experimental research, and sex therapy, specifically in regard to a firmly behavioristic turn that can be observed in all of these realms.

It is clear that Kaplan is ambivalent regarding her orientation to therapeutic treatment, yet she ultimately clings to "atheoretical," behavioristic, and purportedly gender-neutral scientific inquiry in the face of "politics" (another trend that will set the tone for sex therapy and sexual medicine for decades to come). But what may be most important to take from the work of Helen Singer Kaplan is that it very well may have represented one of the last times in the canon of mainstream sexual medicine that the intensely complicated nature of and feedback loops among psyche, body, sexuality, power, trauma, and culture were actively considered—particularly as this project pertained to really grappling with psychoanalysis. Not only this, but it may have also represented one of the last times the sexual relationship between two parties, or the "sexual system" or "erotic environment," was seriously taken into account when considering treatment rather than the sexually dysfunctional individual him- or herself alone.[8] As the North American and European clinic and research laboratory moved away from psychosomatic medicine—the aftermath of Freudian psychoanalysis that is rarely conceived of as legitimate nowadays—they moved toward biologically deterministic explanations for gender-dimorphic patterns of desire, arousal, and sexual behaviors, motivations, and proclivities. This shift is particularly clear in light of the swift and tenacious move toward evolutionary, genetic, and neurobiological explana-

---

8. There are a few noteworthy exceptions to this trend, but these remain the exceptions rather than the rule in mainstream sexual medicine. Here, I am thinking of the early work of the New View Campaign and their four-tiered conceptualization of women's sexuality (Working Group for the New View of Women's Sexual Problems, 2002), and Kleinplatz's "Optimal Sexual Experience" sex therapy (for an overview, see Kleinplatz, et al., 2009; 2018), in addition to the psychoeducation and bibliotherapy of Lonnie Barbach, Betty Dodson, and Gina Ogden. Although these paradigms do explore gendered social relations and power, I argue that in some cases they reify and essentialize gender differences, and also ignore trauma as they jettison psychoanalytic conceptions of desire. Kleinplatz is an exception to this trend with her focus on BDSM, and she also importantly points out that, excluding the trauma-informed sex therapy of Maltz and Holman (1987), most trauma-focused clinicians and theorists have tended to ignore sexuality, while sex therapists have too often ignored trauma and its impact on desire (Kleinplatz, 2018).

tions for these phenomena—articulated in terms of individual disorders and dysfunctions—beginning in the late 1970s in almost all popular, mainstream, and, importantly, well-funded studies on these topics.

(Sexually Dimorphic) Desire in Evolutionary Sexology

In the years following the publication of Kaplan's *The New Sex Therapy* in 1974 and *Disorders of Desire* in 1979, many clinicians and sex therapists began to identify "low desire" as one of the most common complaints their patients presented with[9]—particularly their female patients. Desire began to be examined more closely in this post-psychoanalytic milieu as a key feature of healthy sexuality—although as I will show, beginning with Kaplan and in the decades since then, it was increasingly framed in more rationalistic and cognitive behaviorist terms, and eventually as "incentive" to engage in sex. People, especially women, might *desire to desire*; they may note that they had felt desire previously, perhaps for a specific partner, and now miss it, as this feeling has waned—and this was framed as something they deserved help for. Thus, the notion that having sex (and desiring to have sex) is part of a fulfilling and healthy life, that it is a "right," became more commonplace—aided in large part by the sexual revolution of the 1960s in North America, which provided the backdrop for a newfound interest in sexual desire. The activism of second-wave feminists, including those who designed sexual and reproductive health workshops in the 1970s, also helped foster the notion that women, just like men, might *want* to have sex, and that they should be able to do so. Concomitant with all of this was the notion that *not* wanting to have sex potentially indicated some type of pathology—a trend that paved the way toward what scholars now critique as "compulsory sexuality" (Gupta, 2015). Accordingly, desire disorders began to be added to the *Diagnostic and Statistical Manual of Mental Disorders*—the first diagnosis being inhibited sexual desire (ISD) in the *DSM-III* in 1980, renamed hypoactive sexual desire disorder (HSDD) when it was revised in 1987 (the criterion that the lack of desire must cause "interpersonal difficulty" was then added when the *DSM-IV* was published in 1994). Each of these diagnoses was gender-neutral; men and women could both be diagnosed, although since the inception of ISD, women have disproportionately been candidates for diagnosis.

There has been much antimedicalization and social constructionist feminist critique following the official recognition of these diagnoses through the

---

9. For one example, see the work of Harold Lief (1977).

publication of the revised version of the *DSM-IV*. Antimedicalization feminists have also been vocally critical of the shift toward biological and individual-focused explanations for sexual dysfunctions, with pharmaceutical treatment as the accompanying "state of the art." Much of this type of critique in the last two decades, however, has interrogated medical profiteering by "Big Pharma" within "Viagra Culture" at the expense of other aspects of the medical and scientific discourse—elements that I believe are just as important to examine. For instance, in the backdrop of this individualistic and pharmaceutically oriented shift in sexual medicine, we often see either an explicit lack of theorization for observed gender differences in desire within a cognitive behaviorist framing, on the one hand, or we see an explicit evolutionary psychology theorization, on the other hand—often thrown in at the end of published reports on gender differences in sexual expression rather haphazardly, as if the notion that "our cavepeople ancestors" were rapists and "mate poachers" is completely self-evident. In some cases, this type of evolutionary theorizing guides the research, and in other cases, it seems to be included almost as an afterthought. And in some cases, when the gender differences are not explicitly theorized (as is the case in much experimental sex research that claims to be atheoretical and apolitical), other parties utilize an evolutionary paradigm to make sense of the findings, in light of this absence of theory. In the late twentieth century, into the first two decades of the twenty-first century, there are many examples of journalists, media writers, and pop psychologists "filling in the blanks" of these undertheorized studies—specifically with popular evolutionary psychology explanations. I will examine some of the most noteworthy of these contemporary studies on female sexual dysfunction—and their popular interpretations—in the next chapter. For now, I look at the impact of popular evolutionary psychology motifs on sexology, sex therapy, and sexual medicine more broadly over the last few decades.

In the early 1990s, right around the time the *DSM-IV* was released, many psychologists fully diverged from a psychodynamic framework for sexuality and began to take up a view of human behavior rooted in a model claimed as more "evolutionary" and in line with the theory of sexual selection associated with Charles Darwin. This new metatheoretical framework came to be known as evolutionary psychology (EP) and was not only based on neo-Darwinian models of evolution[10] but also embraced many of the tenets of Edward O. Wilson's sociobiology (1975)—including his analogizing of human

---

10. The EP version of evolutionary theory I describe here has been critiqued as only loosely related to Darwin's actual thought, and some critics, including biologist Stephen Jay Gould and geneticist Richard Lewontin, have further argued that evolutionary psychologists drastically misinterpret modern macroevolutionary theory.

social relations with nonhuman animal behavior. Although EP took off in full force in the 1990s, many of its core features can be traced back to the 1960s and 1970s: its ideas about human behavioral patterns and psychological makeup, with their foundation in natural and sexual selection; the notion that these are based on ancient, evolved adaptations that fostered our fittest human ancestors' survival and reproduction in prehistoric environments; and the theme of similarity between many nonhuman animal species and human societies (especially regarding sexual relations). Early evolutionary psychologists explored themes such as kinship and familial ties (Hamilton, 1964), selfishness and altruism (Dawkins, 1976), and sexual difference (Symons, 1979; Trivers, 1972) and linked these to an evolutionary drive to genetic perpetuity and reproductive success. Today, these ideas still hold much sway among experimental and clinical psychologists who do sex research, even those who do not explicitly identify as evolutionary psychologists.

As sex therapy in its dyad-focused and relational Masters-Johnson-Kaplan formation became less commonly practiced in the 1980s and 1990s, and was increasingly replaced by individualized treatments for sexual dysfunction from the realms of polypharmacy, cognitive behavioral therapy, and, eventually, mindfulness, this popular evolutionary orientation began to impact protocols for managing sexual problems. Notably, the threads of an evolutionary theory of *desire*—a term which would eventually be replaced with notions of sexual "incentives," "motivations," and "information [to be processed]," particularly in the case of women—can be seen in the writings of Masters and Johnson, Helen Singer Kaplan, Harold Lief, and many other researchers beginning in the 1960s and 1970s. But it wasn't until well-known psychologists such as David Buss and Cindy Meston, researchers at the University of Texas at Austin, took up the question of gender differences in sexual behavior in their popular mainstream research agenda that the impact of evolutionary psychology on formulations of healthy and dysfunctional sexuality (and the hetero- and cisnormative assumptions about gender differences therein) would become clear. Take this discussion of "sperm competition" and its impact on sexual decision-making from Meston and Buss's 2007 article, "Why Humans Have Sex":

> From this ["sperm competition"] perspective, a man whose partner might have been sexually unfaithful might seek sex, which functions to displace the sperm of the rival male. Or a woman might deplete the sperm of her partner, leaving few available for insemination of rival women. *None of these hypothesized functions, of course, need operate through conscious psychological mechanisms.* (p. 478; italics added)

There is much to question about this theorization regarding (purportedly universal) reasons people have sex, but what I think is particularly interesting is the last sentence, where the authors posit the existence of a type of evolutionary drive that is said to dictate not only sexual behavior but desire itself. The libidinal unconscious of psychoanalysis has been replaced here by an *evolutionary* unconscious. Ironically, the caveperson unconscious that is theorized here, and that will become the go-to explanation for sexual behavior in mainstream twenty-first-century experimental sexology, is much less open to being affected by the environment (or family, or socialization, or trauma) than the unconscious of psychoanalysis. It is also more difficult to critique, particularly without recourse to the strawman of social constructionism, as it is proclaimed to be presocial or even asocial. It seems ironic that 1970s sex therapists like Helen Singer Kaplan were reticent to talk about desire in psychoanalytic terms and to consider the role of the unconscious, as they believed the Freudian conceptions of these were too rigid (i.e., too wedded to a fixed Oedipal vision of psychosexual development), but that now, today's most renowned sexological researchers regularly explain complex human behaviors and desires via an indestructible and uncritiqueable evolutionary motif. Also of note is that this evolutionary unconscious described by Meston and Buss, in all of its paradoxical presociality (paradoxical in that it does, in fact, rely on a reified and ossified vision of a *past* social world), is also pre-race, pre-class, pre-oppression, and pre-*power*. The most purportedly "natural" thing in the world then turns out to also be one of the whitest, most cis- and heteronormative, and most bourgeois.

This gendered evolutionary unconscious described by Meston and Buss in 2007—to be fleshed out further in 2009 with the release of their popular psychology book *Why Women Have Sex*—relied on much older tropes. Although sociobiological explanations for human behavior and a "gene's-eye view" of evolution (Hamilton, 1964) began to be popularized as early as the mid-twentieth century, it wasn't until the 1990s that EP was linked with cognitive neuroscience via behavioral biology and ethology. In 1994, Leda Cosmides and John Tooby, citing Richard Dawkins (1976), wrote, "Natural selection—*an invisible-hand process*—is the only component of the evolutionary process that produces complex functional machinery in organisms.... [N]atural selection built the decision-making machinery in human minds" (p. 328; italics added). This "invisible [evolutionary] hand," neutrally guiding human psychology and behavior, also purportedly guides human sexual relationships, mating strategies (in addition to "extra-pair" sexual strategies), and the expression or inhibition of dimorphic masculine and feminine sexual desires—all of which are core foci of many evolutionary psychologists and the clinicians, researchers, and sex therapists who are guided by these same tenets.

Why is this extension of evolutionary psychology into sexological research so important to consider? For one thing, this discourse is incredibly pervasive in the popular sphere. Not only did Meston and Buss's 2009 book *Why Women Have Sex* receive much attention, but, because it was written by reputable psychologists at a research university, ideas like those summed up in the book came to be easily interpreted in the mainstream as the simple truth of sexuality, and, importantly, of gender differences therein. In their 2007 precursor article, the researchers claim: "The current research [their own study] provided the most comprehensive examination to date of gender differences in expressed reasons for engaging in sexual intercourse" (p. 499). One of the gender differences they describe through evolutionary psychology discourse is the tendency for men to be more invested in their mate's physical appearance and aroused by visual cues, "since physical appearance provides a wealth of cues to a woman's fertility and reproductive capacity" (p. 499). Accordingly, Meston and Buss cite fMRI studies (conducted by Emory primate researcher Kim Wallen and colleagues) that have provided "neurophysiological [evidentiary] support" for this gender difference in arousal by visual cues via reports of a "greater activation of the amygdala and hypothalamus to visual sexual stimuli in men than in women" (p. 500).

So, another reason why this evolutionary psychology extension into sexological research is important is that evolutionary explanations regarding gender differences in sexual behavior are presented as universal and ubiquitous, particularly when they are supported with neuroimaging and other contemporary medico-scientific technologies (and this is often the case even when subsequent studies do not substantiate the original claims). Meston and Buss (2007) go so far as to say that the reasons they elucidate for why people have sex, including "adventure," "celebration," and "opportunity," "may reflect a fundamental universal core of human sexual motivation" (they do acknowledge that this would "require cross-cultural research to test") (p. 498). This assertion, even with their cross-cultural research caveat, is troubling, particularly as their sample consists of psychology students at the University of Texas who received course credit for completing the researchers' survey, the majority of whom were white, and more than a third of whom identified as "fundamentalists" in regard to their religious affiliation. The mean age of the sample was nineteen years old, and it was almost two-thirds female. Apparently, questions about sexual orientation and sexual identity were not asked at all, and there is no data on whether or not alternative gender or sex categories beyond "male" and "female" were provided as choices on the survey. How much can we really glean about the "fundamental universal core of human sexual motivation" from this sample?[11] The answer to that question apparently doesn't matter much to researchers following Meston and Buss, as the 2007 study is heavily cited in experimental and clinical research to this day.

The myriad problems with evolutionary psychology have been enumerated by other writers at length (for seminal examples, see Gould, 2002; Lewontin, 1991; McKinnon, 2006; S. Rose, Kamin, & Lewontin, 1984), including on account of its lack of generalizability, reliability, and validity, and some scientists have critiqued EP specifically on the basis of its heteronormative ideological assumptions and flawed logic regarding human sexual relations (for examples, see Fausto-Sterling, 1997; C. Fine, 2010; Gannon, 2002; Gowaty, 2000; Liesen, 2007; Travis, 2003). One of the biggest preoccupations of EP researchers and clinicians from the outset has been sex and gender role differentiation via sexual selection and how this is indicated by early hominid behavioral adaptations or evolved mating strategies, which are posited as neurological or "hardwired" (for an example, see Buss, 1994). In this book, an analysis of these themes from EP is crucial for two reasons: (1) These ideas about sexual difference are deployed as theoretical backing within some of the most prolific experimental research on gender differences in sexual behavior and desire, and that research subsequently informs the way sexual dysfunctions are configured and treated. And (2) many of the women I interviewed described how they feel their own desires and experiences have been affected by exposure to these ideas about femininity and gender differences in sexuality. Not only have women's sexualities been influenced via this exposure, but some participants describe how they believe their (in many cases male) partners' attitudes toward sex have also been influenced by these ideas, which has affected the types of sexual experiences the participants are most likely to have with these men. Although my sample was small and thus not generalizable, my qualitative study indicates potential themes that might be salient to other women, and that should be explored in future research. Rather than these evolutionary psychology theories simply explaining universal facts, my data suggest a different potential pathway: that, in some cases, it's the other way around—the circulation of these expert ideas, as pervasive forms of social discourse, affects how women have sex.

There are many examples from contemporary sexological research and related areas that demonstrate the impact of evolutionary psychology. Some of the most well-known of these include Roy Baumeister (2000, 2004), who hypothesizes that women are biologically more erotically flexible and "plastic"

---

11. For a well-known critique in this vein, see Henrich, Heine, and Norenzayan (2010).

than are men; Stuart Brody, who continues to posit that women who experience orgasms from penile-vaginal intercourse are healthier, more psychologically stable, and more sexually functional than women who experience orgasms only from clitoral stimulation (for a recent example, see Brody & Costa, 2017); and Randy Thornhill and Craig T. Palmer, who made the case in their 2000 book *A Natural History of Rape: The Biological Bases of Sexual Coercion* that rape is not only natural and inevitable due to an unalterable biological power imbalance between men and women, but that women in fact evolutionarily *select* for rape behaviors—because these behaviors provide evidence of a potential mate's "strength, endurance, and vigor" (p. 83). These researchers publish in scientific journals and their books are either academic or have wide crossover appeal; additionally, many popular writers, from the early 1990s (e.g., Matt Ridley with *The Red Queen: Sex and the Evolution of Human Nature* [1993]) through to the second decade of the twenty-first century (e.g., Ogi Ogas and Sai Gaddam with *A Billion Wicked Thoughts: What the Internet Tells Us about Sexual Relationships* [2011]) have continued to make the case for sex differences in behavior rooted in evolutionary psychology. These include the notion of hardwired gender differences in stimulation from pornography or other visual cues, to one of the most popular themes, which is the notion that women's sexuality is less "category-specific," "target-specific," or "object-oriented" than is male sexuality. Women have been configured via evolutionary psychology discourse here as more erotically plastic, flexible, and malleable, and more likely to be physiologically aroused by objects and situations that do not align with their stated sexual preferences (they are said to be more likely than men to exhibit subjective/genital "discordance," a concept that will be explored further in the next chapter). In other words, women are less likely to have a distinct sexual orientation than are men. The prominence of these scientists, in conjunction with their popular counterparts, suggests how far evolutionary psychology explanations can travel, and how much they have affected debates about healthy versus dysfunctional sexual desire and behavior—particularly in terms of gender differences—in the last few decades.

Perhaps the irony of the neo-evolutionary psychology turn in sexology is the ways that it hearkens back to the most misogynistic ideas about femininity and human development from psychoanalysis—even as it claims complete neutrality, objectivity, and rationality. In a series of scientific peer-reviewed journal articles published in the earliest years of the twenty-first century, psychologist Roy Baumeister set the tone and the course, in behaviorist and vulgar evolutionary terms, for the now widely accepted notion of the essential "responsiveness" and "receptivity" of female desire. In a particularly well-cited article (to this day) published in *Psychological Bulletin* in 2000, Baumeister made his case for female "erotic plasticity":

> Female sexuality, as compared with male, is more subject to the influence of cultural, social factors . . . [and] male desire is depicted here as relatively constant and unchanging, which suggests a powerful role for relatively rigid, innate determinants. Female sexuality, in contrast, is depicted as fairly malleable and mutable: it is responsive to culture, learning, and social circumstances. The plasticity of the female sex drive offers greater capacity to adapt to changing external circumstances as well as an opportunity for culture to exert a controlling influence. (p. 347)

One of the most interesting—and alarming—aspects of the "female erotic plasticity hypothesis" is that Baumeister seems to have thought he was somehow untangling the "nature/nurture debate" about sexuality in making his argument. This is clear as he goes on: "The present article offers yet another conceptualization of the relative contributions of nature and culture to human sexual desire [as distinct from both the 'social constructionist' and 'essentialist' conceptualizations]. The point of departure is that there is no single correct answer that holds true for all human beings" (p. 347). But clearly Baumeister proceeds from an essentializing, biologically reductive, evolutionary psychology–informed standpoint in making this very claim that women are more open to the influences of "nurture" and "culture" than are men—a reductive, universalizing biology is the very framework through which the disproportionate effect of "nurture" or "culture" on women's sexuality is understood to operate! Baumeister has been critiqued in this vein (see Hyde & Durik, 2000 for an example), but his argument has carried on in many guises, and it set the stage for the contemporary notion that men's and women's sexualities literally exist on different planes, or as different substrates—again hearkening back to the worst of Freud. Or, maybe it makes more sense to say that men are the only ones who can actually *be* sexual, per se, according to this paradigm; women have something completely different going on, and it clearly cannot be defined as *sexual,* proper.

Baumeister's argument for innate female erotic plasticity is hypothesized to be the result of a few potential factors, including the fact that men are stronger and more aggressive and have held power over women over "the course of evolutionary history"; that women play the "gatekeeper role" in sex (it is inherent to the "female role" that women are the ones who decide when sex will happen, meaning sex occurs "in nature" when females "change their vote from no to yes"); and that the female sex drive is simply biologically weaker than the male sex drive. All of these explanations are posed by Baumeister in evolutionary terms, and he produces a lengthy, undertheorized literature review to support these claims. In a follow-up article published in 2004 in the journal *Sexual and Relationship Therapy*, he states that he has become convinced of the final explanation—that the female sex drive is simply "milder" than the male drive, resulting in more flexibility for women, and also providing an array of adaptive mechanisms that will ultimately benefit society. For instance, if women are more erotically plastic, then they will be more willing to change their behaviors to fit with whatever the circumstances require—women thus carry the burden of controlling whether there is more or less reproduction of the human species, they maintain the sex ratio if it becomes unequal, and they protect the population from health risks such as the AIDS epidemic (women are likely to become "less promiscuous" in such a situation). According to this line of reasoning, women were biologically designed to play this malleable role, and are the ultimate protectors of the human race. Quite a burden, indeed.

One more theme from this research is worth mentioning, as it comes to be a common trope across both the scientific and popular literature: feminine "inconsistency." Baumeister focused on how women are more likely to exhibit "attitude-behavior inconsistency" (sexually, they do not always do what they say they want to do, whereas men's sexual attitudes [or desires] and behaviors are more likely to align). Baumeister (2000) states: "One reason for female erotic plasticity is that women's role requires them to participate in sex even when they do not particularly wish to do so. Having sex without desire is one form of inconsistency" (p. 360). This theme of feminine inconsistency between attitudes and behaviors will be extended in the years after Baumeister's initial publication of his female erotic plasticity hypothesis, into new hypotheses regarding feminine inconsistency between the subjective experience of sexual desire and physiological genital arousal—the notion of "discordance," which becomes an important explanation for *either* healthy female sexuality *or* female sexual dysfunction. However, this function/dysfunction distinction really depends on what year it is—both explanations have been posited in the literature, at different times. The broader point is that discordance is understood to occur more frequently in women, across studies. Contemporary sexologists love to talk about this phenomenon and it is often (under)theorized in evolutionary terms.

Although Baumeister was a particularly vocal example, many other psychologists at the turn of the twenty-first century began to make similar arguments, some of which have been framed as "feminist" in the last two decades.

Ideas about female receptivity and responsiveness, for instance, came back full circle in the 1990s and early 2000s, and eventually combined the neutral rationality of cognitive behaviorism with a liberal feminist, "sex-positive" approach. I focus primarily on Baumeister's work here because while he is not a sex therapist, his hypothesis about female complexity/malleability brought together many different strands of thinking on gender differences in sexual desire, right at a time when lines of thought that would inform the next incarnation of the *DSM* were percolating among sex therapists, clinicians, and experimental sex researchers. His combination of a neo-evolutionary psychology gendered framework in the guise of objective neutrality, a lack of any structural theorizing of desire differences or discussion of trauma, along with a cognitive behaviorist focus in terms of treatment for dysfunction, was archetypal of the turn sexology and sex therapy were taking at the time. Importantly, he portends the fallout of this new turn at the end of his widely cited paper (2000): "There are clear and important implications for clinical practice. The greater plasticity of female sexuality suggests that sex therapists should be more effective at treating women than men. In particular, cognitive-behavioral treatments and other social interventions should be much more effective with female than male clients. The relative inflexibility of males suggests that sexual problems may require more physiologically and biochemically-oriented interventions" (p. 370). Remarkably, this comment is situated amidst a discussion of women's lower (than men's) achievability of sexual self-knowledge, their restricted capacity for and more tortuous experience of sexual decision-making, and their greater ability for sexual *compromise*—"women are better able to adjust their preferences and expectations to what is actually available to them, and so a compromise gradually ceases to seem like a compromise" (p. 370). Baumeister can't bring himself to really theorize the effects of social structure—including cisheteropatriarchy—on sexuality, so he leaves his readers with evolutionary explanations for all of these themes, which continue to haunt sexual medicine today.

Men and women are pitted against each other in popular sexual science narratives, from the psychoanalysis of the nineteenth century to the evolutionary sexology and behaviorism of the twenty-first, and now, this conflict is naturalized—and neurologized—as inevitable. The naturalness of gendered conflict is a central theme in popular evolutionary psychology-informed literature on sexuality—in which, again, women's drives are framed as not-exactly-sexual. This theme has been taken up in a variety of popular outlets, and has also been written about by nonscientists, with much import. It could even be argued, as Cordelia Fine (2013) has, that the popularization of these scientific studies perpetuates fallacious "scientific jargon-speak for 'men are from Mars, women are from Venus.'"[12] And importantly, these themes about sexual difference have been popularized amongst the general populace due to the "cross-pollination" of scientific and popular discourses (Angel, 2012, p. 3). In the remainder of this book, I analyze how these discourses affect women's lived sexual experiences and shape their sexual biographies, and it is clear that many women who do not have access to peer-reviewed scientific journals (nor the training required to analyze them) *do* have access to best-selling books, blogs and websites, online and print news outlets, and popular magazines.

The *antagonistic* or *violent complementarity* espoused via evolutionary psychology and its popularized versions is also incorporated in other domains, including in the work of clinicians and researchers involved in designing the recently released *DSM-5*—even though this is perhaps not always intentional. The cross-pollination has a far reach. Sexual dysfunction diagnoses have very real and profound consequences on women's sexual and psychological health—even those who are not clinically diagnosed. In order to ground the themes that emerged in the interviews with my low-desiring participants, I now turn to the immediate context of changes within sexual medicine, sex therapy, and experimental research on sexual arousal—all changes that occurred from the 1990s through the first decade of the twenty-first century, and that set the stage for the introduction of the newest sexual dysfunction diagnosis in the *DSM-5*, released in 2013. This new diagnosis, female sexual interest/arousal disorder, or FSIAD, can by definition be diagnosed only in women. In the following chapter, I unpack the significance and implications of this new gendered diagnostic schema, and show how it is not as "feminist" as it is purported to be (or rather that its feminism is limited by its liberalism).

---

12. In this 2013 essay, Fine hearkens back to the 1992 multiweek best seller about men's and women's innately different communication and relationship styles—*Men Are from Mars, Women Are from Venus: A Practical Guide for Improving Communication & Getting What You Want in Your Relationships*—through which pop psychologist and relationship counselor John Gray rose to fame.

CHAPTER 2

Interest, Arousal, and Motivation in Contemporary Sexology
The Feminization of Responsive Desire

"For men to be clueless about women is, of course, routine. But what the scientists and sex therapists seemed to be suggesting is that a lot of women are also confused," wrote Richard Conniff in *Men's Health* magazine, a few years before the *DSM-5* was released, along with its women-specific diagnosis, female sexual interest/arousal disorder (FSIAD). I include this quote here because it's a good example of how the scientific research that provided the basis for the change in diagnostic criteria has been popularly interpreted. With the institution of FSIAD and its supporting discourses, including their popular interpretations, sexual "responsiveness" was brought forward as a metric for healthy sexuality in women. Claims regarding feminine receptivity over the last two decades have been based, in part, on the findings of experimental research in which subjective accounts of sexual arousal are compared with objective measurements of genital response to sexual stimuli. These laboratory investigations have consistently reported that both sexually healthy and dysfunctional women—particularly those who are attracted to men—exhibit a disconnect or "discordance" between their subjective and objective sexual states, unlike healthy men, who experience more "concordance." Some researchers (e.g., Bailey, 2009) have gone so far as to state that androphilic women (women who are attracted to men) do not have a sexual orientation—they are physiologically aroused by stimuli that do not accord with their stated sexual preferences or identities. Two decades into the twenty-first century, these ideas about innate feminine erotic plasticity, flexibility, responsiveness, receptivity, complexity, and sometimes confusion, continue to proliferate.

In the remainder of this chapter, I examine how racialized, gendered, heteronormative, and cisnormative prescriptions for healthy sex and sexuality have continued to guide research paradigms, diagnostic schemas, and treatment protocols in the twenty-first century—even as the researchers who conduct these studies have sought to distance themselves from their less-feminist and less-progressive psychologist forebears. Regardless of the intentions of researchers, the wide popular circulation of these tropes means that some individuals come to experience themselves as sexually "discordant" or, alternatively, "in sync," and thus live out a medico-scientific production of sexual difference. My research suggests that these discourses of white feminine receptivity and responsiveness may even be incorporated into racially diverse women's sexual self-images and practices—an example of how individuals internalize and live scientific schemas. This stands in contrast to the notion that science simply uncovers the categories as they already exist. Frameworks for mind/body relations continue to rely on antiquated and reductive typologies in the twenty-first century (including when queer and trans folks are the objects of study), and there is still much work to be done to move contemporary sexology away from reifying ideas about "men" and "women," "heterosexuals" and "homosexuals," and even "androphiles" and "gynephiles" that I discussed in chapter 1. Further, contemporary sex therapy regimens are primarily directed toward cis women, who continue to be framed as having less desire (in terms of frequency, intensity, and spontaneity) than cis men.[1] In regard to sexual pathology, whereas men have been perceived as disproportionately likely to suffer from physical ailments such as erectile disorder, women are still often posited as more likely to suffer from psychological blocks to sexual enjoyment—or, in contemporary behaviorist parlance, from "lack of motivation." These perceived differences result in distinct framings and treatments of sexual dysfunction for men and women, with gendered consequences for sexual health, attitudes, and relationships—among both "dysfunctional" and "healthy" populations. And such perceptions also inform how we all—as individuals who can never fully escape binary (in addition to medicalized, naturalized, and racialized) definitions of gender—come to

---

1. Throughout the rest of this chapter, I will not specify that participants in the psychological research I analyze are cisgender, as it is almost entirely taken for granted and assumed by the researchers that participants are cis, and that is what the research is, in fact, predicated on. Further, I argue that, in the contemporary psychological imaginary, the presumed subjects of both theory and treatment are cisgender.

understand our own sexual motivations and behaviors within the logic of the feminized responsive desire framework.

One thing I would like to make clear, however, is this: "Responsive desire" itself is not the problem. All who identify as sexual, or who experience sexuality along a spectrum of intensity, may experience different levels of "responsive" versus "spontaneous" desire at different times throughout our lives and in different relationships (and alone).[2] What I am concerned with is the sleight of hand in which responsive desire has been framed as feminine, while that gendering is simultaneously denied by today's leading scientists, researchers, and clinicians. Perhaps even more importantly, I am concerned with how responsive desire is framed as uniquely feminine in pop psych and media accounts, with dire consequences when men assume women need to be sexually triggered or primed (and when women assume this about themselves). Another issue that I will interrogate in this chapter is how the deployment of responsive desire as feminine has been framed as femin*ist*.

Many women do report having low desire, and want treatment for this, and many women also report a pattern of responsive desire. But we must ask who the women are that report this, and why they experience it. And we must also consider who will be most affected and how when these notions are legitimized as the new "female-friendly" model of sexuality (i.e., an intimacy-based model that is understood broadly as more accurate for women): Models, of course, imply *truth*. The new wave of feminist-identified sex researchers, clinicians, and therapists undoubtedly have good intentions, and have strived to offer a new model of sexuality to contrast with the linear human sexual response cycle (HSRC) of Masters and Johnson. However, in an effort to depathologize women's "low" desire (i.e., "low" in terms of Masters and Johnson's much-critiqued goal-driven model, a carry-over of a caricature of Freudian "sex drive"), these well-intentioned researchers have inadvertently reproduced and reinscribed the notion that women's sexuality is more essentially complex, labile, and responsive or receptive than is men's sexuality. In the process, some antimedicalization psychologist-activists have also diluted their earlier critiques of the older male-oriented sexology by ignoring the role of trauma in configuring women's experiences of sex (including some women's desire for not-so-feminine things), and by instead taking up a "depathologizing" stance that seems to offer the relatively un-nuanced: "Women have lower

---

2. To this end, I agree with many aspects of the incentive motivation model (IMM) of sexual response as it has been outlined by, for example, Toates (2014)—to be explored below. However, current conceptions of responsive versus spontaneous desire, or of "state" versus "trait" desire, which reduce sexuality to "interests," "motivations," and "incentives," sorely lack a psychodynamic conception of both power and trauma as constitutive aspects of desire.

[spontaneous] sexual desire than men, and that's okay, it's actually normal, just leave women alone and stop trying to shove pills down their throats!" Instead of thinking through why some non-asexual women who have low desire are so uninterested in sex that they only do it "for the intimacy," a multitude of researchers and therapists of different stripes have come together under the umbrella of admonishing the strawman of "Big Pharma." This admonishment tends to be framed in the language of "anti-pharmaceuticalization," with the main critique being of the corporate marketing of a drug for female sexual dysfunction—the common rallying cry is "Down with Addyi!" By contrast, I argue that in order to have an intersectional, trans-inclusive, and truly progressive feminist response to the production and treatment of women's sexuality within medicine and science, we need to dig deeper. There is more to the story than simply condemning the evils of the Little Pink Pill—when female sexuality is produced as more fluid, flexible, and complex, that also leaves it open to new forms of management and training. And not all of these new forms of discipline are pharmaceutical. How this situation came to be and its consequences are what I will explore in the following pages.

Seeking Rewards and Intimacy: The New "Female-Friendly" Sexual Response Models

Since the late 1970s, a variety of changes have occurred in the research and treatment of desire disorders, particularly as they pertain to women, who make up the majority of current diagnosees. After an international consensus conference was convened to analyze female sexual dysfunction in 1998, a group of conference participants called for more attention to women's sexual issues by clinicians and researchers, particularly in light of the glut of attention given to male sexual problems such as erectile disorder (ED).[3] The specialists who were involved in the consensus conference—many of whom went on to form the International Society for the Study of Women's Sexual Health (ISSWSH) and some of whom later served on the *DSM-5* sexual and gender identity disorders work group (or who were mentors and close colleagues to those work group members)—set forth new criteria for discerning and treat-

---

3. Today, ED, or "impotence," is generally not categorized as a desire disorder; it is instead more often considered a physical sexual dysfunction. Although ED may be attributed to psychological difficulties, and as such, it still remains in the *DSM-5*, its desire-related manifestation does not reflect culturally common understandings of male sexual difficulty. This shift to configuring ED as a "physiological" rather than "psychological" disorder is a relatively recent trend, as pointed out by Kleinplatz (2011).

ing women's sexual disorders that they hoped would be taken up on a widespread clinical basis (Basson et al., 2001). One of the most notable suggestions for a change in protocol concerned the diagnosis of hypoactive sexual desire disorder, or HSDD. The consensus committee called for the introduction of the criterion of "receptivity" or "responsive desire" for women. This new criterion indicated the group's belief that a woman shouldn't be diagnosed with HSDD just because she doesn't spontaneously desire or initiate sex, but only if she is also unreceptive to her partner's advances. This call also reflected just one more stage in the process of the gendering of sexual desire and behavior within contemporary psychosexual medicine—obviously a process that was connected to a long history of sexual difference frameworks within psychology, but a particular moment that is notable in light of the fact that it was instituted within the new terrain of purportedly apolitical and atheoretical behaviorist psychology, and, eventually, in the name of feminism.

This proposed change was a response to mounting criticisms that the standard conceptualization of sexual response—Masters and Johnson's human sexual response cycle (HSRC), widely publicized in 1966—is based on a specifically masculine version of sexuality and desire. As described in the previous chapter, the HSRC only focused on physiological changes that occurred once sex (specifically heterosexual intercourse) had already begun, and didn't consider the role of desire (or all of the reasons people might engage in sex—now framed in terms of the behaviorist "motivations" and "incentives"). Since the days of Masters and Johnson, diverse figures—from antimedicalization activists to experimental psychology researchers—have argued that women are different from men when it comes to sex and sexuality (Basson, 2000, 2001b; Brotto, 2010a; Heiman, 2002; Tiefer, 2001), although they have posited different explanations for this fact. Many psychologists have argued that this discrepancy is at least in part due to biological differences between men and women, while others—Leonore Tiefer of the New View Campaign being the primary example—have attended to sociocultural factors that affect women's sexual expression. For all of these psychologists, however, the lack of attention to women's specifically feminine sexual problems represents, at best, a serious lacuna in medical practice and research, and at worst, willful (and sexist) ignorance by doctors and researchers.

Rosemary Basson, a clinical professor of psychiatry and the director of the University of British Columbia Sexual Medicine Program, can be attributed with really changing the terrain of the sexual response debates and legitimating alternative models of sexuality in the mainstream. Basson's qualitative work with Canadian women in the late 1990s, along with the findings of plethysmographic research conducted by Dutch researchers during the same period on women's lack of awareness of their own physiological genital response (Laan & Everaerd, 1995, 1998), led her to develop a framework for "responsive desire," which she deemed better suited to describe women's experiences in long-term (cisheterosexual, monogamous, and romantic) relationships. Importantly, she explicitly devised the model as a way to depathologize what she understood to be many women's different (nonlinear and non-goal-oriented) experiences of sexuality, and thus to destabilize the dominance of Masters and Johnson's linear human sexual response cycle. Basson's circular framework is often referred to in both clinical and popular literature as the "arousal-first" model of desire (Bielski, 2015).

Basson's (2000) original model was configured on the basis of four claims: (1) Women are not biologically driven to release sexual tension in the same way men are because they do not have as much testosterone as men. (2) Women experience different motivations to engage in sex than men, including "incentives" and "rewards" that are not strictly sexual in nature and that might be much more important to their willingness to engage in sex than any biological urges to do so (e.g., promoting intimacy, pleasing a partner, preventing relational discord, etc.). (3) Women experience subjective mental arousal that may or may not be accompanied by genital arousal (or they may be unaware of their own genital arousal—that is, they are more likely than men to experience subjective/genital discordance). And (4) women do not always experience orgasms during sex, even if they are orgasmic are not always driven to reach orgasm, and when orgasmic release does occur for women, it may take a variety of forms that deviate from the traditional sexual release model. In the seminal article in which Basson (2000) initially introduced this new model, "The Female Sexual Response: A Different Model," she states: "Sensing an opportunity to be sexual, the partner's neediness, or an awareness of one or more potential *benefits* or *rewards* that are very important to them (but not necessarily sexual), women move from a *sexual neutrality* to seeking stimuli necessary to ignite sexual desire" (p. 53; italics added). In the first decade of the twenty-first century, Basson's model (what I will from now on refer to as her "circular sexual response cycle," in keeping with contemporary usage) acquired widespread support and was utilized by numerous other researchers. Although one article she published in 2001 in the *Journal of Sex & Marital Therapy* argued that the model could also apply to men, and a brief 2008 commentary in the *Archives of Sexual Behavior* reiterated this notion, the rest of Basson's writing on the topic has focused on women, and almost all other scientific researchers who have used it have interpreted and referred to the model as female-specific since its institution (for recent examples, see Giraldi, Kristensen, & Sand, 2015; Ferenidou, Kirana, Fokas, Hatzichristou,

& Athanasiadis, 2016). Recently, Basson has gone on record stating that her model was misconstrued as being for women only (Barmak, 2018), but regardless of whether she intended the model to be a description of women's sexual response, uniquely, it has been framed as such not only by other researchers but also in myriad popular accounts—countless popular articles, sex blogs, and even the r/sex Reddit have portrayed this model of responsive desire as specifically "for women." I would argue there is good reason for this—the model *does* seem to fit women better than men. My concern is how we interpret this phenomenon—why is it that women are more responsive? And even if evidence suggests they are, is it a good idea to codify women's sexuality this way, scientifically? I would suggest that one reason *not* to codify it in this way might be that, because of our Western cultural obsessions with objectivity, the truth of behavior, and evolutionary speculation, we run the risk of essentializing and universalizing femininity with a model like this—albeit in new, more female-friendly guises. And this is exactly what has happened since the turn of the twenty-first century, when Basson first put her model forward.

Beginning in the late 1980s, largely in the Dutch context, another model for sexual response was devised—the "incentive motivation model" (IMM)—which emerged from classical experimental psychology rooted in neurocognitive orientations within a behaviorist tradition. This model has often been cited alongside Basson's model, particularly leading up to the publication of the *DSM-5* in 2013, as an alternative to the linearity of earlier conceptualizations of "sex drive," and often alongside evolutionary psychology explanations for gender differences. The incentive motivation model exemplifies a purposeful shift away from psychoanalytic and psychodynamic theories of desire, and it is also theoretically gender-neutral, as is stated in the work of Dutch researchers Ellen Laan, Stephanie Both, Walter Everaerd, and Frederick Toates; these researchers promulgate the notion that sexual desire (for both men and women) can be "situation-dependent," reflecting different "triggers" (e.g., Toates, 2014). The idea here is that all human sexual desire is responsive, and involves balancing excitatory and inhibitory internal information, on the one hand, with the content and effectiveness of external stimuli, on the other. If the stimulus is "competent," then physiological arousal will be activated and then detected, and the individual will then continue to be motivated to engage in the sexual act—and to do it again, in the future, if it is rewarding enough (including for nonsexual reasons), in a psychophysiological feedback loop.[4] Here, sexual activity can be explained by how motivated an individual

---

4. This model is now often used in conjunction with the information processing model (IPM) of sexual arousal (e.g., Janssen, Everaerd, Spiering, & Janssen, 2000), which focuses on how arousal occurs at the level of the organism. The IPM emerges from contemporary

is to engage in any given behavior, when comparing costs versus benefits, in a "push-pull" framework (the "push" coming from within the individual, and the "pull" coming from the external stimuli)—although some of this calculus is understood to be beyond conscious consideration (hence the importance of noting the evolutionary psychology theory that is often in the backdrop). It is via this model of sexual response that the notion that desire and arousal co-occur, or in many cases that arousal precedes desire, came to be instituted. Eventually, the idea that arousal preceding desire is more descriptive of women's sexuality would be inscribed in the FSIAD diagnosis.

In addition to the incentive motivation model often being discussed in conjunction with Basson's circular sexual response cycle (enter the role of *conscious* consideration of nonsexual rewards potentially received for engaging in sex, particularly for women), most of the research conducted using this framework has been conducted on women specifically.[5] The tendency to apply the incentive motivation model primarily to women raises questions around whether or not the pervasive gendered use of a gender-neutral model has contributed to theorizing male and female sexuality—and masculine and feminine desire—differently. According to researchers who utilize the incentive motivation model in their studies, are women naturally and essentially more sexually responsive or receptive than men? Or are men likely also receptive, but enough research simply hasn't been conducted on them to warrant the label of "responsive desire"? The answer to this distinction is not always clear

---

neurocognitive emotion research, which describes a hierarchically organized system in the organism in which involuntary, automatic, and autonomic response to sexual stimuli occurs first (through a proximate or "direct" neural pathway), followed later, or separately, by voluntary, conscious, and controlled appraisal in which meaning is conferred to sexual stimuli. This meaning or conscious arousal involves more elaborate cortical processing (through a distal or "indirect" neural pathway). Although this is another model in which gender differences have been suggested, for example in terms of the multiplicity and importance of sexual "meanings" appraised at the emotional or "felt" level, a full discussion of the IPM is beyond the scope of my argument for this chapter. Similarly, the dual control model (Bancroft, Graham, Janssen, & Sanders, 2009) and *state* theory of sexual desire, response, and arousal (as opposed to an interpretation of these phenomena as sexual *traits,* which are more stable and fixed than sexual *states*) are both alternatives to "drive" models of sexual response that will not be explored fully here as they did not play a key role in the gendering of conceptions of low desire during the period that I analyze.

5. In an interesting twist, Both and Everaerd (2002) penned a response to Basson (2000), supporting her paradigm of sexual responsiveness but questioning the notion that it is uniquely descriptive of women. Despite this, in the decade following that exchange, the incentive motivation model also was much more frequently applied to women, including by some of the original Dutch researchers who moved the model forward (see Laan & Both, 2008 for an example of this gendered application of the IMM in experimental work).

for the very psychologists who utilize the model.[6] It is clear, however, that this "cost-benefit," "rational-motivation," or "incentive-reward" model is, at least in application, thought to be particularly suited to explaining women's complex and responsive sexuality. Why else would women be almost exclusively sampled as participants for these studies? And why have so many studies on women's responsive desire been conducted in the last twenty years? The disproportionate application of the model and associated concepts to women, and the sheer number of studies conducted on women's responsive desire, particularly in the first decade of the twenty-first century, has undeniably perpetuated the notion that women have a completely different sexual reality than do men. Certainly many women do have different experiences of sex than men, and I also emphasize that point, but my biggest concern with the use of the incentive motivation model to disproportionately describe women's desire is that these studies often then lead us to biological, evolutionary explanations for this fact (even if these explanations just "fill in the gaps"). As it is a cognitive behaviorist model, this explanation also leads us away from considering power—both as a coercive mechanism and in its inflection as desire. This is because even as the incentive motivation model is rooted in what researchers refer to as a "biopsychosocial" framework, their lack of structural theorizing—and their emphasis on the "push" of internal biological data that come into contact with the "pull" of the external environment—leaves us with no analysis of the vicissitudes of desire, and instead with the image of a neutral biological organism reacting to its neutral environment. But what happens when the environment *pushes* one to engage in sex? Or when the internal psychic experience (e.g., trauma) *pulls* us back in? Or: Is it even useful to consider internal and external stimuli—and pushing and pulling—as separate phenomena?

6. Some researchers have emphasized that men may also be sexually receptive and responsive (for examples, see Janssen, McBride, Yarber, Hill, & Butler [2008]; Goldey & van Anders, [2012]; and Murray [2019]). This contrasts with much of the literature up to this point, though, including the seminal articles by Basson and more recent experimental studies that suggest ("androphilic") women's sexuality is uniquely responsive and discordant. There is much slippage between Basson's model and the Dutch incentive motivation model, and there is a lack of consensus among researchers themselves regarding whether the incentive motivation model is more appropriate for women. Some researchers suggest conflicting stances in this regard, and sometimes in the same article (see Chivers & Brotto, 2017 for an example of a publication in which conflicting stances on the "truth" of women's responsive desire are posited—in some places in this article, the authors suggest that women's sexuality is unique and that its study requires a "gendered approach" [p. 19]; in other places, the authors argue that men and women are similar sexually, including in terms of [responsive or state-dependent] sexual desire [p. 15]. Contradictions abound even in the discussion of state versus trait desire, however, as the authors also suggest that using state-dependent or context-focused [responsive] measures to assess desire is more appropriate for women).

To be clear: I recognize the importance of representing and attending to diverse models of sexuality that provide alternatives to Masters and Johnson's four-staged HSRC model of human sexual response. However, it is necessary to analyze and interrogate the long-standing cultural obsession with women's sexuality as a deviation from this linear model. What are the potential consequences of marking this kind of deviation as uniquely and innately feminine, and treating it as such? Advocates of alternative models for female sexual response argue that many women's general state of sexual neutrality, their need to be sexually triggered due to their receptivity or responsiveness, and the importance of nonsexual incentives regarding their participation, interest, or "willingness" to engage in sex must be taken into account when assessing women's desire—specifically in terms of whether or not they are to be diagnosed as dysfunctional. A crucial aspect of these models is the notion that for women, physical arousal is often antecedent to or unaligned with a conscious or stated interest in sex. While some of what is put forward here may in fact be true about women (and, indeed, scientific data certainly suggest that it is), that is not the same as saying that it is *natural* for women to experience sex in this way. The problem with these feminized models of receptivity, then, is that they do not take into account *how women got this way* (bracketing the models that vulgarly explain this phenomenon via evolutionary psychology tropes, which argue that receptivity is an adaptation to cave-rape, and/or a mating strategy). By failing to account for or theorize many women's receptive sexual response patterns in explicitly sociopolitical terms, these models gloss over the very inequalities within cis-/heteronormative sex relations implicated in women's "alternative" (i.e., discordant, responsive, receptive, plastic, flexible, complex, complicated, circular, etc.) forms of sexual response. To this end, as these researchers have sought to normalize women's responsive desire, I want to trouble that normalization. If the reasons for women's responsiveness include lack of sexual agency, regular experiences of coercion, or lack of access to pleasurable sex, then this receptivity, and the framework that naturalizes it or puts it in the terms of "incentives," "rewards," and "motivations," *is not normal*. Or: It is normal only insofar as gender inequality in sex is normal. Further, many of the low-desiring women I interviewed suggested that their own experiences of desire do not align with the receptivity framework, or, in some cases, throw its very premises into critical relief—they are very aware of the concessions they've been expected to make sexually, and they want something better. In some cases, that might mean actively playing with the power inequalities they experience in a cisheteropatriarchal society and making them into the stuff of domination and submission fantasies, into the stuff of hot, sexy desire—not "motivation" or "interest."

Measuring the Gap: Plethysmography and Mind/Body Disconnects

Much contemporary experimental sex research seeks to measure gender differences in sexual behavior and response, particularly in terms of subjective/genital "concordance" and "discordance" (for examples, see Chivers, 2010, 2017a, 2017b; Chivers & Bailey, 2005; Chivers, Seto, & Blanchard, 2007; Chivers, Seto, Lalumière, Laan, & Grimbos, 2010; Heiman, 1977, 1980; Laan & Everaerd, 1995, 1998), and findings have been used to support the necessity of alternative sexual response models for women. In 2004, Meredith Chivers and colleagues coined the terms "category-specificity" and "category *non*-specificity" (used interchangeably later with "target-specificity" and "target *non*-specificity"[7]) to describe whether a male or female laboratory subject's objective, physiological, genital arousal matches that same individual's subjective account of how turned on they feel by the "categories" they claim to prefer. Frequently, gender is measured as the category of interest—that is, does the person's physical sexual response align with who they say they are attracted to, in terms of gender? Are there significant differences for men versus women in this regard? In order to assess this gap (discordance) or alignment (concordance), researchers use vaginal photoplethysmography (traditionally, a vaginal probe that measures blood flow in the vagina or vaginal pulse amplitude [VPA] is used, although more recent studies also sometimes use a labial thermistor clip to detect blood flow and temperature changes in the vulva or clitoral photoplethysmography to measure blood flow in the clitoris[8]) and penile plethysmography (using a phallometric gauge that similarly detects penile blood flow or erection) and compare physiological measures to subjects' stated arousal as discerned by an "arousometer" that they move with their fingers to indicate how turned on they feel. The assessment is usually made while subjects watch pornography or neutral films in a clinical environment. Such devices were popularly used by Masters and Johnson and even before them, beginning in the 1950s and 1960s, with more sophisticated volumetric tools developed in the 1970s. Since the earliest days of this research, women have been shown to be less category-specific than men in terms of

---

7. Lalumière (2017) has made a case for using the term "cue-specificity" as a measure of the intensity or degree of response discrimination to any given sexual cue and comparing this with level of concordance; this was proposed as a solution to perceived measurement problems regarding sexual orientation.

8. See Huberman & Chivers (2015) for an example of a study that uses labial thermography and Suschinksy, Dawson, & Chivers (2020) for an example of a study that uses clitoral plethysmography.

their physiological response, and to exhibit more discordance between physical and psychological arousal states.

Famous for popular assessments that associated her with the notion that "women get turned on by everything, including bonobo porn!" (as was suggested by Andy Newman in 2008 and Daniel Bergner in 2009, writing for the *New York Times*), Meredith Chivers, a sexologist at Queen's University in Kingston, Ontario, has become the icon of this contemporary research. In the first decade of the twenty-first century, Chivers published multiple articles on the *lack* of "category-specific" sexual arousal in women (some studies suggested that women are even physically aroused by nonhuman primate sex—hence the above quote about bonobos; see Chivers et al., 2007) in addition to the *presence* of category-specific arousal in trans women or "transsexuals,"[9] with J. Michael Bailey and Ray Blanchard, among other evolutionary sexologists.[10] Chivers and Bailey, along with colleague Gerulf Rieger, also coauthored an article in 2005 arguing that "true bisexuality" in men does not exist (based on phallometric measures of physiological arousal, which were said to suggest that men are physiologically either gay or straight—because they reliably experience erections in response only to either men or women; see Rieger, Chivers, & Bailey, 2005). This last study was picked up by several popular news outlets around the same time (e.g., "Straight, Gay, or Lying?" by Benedict Carey in the *New York Times*), and has remained controversial, even after a later study coauthored by Bailey (see Rosenthal, Sylva, Safron, & Bailey, 2011) confirmed that (surprise!) some bisexually identified men are, in fact, bisexual.

Studies featuring plethysmography span decades (Geer, Morokoff, & Greenwood, 1974; Heiman, 1977; and Hoon, Wincze, & Hoon, 1976 are some of the earliest big publications on gender differences in genital/subjective

---

9. In the seminal study in which the term *category-specific arousal* was coined (Chivers, Rieger, Latty, & Bailey, 2004), trans women, who are referred to as "male-to-female transsexuals," were grouped with cis males based on similarity of genital arousal data, and this was used to suggest the possibility of a "true sexual dimorphism" in arousal patterns (p. 737). The authors state: "Our finding that male-to-female transsexuals show a male-typical [sic] pattern . . . helps to rule out some possible explanations. [Cis]women's nonspecific pattern might not be fully explained by their lack of visible genitalia because transsexuals show a category-specific pattern despite a similar lack. Transsexuals reject the male gender role into which they were socialized yet continue to show the category-specific pattern of arousal that is characteristic of their genetic sex" (p. 742).

10. Bailey and Blanchard became infamous in the late 1990s and early 2000s for their controversial theories of the two pathways to "transsexualism" in male-to-female individuals, which include either "extreme homosexuality" or "autogynephilia" (i.e., the self-obsessed and narcissistic fantasy of themselves as women, which constitutes a paraphilia). See Bailey (2003) and Blanchard (1989) for more on this notion that "some transsexuals [transgender women] are the most feminine of males" (Chivers et al., 2004, p. 742).

concordance). And even before the newer wave of psychophysiological sex research on women's discordance, arguments about how the "truth" of sexual desire could be discerned by comparing subjective accounts to physiological measures were put forward by Czech sexologist Kurt Freund, who utilized phallometry as a type of sexual polygraph for men; the penile strain gauge was initially used to determine whether a military conscript for the Czech army was heterosexual or homosexual (i.e., to identify men attempting to avoid service by claiming they were gay). The claim here is that men, unlike women, are *very* concordant—their erections are a good measure of what they are subjectively turned on by. Later, these measures were used in conjunction with conversion therapy under a behaviorist paradigm; via the logic of what Waidzunas and Epstein critically refer to in their 2015 article "For Men, Arousal Is Orientation" as a *technosexual script*, the "truth" of desire was deciphered (or rather produced) via phallometry, so that so-called abnormal sexualities could be changed. Although I focus here on category-specificity as it has been gendered in contemporary research using plethysmography, similar methods of making this determination have been used not only to assess heterosexuality and homosexuality in all-male samples but also as forensic evidence for pedophilia and other sex crimes, as physiological arousal to images of children is said to be an important predictor of reoffense (this work is pioneered today by experimental researcher Michael Seto). The newest research on women's discordance and lack of category-specificity is thus one moment in a long line of technoscientific research in which subjective and objective accounts of desire are measured against each other. The difference is that in the past, the focus was on physiological arousal as a proxy for desire in men (and it still functions this way in research on men), and now, a disjuncture between subjective and objective accounts in women is the focus. Notably, the new wave of feminist-identified sex researchers who argue for the normalcy of a feminine disconnect have seemingly made this case in order to rescue women from the problematic linear model of "arousal equals desire." However, in doing so, they have reified feminine sexual complexity and confusion—and the legacy of using plethysmography as a method of telling the "truth" of sexuality continues, albeit in new forms. That is: The mind/body disjuncture itself has become the truth of women's sexuality, and the gendered and forensic history of the plethysmograph tells us the truth of sexual difference.

After publishing prolifically with Bailey, Blanchard, and others, Chivers quickly moved into the role of a true trailblazer in the study of the complexities of women's desire. During the summer of 2019, the Queen's University website stated: "The results [of Chivers's] research have exposed a disconnection between women's minds and bodies, making it clear that there is still much to be understood about female sexuality." A multitude of popular outlets have also taken interest in the "new science of female sexuality"—Chivers is one of a few women sex researchers consistently cited in the media. In 2010, she conducted a meta-analysis along with four colleagues (Chivers et al., 2010) to assess continuity in observed differences in male and female sexual response. This meta-analysis asserted a statistically significant gender difference in sexual response across multiple studies over decades, and suggested that men demonstrate more subjective/genital concordance than women, and also greater category-specificity in terms of their response. In the years prior to the release of the *DSM-5*, this research was used alongside the new alternative sexual response models to support the idea that women's sexual response is organized fundamentally differently than men's sexual response.

In more recent research of this type, it has been suggested that certain women are more concordant than others.[11] Chivers (2017a) suggests that "gynephilic" women (women who are attracted to women, but who do not necessarily self-identify as lesbians) have the highest rates of concordance among women, along with "ambiphilic" women (women who are attracted to both men and women but who don't necessarily self-identify as bisexual), who also demonstrate higher rates of concordance across recent experimental studies (and interestingly, physical response to female stimuli specifically). In her award-winning 2017 review of the existing scientific theory on women's category non-specificity and discordance, Chivers concludes that it is "androphilic" women—and especially those who are exclusively androphilic—who demonstrate the lowest rates of category-specificity in terms of gender preference. This means that women who are attracted to men, and especially those who state that they are exclusively attracted to men (but who don't necessarily identify as heterosexual), experience the biggest gap between their subjective preference and genital response. It is these women who are most likely to demonstrate strong genital response to pornography featuring individuals of any gender, engaging in almost any sexual act (or in some cases nonhuman animals engaging in sex or even humans not engaging in sex but doing other things, including "violent nonsexual" acts), yet not self-identify as feeling "turned on." For these women, stated sexual preference does not align with who or what physically arouses them. Chivers (2017a) offers ten hypotheses

---

11. For instance, Chivers, Bouchard, & Timmers (2015) suggested that gynephilic women are more likely than their androphilic counterparts to be category-specific, and Velten et al. (2016) suggested variability in sexual response across female subjects. In one study, men and women were said to be more similar in terms of desire when desire was measured as emergent (as a state) rather than stable (as a trait) (Dawson & Chivers, 2014).

for why this may be the case, some of which derive from evolutionary psychology and brain organization theory. These include

- the "preparation hypothesis"—women get turned on by everything as a "low-cost" adaptive evolutionary protective mechanism so they don't experience physical harm during rape;
- the "fertility-dependent change" hypothesis—women's greater receptivity is related to hormonal shifts due to their menstrual cycles (ovulation);
- the "neurohormonal hypothesis"—lack of prenatal androgen exposure results in a gender-nonspecific response; and
- the "non-sexual motivations interact with stimulus prepotency hypothesis"—intrasexual competition over millennia has resulted in women's scrutiny of female competitors for male mates, resulting in nonspecific patterns of physiological arousal.

Out of her ten hypotheses, three suggest broadly social reasons for gender differences in desire patterns, or androphilic women's lower rates of concordance. One suggests that it may be possible that women who are attracted to men don't get as much out of their sexual interactions with men (i.e., in terms of orgasm), and thus they do not select strongly for "male cues" (p. 1174) (as opposed to gynephilic women, who receive more rewards from having sex with women, and thus are incentivized to select for "female cues"). One hypothesis is grounded in theory of mind, and describes women's potential capacity to identify with the pleasure of other women as a source of their plasticity. Another hypothesis acknowledges that women who are attracted to men may get physically turned on by other women because of the widespread objectification of women's bodies in the media, such that women are accustomed to seeing other women's bodies sexualized and have thus come to respond to them sexually, inadvertently and neurologically. I am excited to see Chivers engaging with ideas such as these, and I hope she will go even further, and consider socialization as a deeper and more complex process, rather than leaving even this social analysis within the realm of a reductive biology that ignores trauma. This review of the existing psychological theory on female discordance seems to be a positive harbinger of potential change in mainstream sexology, and it makes me hopeful that some researchers are considering explanations for phenomena outside of evolutionary psychology narratives (for an example in this vein, see Suschinsky et al., 2020). But, in light of the history of how volumetric tools have been implemented to tell the truth of desire, I worry about how they are still being used to construct a new model for women's sexuality, one that will invariably produce feminized populations (even if those populations are now more internally diverse—i.e., the terms *androphilic, gynephilic,* and *ambiphilic* still leave us tethered to old categories via their very methodological construction).

Chivers has publicly stated that women's intense, rapid, and automatic physical response to a multitude of sexual stimuli should not indicate that they are consenting to sex, nor that they ought to, and also that their non-categorical, non-gender-specific, and discordant physiological arousal does not indicate anything about their sexual identities or subjective desires per se. Her work, and the work of other sexologists within this realm, has been used to argue a variety of things about women's peculiar sexuality, along a polarity. In some instances, this research has been used to support the program of women's sexual liberation—if it's natural for women to get turned on by everything, then it should be permissible for women to pursue sex with women (and men) and get in touch with their essential queerness and fluidity as it is demonstrated via their natural state of discordance (Chivers, 2017b describes a reporter suggesting this notion to her about her own research). On the other hand, and more frequently, this research has been used to support the idea that women are "lying" about their sexualities, or that they are just disconnected from the "truth" of their desires. This line of thinking has been suggested by multiple popular evolutionary psychologists, along with journalists, other popular writers, and media pundits. For example, popular evolutionary psychologists Ogi Ogas and Sai Gaddam, in their 2011 book *A Billion Wicked Thoughts: What the Internet Tells Us about Sexual Relationships,* link women's subjective/genital discordance to innate masochistic feminine desire, arguing that this must be rooted in differences in male and female brains, and cite Chivers's research as evidence for women's evolved desire to be dominated by men (even if they don't know it). As is likely clear to readers at this point, this is an example of the line of thinking that I am most concerned with in this book, as it raises huge red flags around consent, potentially sets up women for coercion, and thus may continue to pave the way for a misogynistic anti-feminist backlash in the post–#MeToo era. Chivers (2017b) has stated that this argument about women's innate mendacity or biologically ordained sexual confusion is not the intent of her research, that she hopes instead her work will help women feel relieved to know "their unbidden physical response is measurable and demonstrated by other women" (p. 1216), and that it will inspire women to explore their "internal playground" (as cited in Martin, 2018, p. 46). Still, I am wary of the results of these studies being disseminated and popularized, particularly in light of the pairing of findings with evolutionary psychology explanations, in a world in which openness and flexibility are made modulable—and given how plethysmography and similar sexual truth-telling technologies have been used in the recent past. How are "women," as a category, made and remade through this type of research? What feminized populations are produced—and how are they left otherwise unmarked? And how does this research feed into broader retrograde, misogynistic, and potentially dangerous notions about feminine confusion and complexity? These questions are particularly salient when considering the types of diagnoses and treatments this research is used to support. Using a plethysmograph at all raises the question of the truth and who or what is to be trusted, and it also reifies mind/body dualisms. This is the case even when the research is conducted by self-identified feminist (and self-identified queer) researchers.

Beyond these conceptual concerns, there are some serious methodological issues at stake. It is unclear how most of this lab-based research could assess anything approximating the intense, powerful, sometimes fragile, and very personal experience of desire, as these studies utilize questionably operationalized variables to quantify this phenomenon and are performed in manufactured experimental settings.[12] The sample sizes in these studies are often small and homogenous (race, socioeconomic status, and other important demographic data have traditionally not been gathered or at least not disclosed, although some more recent studies are reporting more on racial identification of participants), which makes any statistical findings unreliable, at worst, or low in power, at best. Volumetric measurements are assessed in a lab, while participants are exposed to a variety of different types of pornography, neutral stimuli, and sometimes "non-sexual stimuli with positive or negative valences" (Suschinsky et al., 2009). Participants in one such study were asked "to respond to the films as naturally as possible, and to avoid contracting their muscles, manipulating their responses, touching their genitals, moving, or talking during the films" (Suschinsky et al., 2009, p. 563). The pornography in any given study might include male-female, male-male, and female-female sexual encounters; women and men exercising in the nude; sexual coercion and rape scenes; and sometimes nonhuman animal sexual encounters (Chivers & Bailey, 2005; Chivers et al., 2007). Some studies have attempted to find erotica that is "woman-friendly" (higher in "intimacy," etc.) to use with women samples (Laan & Both, 2008). But of course, the stimulus used in any given study depends on what facet of sexual arousal or "category" it is that is being measured (this may be gender differences in masochism, sociosexuality, etc.).

---

12. For a useful critique of the methods of lab-based sex research and "volunteer bias," see Ussher (2017). It should also be noted that some researchers are now attempting to gather data on how similar their clinical research populations are to the general public, and thus how much bias they need to account for—and ideally correct for (Dawson et al., 2019).

As my primary concern here is to expose the ways that men's and women's sexualities are produced as categorically different via this research, I will not extensively attend to the obvious critiques of the research methods being discussed. But beyond the issues with inadequate sample size, homogeneity, and potential problems with reliability, validity, and conceptualization and operationalization of assessment measures, there are myriad irresolvable issues regarding the generalizability of the experiments, including the fabricated and isolated nature of the experimental setting and the fact that it is divorced from any environment in which sexual activities would normally take place (the lab itself may be distracting, or arousing); that a device is attached to the genitals throughout the experiment, which may produce discomfort or enjoyment outside/beyond the audiovisual stimulus and is thus a potential intervening variable; that the neutral or any of the experimental audiovisual stimuli—combined with the situation in which they are viewed—may produce enjoyment, displeasure, or other affects outside/beyond their intended effects on the participants (in some studies, participants are shown more than fifteen pornographic video clips in succession, and sometimes the same ones are shown more than once); the fact that there is no standardization across various volumetric instruments and thus no standard unit of measurement by which to reliably compare across populations; and the fact that a complicated phenomenon such as desire is being measured by comparing "minds" to "bodies" and quantified at all. There are other extra-experimental dynamic and contextual issues—such as individual life history; race or ethnicity; cultural background; socioeconomic status; sexual history, including possible trauma or abuse; relationship status and quality; disability and mental health status; and other interpersonal issues—that seem to be rarely taken into account in this research, and that invariably affect the outcomes of these studies (or, if any of these data are collected, they are generally not publicized in the written reports). Thus, even if the intention is not to do so, this research leaves objective and subjective arousal as proxies for desire, the vicissitudes of which clearly cannot be captured in an experiment. However, it is interesting to consider what unintended effects the experiments may have on subjects, in terms of desire and arousal, that are not accounted for in the design.

Volumetric research has also been used to make arguments about the connection between female discordance and sexual dysfunction, with most studies suggesting that women who experience low desire and arousal are even more discordant than sexually functional women (Chivers, 2010). Accordingly, "women with sexual arousal problems report lower subjective sexual arousal to sexual stimuli in the laboratory, but do not show significantly lower genital responses when compared to women without sexual arousal problems"

(Chivers, 2010, p. 412). Here, it seems that the diagnosis of sexual dysfunction in women is tied to their lack of awareness regarding their bodily state, as receptivity and responsive desire are increasingly normalized for women. If both sexually functional and dysfunctional women are said to experience a disconnect between their psychology and physiology, is the difference that a normal (i.e., responsive) woman can recognize and be receptive to her (always already aroused) physical state, whereas the task of recognizing and being receptive to her body is more difficult for a sexually dysfunctional woman?

One recent study suggests that mindfulness-based sex therapy (MBST, to be explored in the next section of this chapter) is a potential way to bridge the gap:

> A top-down mechanism in which women deliberately focused attention on emerging, moment-by-moment sensations over the course of treatment, likely led to their contemporaneous detection of genital arousal in the laboratory setting, thereby increasing sexual concordance.... [G]iven evidence that negative affect during sexual encounters may significantly predict sexual difficulties (Nobre & Pinto-Gouveia, 2006), it is possible that women experienced an improved ability to regulate such emotions and thereby tune into and accept their visceral sensations. (Brotto, Chivers, Millman, & Albert, 2016, p. 1918)

Although this study ultimately concludes that improved concordance manifests as increased subjective arousal predicting increased genital arousal, the mechanism of improvement lies in women being more "in tune" with their bodies. And according to some of the most recent studies, women with desire problems are now—perhaps predictably—*too* concordant. Suschinsky et al. (2019), for instance, report that low-desiring women are actually more concordant than women with normal levels of desire—is it that these women need more mental stimulation to motivate themselves to have sex, because they are not attuned enough to their bodies? Is the assumption that these low-desiring women are unreceptive and unresponsive to their aroused genitals, too caught up in their heads—and this now puts them in the category of dysfunctionality? If this is the case, is discordance now understood to be healthier for women? Is receptivity now women's natural, healthy state?

Recent developments in the empirical investigation of sexual response include a multitude of techniques utilized to assess dysfunctions and gender differences, including tests of visual attention to sexual stimuli via methods like eye-tracking (for an example, see Dawson & Chivers, 2018). In particular, neuroscientific imaging techniques such as fMRI and PET are used more and more frequently to explore sex differences in desire and have affirmed the same conclusions regarding discordant female sexuality as have other types of experimental psychological research (Karama et al., 2002; Maravilla & Yang, 2008; Safron, Sylva, Klimaj, Rosenthal, & Bailey, 2019). Researchers have argued for a number of sex differences in arousal-related brain activity. For example, recent studies purport that during the processing of sexual stimuli, brain areas associated with emotional inhibition in the anterior cingulate cortex are activated among women, whereas men have greater control over their genital response as demonstrated by activity in the prefrontal cortex (Laan, 2007 as cited in Chivers et al., 2010; Laan, Scholte, & van Stegeren, 2006); the level of perceived sexual arousal is significantly higher in male than in female subjects as indicated by hypothalamic activity when viewing visual erotic stimuli in a lab setting (Karama et al., 2002); and differences can be observed among men and women and between healthy women and those with sexual interest/arousal disorders based on "overall brain activation" as determined by fMRI (Maravilla & Yang, 2008). In addition to experiments that directly compare men's and women's neural sexual processing, other studies examine sex differences by analyzing neural correlates of parental and romantic love (Bartels & Zeki, 2000, 2004) and conclude that women and men also differ in these realms. What can be gleaned from these studies is questionable at best, as many unstated narratives about sex differences in cognition, sexuality, and desire abound and inform hypotheses and experimental design—before the research has even begun. In any case, this research, along with the psychophysiological studies described above, has exploded in recent years, and has reinforced the purported need for an alternative model of sexual desire for women, including in the rhetoric of the *DSM-5* low-desire diagnoses—which are now different for men and for women.

Frigid or Burning Up? Gendering Low-Desire Diagnoses and Sexual Dysfunctions in the *DSM-5*

At the end of the first decade of the twenty-first century, the new alternative response models and the results of plethysmographic studies were in the sexological spotlight. All signs were pointing to the need for a new framework for understanding women's sexuality, and for diagnosing women's unique sexual difficulties. Accordingly, in her description of the rationale for changes to the low-desire diagnosis for women in the *DSM-5,* powerhouse sex therapist, researcher, women's health expert, and mindful-sex guru Lori Brotto (at the time also a member of the *DSM-5* sexual and gender-identity disorders work group and a close colleague of Rosemary Basson) made a case for the normalcy of responsive female desire. In a research review and explanation of the proposed criteria for a new low-desire diagnosis for women, Brotto (2010a) highlighted the utility of the incentive motivation model in considering women's desire patterns and further solidified the notion that women are more likely to experience this responsive, receptive, or "triggerable" desire, in addition to experiencing less "target specificity" than men when it comes to their physiological arousal, and more genital/subjective discordance. Brotto, along with Cynthia Graham (another member of the *DSM-5* sexual and gender-identity disorders work group), stated that research verifies that many women have a hard time distinguishing arousal from desire, or that these states tend to co-occur in women (see Brotto, 2010a; Graham, 2010). All of these ideas resonate not only with the alternative response models and psychophysiological research that had become so popular in studying women's sexuality in the 1990s and early 2000s, but they also have an unfortunate resonance with some of the foundational tenets of evolutionary psychology—that male and female sexuality are organized very differently, constructed via entirely different schemas, and seemingly existing on different planes of reality. Brotto's and Graham's discussions of the rationale are thorough and evidence-based; it is clear that they do not identify as evolutionary psychologists, and instead draw from quantitative and qualitative data drawn from clinical and community samples. But the framing of women's sexuality in Brotto's 2010 rationale, for instance, sounds too much at times like Baumeister's (2000, 2004) female erotic plasticity hypothesis and other arguments for evolutionary gender differences in sexual desire. She utilizes Basson's circular sexual response cycle and the incentive motivation model to describe female interest and motivation for sex, and cites Meston and Buss (2007) in a description of the nonsexual, intimacy-oriented nature of these rational feminine incentives. And there is little attention paid to power dynamics that may influence these phenomena, even as the intended point of the diagnostic change is to recognize the variability in women's sexuality, and to depathologize women's responsive desire. This is another place where we see an evolutionary psychology hangover, even as the feminist-identified researchers of this era (who are now some of the most reputable and well-known in the world) seemed to have genuinely sought to understand, explain, and accommodate women's distinct experience of sex.

After several decades of research on women's lack of target-specific physiological arousal and their subjective/genital discordance, hypotheses about women's innate erotic plasticity and lack of sexual orientation, plenty of other evolutionary psychology tropes about an overriding drive to motherhood, and the institution and deployment of a few different alternative models for female sexual response guided by the tenets of classical and operant conditioning and behaviorism, we arrive at the newest instantiation of female sexuality with the release of the *DSM-5* in 2013. In this latest edition, low female desire is diagnosed as female sexual interest/arousal disorder (FSIAD), which took the place of hypoactive sexual desire disorder (HSDD) in women and also incorporated the *DSM-IV* diagnosis of female sexual arousal disorder (FSAD). The revision subsumes the following criteria:

> Lack of, or significantly reduced, sexual interest/arousal as manifested by at least three of the following:
>
> 1. Absent/reduced interest in sexual activity.
> 2. Absent/reduced sexual/erotic thoughts or fantasies.
> 3. No/reduced initiation of sexual activity, and typically unreceptive to a partner's attempts to initiate.
> 4. Absent/reduced sexual excitement/pleasure during sexual activity in almost all or all (approximately 75%–100%) sexual encounters (in identified situational contexts or, if generalized, in all contexts).
> 5. Absent/reduced sexual interest/arousal in response to any internal or external sexual/erotic cues (e.g., written, verbal, visual).
> 6. Absent/reduced genital or nongenital sensations during sexual activity in almost all or all (approximately 75%–100%) sexual encounters (in identified situational contexts or, if generalized, in all contexts). (American Psychiatric Association, 2013, p. 433)

Whereas FSIAD is a female-specific diagnosis, low-desiring men are still diagnosed with HSDD (now *male* hypoactive sexual desire disorder, or MHSDD) under this new protocol. For comparison, I include the entry for MHSDD here, for which there is only one diagnostic criterion:

> persistently or recurrently deficient (or absent) sexual/erotic thoughts or fantasies and desire for sexual activity. (American Psychological Association, 2013, p. 440)

Regarding the new terminology for FSIAD, Brotto (2010a) reported that "interest" is a better descriptor than "desire" because it "emphasizes a broader construct than the more biological 'drive' connotations of sexual desire and it [a diagnosis of low sexual interest] reflects the lack of motivation [to engage in sex]" (p. 234). In this discussion of the diagnostic criteria, she does acknowledge that "interest" may not be an ideal term, given that some may feel that it is "devoid of any sexual meaning" (p. 234).

Given the moment in which this diagnosis was instituted, in light of the incredible popularity of plethysmographic research (the notion of female discordance is now a scientific truism), and the new sexual response models, it is appropriate to ask: What assumptions about female sexuality appear to undergird the FSIAD diagnosis? And what happened to desire here? Further, how did we end up at a place in the beginning of the twenty-first century wherein cognitive rational behaviorist models of sexuality seem more appropriate for women, whereas more traditional drive models continue to be applied to men? As a reminder: Interest (a stand-in for "desire" but with connotations that imply cognitive, incentive-based, and reward-seeking behavior—a rational construct that is quite different from traditional formulations of the lusty and impetuous nature of desire) and arousal (physiological changes in genital response, including vaginal vasocongestion and lubrication) are understood as often out of sync for women, are often scientifically framed as unrelated facets of women's sexualities, yet are simultaneously merged in this diagnosis. In fact, the merging of HSDD (low desire) and FSAD (low arousal) was based on research that suggests that many women have a hard time distinguishing arousal from desire. The architects of FSIAD have stated that what is actually being merged here is "desire" and "*subjective* arousal" (one's own experience of one's physiological arousal). But if research suggests that women tend to be unaware of their own physiological response, then, according to this logic, under what circumstances would they even *have* "subjective" arousal? The endless parsing of terms feels contradictory and the addition of *subjective* as a qualifier to *arousal* only solidifies the notion that confused, complex, discordant women need to be triggered to experience a sexual subjectivity that is not fully theirs to begin with.

These contradictions and paradoxes are alarming, and I worry that, even if it is unintentional, bringing together desire and arousal in this diagnosis, and highlighting "receptivity," potentially perpetuates the notion that, for many women, it is actually the case that arousal precedes and perhaps even governs sexual willingness or interest—or at least that it does in sexually functional women. At the same time, the framing might lead one to believe that willingness and interest are often nonsexual experiences for women, and that if they do precede arousal, are in many cases cognitive or rational in nature, divorced from the sexual body and divorced from an agentic want or need for sex itself (outside of a woman's partner's wants and needs). Amidst these tortuous narratives of feminine interest and motivation, physiological response, and subjective arousal, *desire*—seemingly now passé, or even offensive—is increasingly left out of the discussion completely. But how and why did a term associated with *wanting* become such a dirty word?

While the presumption of a singular, decontextualized, biologically based, testosterone-driven desire or "sexual urge" (Brotto, 2010a, p. 227) is arguably hegemonic and certainly worth questioning, setting up a binary between this masculine "urge" and an incentive-based feminine sexual "interest," "responsive arousal," or set of "motivations" may be equally problematic. For one thing, a now-codified notion of healthy feminine receptivity implies that the woman who suffers from FSIAD (or at least a diagnosee who fits criteria #1 and #3) is potentially dysfunctional for being uninterested in creating intimacy through sex with her partner, and she runs the risk of being pathologized for being unreceptive to his attempts to initiate sexual activity—or, even if not diagnosed, she may understand herself this way. For another, it insinuates that it is abnormal for a woman to *not* be concerned with the rewards she would otherwise receive by placating her partner or by laboring sexually to create a conciliatory environment in the relationship.[13] Even if these ideas are not directly spelled out in the diagnosis, it is easy to see that the trajectory of how this diagnosis came to be tells a different story, and the concern that women and men may interpret the diagnosis to suggest these things is thus warranted.

FSIAD was borne out of the desire to stop pathologizing women for not having a linear sex drive, in accordance with the purportedly male-oriented mandate of Masters and Johnson's human sexual response cycle. It was borne out of an attempt to reassure women that their responsive desire is normal, that they are not dysfunctional just because they don't have spontaneous desire. But does the newest framing of women's sexual response promoted in this diagnosis simply create a new set of criteria against which women will measure themselves? If women are not receptive, responsive, or triggerable, will they feel pathological? Like they are failing?

The researchers charged with creating this diagnosis have stated that the polythetic criteria of the diagnosis allows for the possibility of (a lack of) either spontaneous or responsive desire, and that the multiple criteria account for the variability in women's sexuality (Graham, 2016). I acknowledge their

---

13. According to the new *DSM-5*, women will only be diagnosed with FSIAD if their low desire causes them "clinically significant distress," thus ruling out those who are asexual. This is arguably an improvement over the old criterion of "interpersonal difficulty," but I suggest that "significant distress" in many cases may very well be caused by "interpersonal difficulty" (i.e., a [tacitly male] partner's frustrations over his female partner's lack of desire, or, rather, his own lack of sexual satisfaction on account of this, not to mention a woman's potential feelings of inadequacy for not being responsive enough when sexuality feels so compulsory in Global North societies).

intentions, but again, my point here is not to suggest that those who designed the diagnosis are malicious misogynists, but rather to outline the troubled trajectory of research (including research conducted in the name of feminism) that led up to FSIAD's institution, to highlight the scientific background (i.e., apolitical/atheoretical behaviorism combined with evolutionary psychology) within which it resides, and to point to the way this diagnosis clearly looks on paper. Further, the polythetic diagnostic criteria that are meant to suggest the variability in women's desire reify the notion that women's sexuality is complex and complicated—which may very well be true for some women. But, if it is true, we have no good explanation in the *DSM-5* or its supporting discourses for why it is the case. What we do have, however, is one diagnosis that *looks* quite complex and confusing (the one for women), juxtaposed next to another that is very streamlined and simple (the one for men).

Many gendered assumptions are directly spelled out in the language of the full FSIAD diagnostic entry, and this contrast between textual instantiations of masculine and feminine desire is particularly evident when comparing FSIAD to MHSDD.[14] The terms *interest* and *responsiveness* are not used in the MHSDD "Diagnostic Criteria" at all, whereas in the section entitled "Diagnostic Features" (which directly follows the "Diagnostic Criteria" for all diagnoses in the *DSM*) in the entry for FSIAD, these terms are articulated throughout:

> In one woman, sexual interest/arousal disorder may be expressed as a lack of interest in sexual activity, an absence of erotic or sexual thoughts, and reluctance to initiate sexual activity and respond to a partner's sexual invitations. In another woman, an inability to become sexually excited, to respond to sexual stimuli with sexual desire, and a corresponding lack of signs of physical sexual arousal may be the primary features. (American Psychological Association, 2013, pp. 433–434)

Here, the notion that even women with "normal" levels of interest and arousal are presumed to not feel sexual until their partner "invites" them to "respond with desire" is instantiated. In contrast, in the MHSDD diagnosis, sexual "receptivity" or "responsiveness" to a partner's advances are not discussed in the beginning of the entry in either the "Diagnostic Criteria" or the "Diagnostic Features" sections, and are instead not mentioned at all until the "Asso-

---

14. For men, desire and arousal disorders were retained as separate entities, although it is worth noting that Brotto (2010b) suggested they may be brought together, and that responsiveness may also be normal for men. It is unfortunate that Brotto's recommendations were not taken up in the final version of the *DSM-5*. More recently, Murray (2019) has suggested the need for a different framework for men's sexuality and desire.

ciated Features Supporting Diagnosis" section, much later on in the entry. When these constructs are introduced, it is with a qualifier regarding men's situational *preference* for their partner to initiate sex (thus their own responsiveness is not framed as a core component of male sexuality):

> Although men are more likely to initiate sexual activity, and thus low desire may be characterized by a pattern of non-initiation, many men may prefer to have their partner initiate sexual activity. In such situations, the man's lack of receptivity to a partner's initiation should be considered when evaluating low desire. (American Psychological Association, 2013, p. 441)

Later in the entry, in the "Gender-Related Diagnostic Issues" section, this notion of "initiation" or "invitation" as a thoroughly masculine sexual trait is rearticulated very clearly:

> In contrast to . . . sexual disorders in women, desire and arousal disorders have been retained as separate constructs in men. . . . [M]en do report a significantly higher intensity and frequency of sexual desire compared with women. (pp. 442–443)

Throughout the diagnostic terminology, the disproportionate use of the language of the incentive motivation model specifically for women is evident. Elements of the feminized receptivity discourse of Basson's circular sexual response cycle for women, in addition to notions of gender differences in subjective/genital concordance, have also been imported into the diagnosis. Men's and women's sexual dysfunctions—and thus their healthy states, as counterparts—are framed as disparate. If we trust that Basson's clinical research and Chivers's experimental research are scientifically valid and replicable, we might still ask: Where do these gender differences come from? How do they manifest? And what do they indicate in terms of treatment for sexual problems—for cis and trans men and women, for agender and nonbinary individuals? For queer- and straight-identified folks?

There are many other important divergences in the diagnoses of MHSDD and FSIAD, including how sexual and erotic thoughts or fantasies are framed in each (these are framed as more central for men), what constitutes an "adaptive response to adverse life conditions" and would thus preclude a diagnosis (the example offered for MHSDD is of a man whose desire has suffered because his partner becomes pregnant at the same time that he is planning on ending the relationship [!], while no example of an "adaptive response" is offered for women), and the role of psychophysiological data in understanding dysfunction (for FSIAD, plethysmographic research is cited that suggests that dysfunctional women, like normal women, have high rates of physiological arousal even if their subjective arousal does not match this state; postulations about male concordance are thus insinuated by proxy, but are not explicitly included in the MHSDD criteria). Further, "*severe* relationship distress," such as "partner violence," is mentioned as a possible reason to not diagnose a woman with FSIAD, but this arguably neglects many forms of complex, everyday, banal, and insidious traumas (Cvetkovich, 2003) that may be comorbid with low desire yet are not discussed in the diagnosis (for more on the important role of trauma in sexual desire and its dysfunctions, see Spurgas, 2016a, 2016b and chapters 4 and 5 of this book).

In the wake of and leading up to the publication of the *DSM-5*, many clinicians expressed concerns about the "lumping together" of arousal and desire for women, and also of what they saw as an "ideological" importing of Basson's circular model into the female-specific diagnosis (see Balon & Clayton, 2014; DeRogatis, Clayton, Rosen, Sand, & Pyke, 2011). In addition to doctors and sexologists being divided on the new diagnosis and associated framework, sociologists, therapists, and other scholars have also registered concerns about the naturalizing of women's responsiveness. Narratives about an essential feminine proclivity to seek out sexual rewards and benefits may be harmful to women who identify as having low desire, a point that Tyler (2009) has elucidated. Regarding the formulation of feminine receptivity as a "willingness to proceed [with sexual activity] despite absence of sexual desire at that instant" (as cited in Basson, 2002), Tyler (2009) makes the case that "using receptivity as a benchmark for women's sexual desire may actually reinforce male sexual demands, and promote coercive sex in heterosexual relationships" (p. 41). Przybylo (2013) has made similar points regarding the precarious position that the notion of low female concordance puts asexual women in, specifically stating that this "sleeping beauty model" of receptive female sexuality "suggests that women are in a sense incapable of being asexual" (p. 236)—as they are understood to be always on the precipice of noticing, and perhaps pursuing, their physiological arousal, thus disqualifying them from a "true" asexual identity. And Flore (2016) describes the FSIAD diagnosis itself as a framework for sexual training, as a way for patients to fashion their own sexual subjectivity, with the burden of this management falling on women.

Kleinplatz (2011) has also expressed concerns about the resignation of women to substandard sex that they do not really want to engage in. She states, "We often proceed as if low frequency of desire were evidence of psychopathology whereas it may instead be evidence of good judgment" (p. 7). She goes on to describe how patterns of low desire can become relationally sedimented for women, through distasteful and unsatisfying experiences with sex, and how women ultimately learn that they should be receptive to their partners' advances:

> The usual pattern . . . involves increasing episodes of mediocre sex, leading to lowered arousal during sex, which results in low satisfaction after sex. . . . [M]any [women] choose to continue engaging in sex out of commitment to relational harmony . . . even though this entails having sex without sexual desire. Or sometimes, they follow the "just do it" approach because they have read that women's desire tends to be receptive rather than coming from within (p. 8)

Here, Kleinplatz elucidates the ways this pattern of sexual servicing comes into existence in a heterosexual relationship, throwing the circular sexual response cycle into stark relief. She frames this not in terms of coercion per se, but contributes a sad vision of extremely bland and thoroughly annoying, frustrating, and lackluster sex that some women feel they must endure to make their partners happy. Rather than attributing this notion of sexual service to women's natural receptivity and responsiveness in essential or biological terms, or sugar-coating it by suggesting it as a normative way for women to enjoy sex more, Kleinplatz exposes how women *learn* to provide sexual services to their male partners, and explains why this leads to unenjoyable sex for both parties. Thus, she provides a much-needed corrective to the dominant discourses about responsive feminine sexuality.

Louise, a psychologist and activist I interviewed, also contributed a critique of Basson's circular sexual response cycle:

> I don't feel that it's an escape from the box. I think it's probably a more female-friendly box, but I think it's a box. It doesn't describe a lot of women I know who have a different thing going on, and I think it's too prescriptive, as in really not as descriptive as you would think—it's more *pres*criptive. I think it's become popular because it sounds good, but it's too narrow, it doesn't take enough factors into account, it doesn't take enough diversity into account, diversity that I understand to be part of people's sexual makeup. . . . I'm not crazy about her [Basson's] model, and I'm not crazy about any model, because I don't think there is a model.

Beyond these practical and clinical critiques of responsive desire as they pertain to heterosexual relationships and women's sexual identities, I am concerned with the overarching tales that this logic promotes and deploys regarding femininity, female sexuality, and heteronormative gender relations more broadly—including with how these might affect individuals of diverse gender identities, sexualities, and lifestyles.

Two of the low-desiring women I interviewed for this study had been treated in a program designed to help women with female sexual dysfunctions, including vulvodynia and comorbid HSDD in women (their treatment was prior to the publication of the *DSM-5* and thus the institution of the FSIAD diagnosis). One of these participants, Astrid, had deep criticisms of the program, and specifically of aspects of the treatment protocol that were clearly implementations of Basson's circular sexual response cycle and incentive motivation model as these are applied to women:

> That's where I began to hear about this cycle. . . . [T]hey explained that in the course of a normal relationship, a heterosexual relationship *just understood*, that perhaps when you first start out that both the man and the woman might experience this "spontaneous desire" for sex with each other but as time would go on the man might still experience that but the woman would no longer experience the spontaneous sexual desire but what she would experience instead would be sort of a *willingness* to engage in sex. So like for reasons of increasing the intimacy levels or whatever, like "we get to cuddle at the end" and stuff, that we would have been willing to respond to the advances of our husbands or the men in our lives, and that this is kind of how normal relationships go.

In Astrid's comments, the heteronormative bias of the feminized responsive desire framework—as it is produced through sexual difference narratives in evolutionary sexology, alternative female sexual response cycles and diagnoses, and clinical protocols that treat women based on ideas about their essential "discordance"—is clearly exposed. It is also clear how, through this treatment program, women were taught what the normative framework for female desire is—a framework that is based on receptivity, responsiveness, and a willingness to be seduced or coaxed into sex by an initiating male partner. They were also tacitly taught that the kind of sex they were *not* going to naturally or spontaneously desire, but that they should be receptive to engaging in for their male partner's benefit, likely involved penetrative intercourse with accompanying male pleasure (and male orgasm). Thus, women in this program were taught not only what their own desire (or lack thereof) should feel like, but what kind of sex they were meant to be engaging in, and for whose enjoyment.

These clinicians' and patients' critiques of FSIAD and its associated discourses support my previously stated concerns about the trajectory of the new science of female sexuality and the feminized responsive desire framework. Here, an emphasis on feminine responsiveness, receptivity, flexibility, and complexity does not sound so liberating for women. This is particularly so when feminine complexity and flexibility are juxtaposed against masculine desire's stability, constancy, activity, and (dependable) spontaneity. Many of those who have argued most vehemently for a different model of female sexual response have done so in order to challenge the rigidity and normativity of earlier conceptions of desire: something it has been argued time and again that women simply do not *have* in the same way that men do. FSIAD reinforces this notion of feminine lack. In the new FSIAD diagnosis, we see the formulation that for women, sexual interest often follows physical arousal, desire is no longer even part of the equation, and, for more than a quarter of the premenopausal female population in the US (Laumann, Paik, & Rosen, 1999; West et al., 2008), getting the psyche in line with the body during any given sexual experience may require quite a bit of coaxing. So, although a critique of the traditional, linear HSRC may be timely and worthwhile, it is important to consider the retrograde gendered implications of this diagnostic shift—particularly in light of the rising prevalence of experimental research on gender differences in sexual behavior and desire, the deluge of media spotlighting of and public attention to women's responsive desire, and the explosion of treatment protocols for female patients who present with desire troubles. In the twenty-first century, these protocols extend well beyond the clinic.

Bringing Bodies and Minds into Line: Brain Drugs and Mindfulness-Based Sex Therapy

Since the blockbuster success of Viagra—the little blue pill to enhance erection, rolled out by Pfizer in 1998 in the US, with many other locales soon to follow—there has been increasing investment in treatments for "female sexual dysfunction," or FSD. This amorphous catch-all category, and how it came to be, has been critiqued extensively elsewhere (for examples, see Cacchioni, 2015; Kleinplatz, 2018; Kleinplatz et al., 2020; Moynihan, 2005; Moynihan & Mintzes, 2010; Tiefer, 2006, 2012). But the most important part, for my story, is how the aspect of female sexuality that was eventually determined to be the most useful to home in on, invest in, and ultimately modulate is low desire. Over the last several decades, low desire has increasingly been framed as women's number-one sexual problem.

In 2010, the neuro-drug flibanserin went through US Food and Drug Administration (FDA) trials but was not approved (D. Wilson, 2010), in part due to protest by a critical outpouring of members of the anti-FSD New View Campaign[15] along with other antimedicalization activists who argued that the drug had been created to fix a problem that didn't exist, solely for the purpose of making a profit (for these activists, it was the quintessential modern example of "disease-mongering"). But a few years later, in August 2015, flibanserin was finally passed by the FDA, due in part to a purportedly "grassroots" movement of women advocating gender equality in regard to pharmaceutical treatments for sexual problems—many of whom had been paid by Sprout Pharmaceuticals, the company that then bought the rights to the drug. Flibanserin, now brand name Addyi, is a neurotransmitter drug that works on the central nervous system, specifically by decreasing serotonin uptake while increasing dopamine and norepinephrine, purportedly enhancing libido in women (Stahl, Sommer, & Allers, 2011). Newer additions to the neuro-pharmaceutical lineup are Lybrido and Lybridos, which are currently still undergoing field trials (Bergner, 2013a). And most recently, in the summer of 2019, bremelanotide (brand name Vyleesi), which works by activating melanocortin receptors in the brain, was also approved by the FDA. Pharmaceutical treatments for women's desire problems have been referred to as "pink Viagras," but to analogize these treatments with Viagra is inappropriate for a number of reasons. Conceptually comparing the ways the drugs work illustrates the differences.

In their critiques of the cultural and medical fixation on Viagra in the early 2000s, Mamo and Fishman (2001) and Loe (2004) elucidated the compulsory heterosexuality prescribed by pharmaceutical technologizing of the male erection. They argued that by focusing all attention on the mechanical workings of the penis—or lack of this function, in the case of erectile disorder—Viagra and the culture surrounding it perpetuate the notions that male desire never falters and is available in a never-ending supply. Thus, Viagra posits male sexual problems as generally physical rather than psychological, and concomitantly legitimates heteronormative penile-vaginal intercourse as the proper, healthy, and ideal way to have sex.

Much of the feminist antimedicalization critique that was once (in the 1980s and 1990s, specifically) directed at deconstructing *DSM* diagnoses, associated gender-essentializing research on sexuality, and other pathologizing medical discourses has now been redirected somewhat myopically toward attacking the pharmaceutical industry (Angel, 2012, 2013; Spurgas, 2013a, 2013b). Leading up to the publication of the *DSM-5*, there was no antimedi-

---

15. "FDA Hearing on Flibanserin," New View Campaign website: http://www.newviewcampaign.org/flibanserin.asp

calization activist critique of the new feminized sexual response models or impending FSIAD diagnosis, and all of that energy instead went to tearing down Big Pharma. However, it seems self-evident that if sexual responsiveness is now part of the framework for healthy sexuality in women, and via the logic of plethysmographic studies and the circular sexual response cycle women are understood to be always already aroused/arousable (physiologically)—they just have a hard time getting "motivated" and are thus often discordant—then altering their brain chemistry via drugs would be an obvious targeted treatment option. Popular medical discourses concretize the notions that Viagra brings the (disordered) body into line with the (intact, normal, and sexually healthy/functioning) mind for men, while neurotransmitter drugs like flibanserin bring the (disordered) mind into line with the (intact, normal, and sexually healthy/functioning) body for women. In men, the problem is framed as hydraulic, mechanical, and easy to fix, whereas in women the problem is in the organization or design of the system itself: There is a computational error. Thus, that flibanserin (a drug that had previously been used as an antidepressant) is sometimes referred to as the "pink" or "female" Viagra is actually very misleading, as the mechanism of action is entirely different.

I think it is more useful to critique the gendered foundation upon which these sexual dysfunction drugs operate than the marketing of the drugs or corporate "profiteering." I say this for a few reasons: (1) Critiques of capitalism are certainly warranted (this book includes that type of critique), but there is much more to be wary of under capitalism than "corporate industry" (e.g., neoliberal governmentality and regimes of biopolitical self-enhancement). (2) These critics don't consider the queer off-label ways that drugs are taken beyond their intended use (e.g., gay men who use Viagra to maintain erections for longer—see Race, 2009 for more on this). (3) Building on the last point, these critiques assume a natural body that is modified by drugs in a way that other techniques (such as mindfulness) do not modify that body, and that drugs are somehow more "harmful" to that body. And (4) these critics position women in such a way that they must not engage in drug treatment if they are to be "good feminists." It is thus a purist argument. More than that, it has functioned as a strawman so that critics of a variety of stripes could band together "against FSD" (anyone who is "anti–Big Pharma" is now an "activist" and a "feminist"), and in this way, it has diluted robust dialogues around the medical construction and management of women's sexuality.

In fact, flibanserin's mechanism of action functions fully within the logic of female receptivity that I have been outlining. This may seem paradoxical, as there has been much activist outcry against the drugs by the same people who support the feminized responsive desire framework. But I want to place the development of neuro drugs to enhance women's desire squarely within the rest of the history I have put forward in this chapter. It is part and parcel of the shift, since the late 1990s, toward measuring the gap between women's subjective and genital arousal (with the physiological generally understood to be fully functional and ready to go even as motivation might lag), toward conceptualizing women's sexuality as on a completely different plane than men's sexuality (and often in apolitical, atheoretical, or biologically essentialist terms), and toward postulating evolutionary psychology–derived explanations for gender differences in sexual "interests," "motivations," "incentives," and "rewards." Flibanserin and the feminized responsive desire framework are two sides of the same coin.

In addition to pharmaceutical management of female sexual dysfunction, other therapeutic treatments are becoming more and more popular. As psychoanalytic and psychodynamic explanations and treatments for sexual problems have fallen out of vogue in the past decades, cognitive behavioral therapy (CBT) techniques have taken their place. CBT is a psychotherapeutic theory and practice in which goal-oriented, explicit, and systematic procedures are utilized to change one's thinking or relationship to thinking, so that behavioral changes may follow. It can be conceived as a method of self-directed behavioral training. While CBT has been used to treat sexual dysfunction, mindfulness-based techniques are increasingly used today. Both techniques focus on awareness of thoughts, feelings, and bodily sensations, but they proceed from slightly different principles. While CBT is geared toward defusing and ultimately changing negative or biased thoughts, mindfulness-based techniques focus on helping patients sit with negative thoughts "nonjudgmentally" while eventually letting them pass, rather than attempting to change them. Mindfulness has been described as the "third wave" of behavior-based therapies (Brotto, 2011), with its focus on awareness, bodily attunement, and acceptance.

Mindfulness as part of a scientific and medical enterprise made its popular entrée in the North American scene in the 1990s, and fully took off with the publication of Jon Kabat-Zinn's *Full Catastrophe Living: How to Cope with Stress, Pain and Illness Using Mindfulness Meditation* in 1990. Kabat-Zinn had been developing his approach to mindfulness and applying it with patients with chronic pain, stress, anxiety, and depression since the late 1970s—in a protocol now known as mindfulness-based stress reduction (MBSR). By allowing patients to sit with their pain and acknowledge it nonjudgmentally, this technique was shown to be effective at reducing the accompanying negative affects associated with pain (if not pain itself) and with helping sufferers cope. The technique was implemented more fully for depression with the publication of Segal, Williams, and Teasdale's *Mindfulness-Based Cognitive*

Therapy (MBCT) for Depression in 2001, and it has also been applied to the treatment of borderline personality disorder (BPD) and associated symptoms via dialectical behavior therapy (DBT). In her 2018 *Better Sex through Mindfulness: How Women Can Cultivate Desire,* Lori Brotto, of the DSM-5 sexual dysfunctions work group, describes how she learned about mindfulness at the turn of the twenty-first century and began strategizing how it might be applied to women with low desire and other sexual disorders. Over the next couple of years while working alongside Rosemary Basson at the University of British Columbia, Brotto would design one of the most successful contemporary nonpharmaceutical treatments for sexual difficulties in women. And in a milieu in which it seems that one can only be either on the side of "Big Pharma" or against it when it comes to the treatment of female sexual dysfunction, Brotto's technique was lauded—and has been branded as a feminist alternative to the "little pink pill."

The protocol, now known as mindfulness-based sex therapy, or MBST, emphasizes the notion of "being in the present" and is rooted in the concept of mindfulness as it appears in Buddhist spiritual practices (in addition to Kabat-Zinn, Brotto references the work of Buddhist monk Thich Nhat Hanh as an important inspiration). Many of the other practitioners who were involved in designing FSIAD and/or who have conducted plethysmographic research or research on the circular sexual response cycle for women have supported the use of MBST as a therapeutic tool to improve the low-desiring woman's sexual response. MBST is often used within a therapeutic setting involving multiple women who experience low desire or other sexual dysfunctions, in the context of psychoeducational (PED) interventions that may integrate elements of sensory training, body scans, and mindfulness meditation (Brotto, Basson, & Luria, 2008). Patients engage in "self-observation" and "touch" exercises as homework assignments that challenge them to imagine themselves as "competent, sexual, feminine, and sensual" (Brotto, Krychman, & Jacobson, 2008, p. 2743). They also engage in group activities, some of which involve concentrating on the sensual qualities of an object, such as a penny or a raisin, over a period of several minutes, in order to train themselves to remain focused on one thing, in the present, and to notice it in a new way.

Via MBST, women are taught to utilize these meditation and mindfulness techniques to become more aware of their physiological arousal, most often in the context of heterosexual relationships where female desire has waned, thus creating problematic "desire discrepancies." They may use a variety of sensate-focus-style techniques to bring their bodies and minds back into line—in fact, Brotto has explicitly stated that Masters and Johnson, with their tool of sensate focus, were really the first to apply mindfulness in sex therapy (Brotto,

2018). What is interesting now is that women are expected to, at least as a first step, do this work on their own rather than with a partner—so sensate focus has become individualized here. Brotto also links MBST specifically to Basson's circular sexual response cycle (this model and women's responsive desire are generally themes at the mindfulness sessions and are taught to participants) and to plethysmographic research that highlights female genital/subjective discordance, and she states that part of the goal of mindfulness is to help women "tune in" to their physiological arousal, in order to ignite or "cultivate" their own responsive desire. In her 2018 popular self-help book, she states:

> We have evidence that, in general, women's concordance between their self-reported and physical sexual response is low, and that training in mindfulness significantly increases the degree of mind-to-body communication and improves self-reported interoceptive awareness. . . . [M]indfulness teaches women to become more aware of their internal bodily sensations, including sexual sensations, and this may improve their motivations for sex and increase their tendency to notice sexual arousal and have that arousal trigger sexual desire. (p. 154)

Meditation has become a very popular technique for naturally or holistically treating all types of ills today and is clearly effective for many ailments. But my data raise concerns that utilizing mindfulness in this particular fashion potentially sets up women to push through or at least accept traumatic feelings and even to have sex in the name of being responsive and receptive, and promoting relational harmony (M. Barker, 2013 also raises this concern). This line of research, diagnosis, and treatment protocol together exemplify how women's sexuality is configured within contemporary sexual medicine and outside of it in alternative and self-help health spheres, a deployment that arguably perpetuates the naturalization of female receptivity and the notion that women should work on themselves sexually. CBT is explicitly intended to challenge "irrational" beliefs about sexuality. As the third wave of behavioral therapy applies to sex, mindfulness-based sex therapy is intended to increase sexual interoception, or one's ability to perceive one's own embodied sexual response, including genital arousal "in the present," rather than becoming consumed with negative thoughts about the past, future, or any other distractions (including, implicitly, past traumas or experiences of violence). Chivers and Brotto (2017) state: "Mindfulness training induces functional changes in the insula (an area of the brain associated with awareness of body states), and it decreases activation of the amygdala and areas of the ventromedial prefrontal cortex (Holzel et al., 2011) associated with emotions" (p. 17). Brotto has elsewhere been quoted as stating that mindfulness-based sex therapy can change the very "structure of the brain" and its processes, and that in this way, it is similar to the drug Addyi.[16] Thus, while MBST is popularly framed as more female-friendly than taking a drug to increase one's desire, I wonder how similar the two actually are. In both cases, sexual problems are individualized[17] and women ostensibly alter their brain chemistry in order to get in touch with their natural and free-flowing objective physiological arousal from which their minds have become disconnected. The burden of working on sex falls on women, and, in the case of mindfulness meditation, there's actually quite a bit of work to do.

Kelly, one participant in my study, succinctly explains the problems with using behavioral techniques in a clinical setting as a form of receptivity management. In the program she attended to treat genital pain and low desire, she had been encouraged to utilize both vaginal dilators and mindfulness (MBST was in its nascent stages when she was in the program) to ease her pain and enhance her desire:

> The idea was [to use behavioral techniques] so that I could continue to have sex, which is kind of weird because if I didn't want to have sex, why am I doing exercises so I can continue doing it? So that was kind of strange—and male-focused! Because if I wasn't enjoying sex at the time, then it's something that I'm doing almost just so that my boyfriend can still have sex with me; it wasn't something that would help me with my own pleasure.

Astrid further describes her experience with being instructed to relax and be responsive toward her male partner, and to use behavioral techniques to do so:

> So [the idea was that] like in the beginning, you have mutual desire that's like, you see each other and you desire each other, but as things go on the dude still has that but the lady doesn't have that anymore, and so she's I guess like more willing to be seduced. . . . [Later in the course of the program,] the men [male partners] were given a chance to talk about how frustrated they

---

16. Video interview on Dr. Justin Lehmiller's Sex & Psychology blog: https://www.lehmiller.com/blog/2018/4/23/better-sex-through-mindfulness-an-interview-with-dr-lori-brotto-video

17. See K. Barker (2014) for a discussion of mindfulness meditation as "do-it-yourself medicalization of every moment" and Gregg (2018) and Purser (2019) for further critiques of mindfulness as part of the neoliberalization of self-care under late capitalism and for discussions of how the technique is often used to individualize care in the name of productivity.

were, then they were educated in this "response cycle" thing. . . . [T]hat's exactly what they were taught about, that we had also been taught about: "Well, you might feel spontaneous desire for her, but she may need to be coaxed into it" kind of thing.

Here, we see these ideas that are put forward in the feminized responsive desire framework—including notions of women's complexity, their receptivity or responsiveness, and a feminine desire that is motivated primarily by cost-benefit analyses for nonsexual rewards—thrown starkly into the spotlight via the technique of MBST. Kelly's and Astrid's comments make it clear that although all of this research and treatment is done in the name of helping women, in some cases, it becomes a prescription for work and even coercion, it further confuses the murky notion of consent, and it encourages women to assume that there is a specific way they should be having sex and that they should be having sex for specific reasons. Using MBST in this way thus has the potential to compound women's existing sexual traumas, or even to retraumatize them, iatrogenically.

Brotto herself acknowledges that sexual dysfunction is highly correlated with sexual trauma (which is notable given that post-traumatic stress disorder [PTSD] is not discussed as comorbid in the FSIAD diagnosis—a point I have discussed at length elsewhere; see Spurgas, 2016a and also Yehuda, Lehrner, & Rosenbaum, 2015 for more on this comorbidity). In a 2012 article that analyzes the relationships between sexual dysfunction and childhood sexual abuse, Brotto, Seal, and Rellini state: "Despite the presence of (sometimes strong) physical sexual sensations, her mental awareness may have deliberately gone to a nonsexual fantasy world, leading to repeated experiences of physical arousal paired with dissociation" (p. 2). Here, the fact that sexual trauma often leads to dissociation in sexual abuse survivors is a critical counterpoint to the notion that women—particularly androphilic women—are "naturally" discordant. And the treatment options become even more suspect when we question whether discordance is (at least in some cases) the product of trauma or whether it is part and parcel of "natural feminine receptivity." This requires critical ethical consideration, especially when one of the most popular techniques for remedying women's discordance (or maybe it's dissociation?) is now most certainly MBST.

While the benefits of being "in the present," mindful, and attuned to one's body and experiences are undeniably beneficial to some women (and men) broadly, the pairing of a technique such as this with discourses of female receptivity—receptivity of the psyche to the body, and receptivity of a woman to her initiating partner—is potentially harmful. It is because men and women are posited as inherently different kinds of sexual beings that the use of CBT and MBST techniques to alter sexual experience becomes worrisome. In assessing these technologies and their use in the current moment, we must responsibly inquire: What are the goals of these techniques? What is the underlying theory regarding masculine versus feminine sexuality that is espoused within this framework? What forms of desire are encouraged, and which escape, or which are produced but go unaccounted for or are neglected in these interventions? MBST is increasingly used in therapeutic settings in which women learn to maintain awareness and eventually let go of the "negative" thoughts that might prevent them from harnessing their responsive desire or from taking advantage of an opportunity to be sexual in their everyday lives (for instance, when stimulated by an initiating partner). Brotto (2018) uses the word *training* throughout her book to describe the practice of learning mindfulness. How is this technique a type of gendered desire training, and what are women being trained (and training themselves) to experience or to engage in? To enjoy? To ignore? And to what end? Within a framework in which feminine desire is discursively absent; in which "interest" is framed as cognitive, rational, and a cost-benefit analysis; in which "arousal" is often read as physiological; and in which interest and arousal are posited as often out of sync for women—mindfulness appears to be more about bringing the frigid mind into line with the lustful body than with simply bringing the two into harmony. This arrangement lends itself too easily to a potential service requirement of the feminine to their tacitly masculine partners, and betrays the assumption that, within these discourses, the truth of (feminine) desire is produced as originating in the aroused body—or possibly outside of it, in the (cis male) partner and his sexual needs or more broadly within normative and compulsory heteropatriarchal conceptions of sex.

Implications of Shifting Diagnoses: Behaviorism and Sexual (Self-)Management

In an effort to free female desire from the prescriptions of linear, goal-oriented "drive" or "deficit" models, the contemporary science of female sexuality has created a new set of prescriptions. This was not the result of malintent of any specific actors, but rather the result of a variety of discourses and practices coming together in a specific moment to form the feminized responsive desire framework. A taxonomy for healthy and dysfunctional feminine desire is produced via FSIAD, in the new sexual response models, via plethysmographic research on female discordance, with new drugs and mindfulness treatments for desire cultivation, along with activism to promote a new view of women's sexuality—and, taken together, all of this has made femininity newly productive and moldable in the twenty-first century. The gap of feminine discordance itself is now a site of modulation, and *receptivity* and *responsiveness* are the new bywords of sexual production—or sexualized social reproduction—under neoliberal capitalism. Femininity here is complex and complicated, responsive and receptive, discordant and disconnected—and thus perfect for mining, cultivating, and putting to work. This is the heart of the biopolitics of femininity.

How bodies, lives, and relationships are modulated and made productive through the biopolitical discourses of public health, epidemiology, psychiatry, medicine, and technoscience is of key concern in understanding biopolitics. For Foucault (1978), the most important site of modulation through these discourses is unequivocally human sexuality. We can understand sex as the nexus between the public and private, the population and the individual, the species body and the body-as-machine. In his discussion of the deployment of sexuality, Foucault (1978) elucidates a shift from the disciplinary or "deductive" (p. 136) power of the sovereign to the "regulatory control" (p. 139) of a cluster of powerful relations that took the form of an apparatus of governmentality, or what Deleuze (1992) would later call a "control society." One of the most important characteristics of this shift is that regulation is no longer focused on the domination and punishment of the individual transgressor, but is rather framed as a means of protecting the larger populace from "biological dangers" (Foucault, 1978, p. 138) that, if not preemptively guarded against, could potentially destroy the human race or species body. This guarding must come in the form of both surveilling and policing others—in addition to ourselves. Foucault (2000) and followers of his later work have emphasized that within this shift to governmentality, prescriptions for how individuals can and should regulate their own behavior are brought to the fore, and these prescriptions for leading a healthy and productive lifestyle are always asymptotic (they are impossible to reach, and thus we are always striving to be better citizens within a framework of constantly shifting prescriptions). The speculative logic through which debilitated sexuality registers as a biological danger also has a flip side, wherein sex is framed as a site of optimization useful for securitizing populations and for generating productive subjects, perpetually in search of "the good life" (Berlant, 2011).

In this case, the best life is always sought, as subjects maintain optimism regarding how good sex could or should be (i.e., it can always be better). Our contemporary cultural formulations of these mechanisms of (self-)control and (self-)optimization are evidenced by a proliferation of media accounts that espouse a keen interest in healthy sex as a mode of producing healthy citizens, and we see these accounts particularly in women-targeted magazines and on self-help websites (for an example, see Jones, 2011). These regimens are not purely medical—they may come to us increasingly in the form of "alternative" medicine and "lifestyle" medicine (Clarke et al., 2003; Frank & Jones, 2003). The feminized sexual self-optimization that I describe in this book resonates with notions of compulsory sexuality (Gupta, 2015; Gupta & Cacchioni, 2013) and its adjacent aspects, including compulsory heterosexuality (Rich, 1980), compulsory able-bodiedness (McRuer, 2006), and other sexualized, gendered, raced, and otherwise embodied citizenship protocols (Ahmed, 2010; Barounis, 2019; Borck & Moore, 2019; Cacchioni & Wolkowitz, 2011; Cossman, 2007; Preciado, 2013; Repo, 2016). The racialization of regimes of sexual difference must also be forefronted (Schuller, 2016; Snorton, 2017)—as the receptive femininity that is prescribed here is not only cisgender and heterosexual but also white and bourgeois.

In her discussion of erotic and orgasmic reconditioning via behaviorism in the 1950s (and its infamous use to reconfigure the sexual orientation of gay men), Jagose (2013) describes how, given its relatively short duration of active use, the protocol would have seemed more like a passing fad, "if its fundamental learning principles and clinical techniques were not still being keenly pursued in relation to two vastly different demographic profiles, the wholesale behavior modification of which is widely seen as a *social good*: sex criminals and heterosexual women" (p. 123; italics added). Here, Jagose alludes to how behaviorist sex therapists such as Masters and Johnson trained women to have coital orgasms. The women, of course, wanted this treatment—they sought it out. While the behaviorist protocols of today, including MBST, do not seek to train women to have vaginal orgasms, they do capacitate femininity—they seek to make otherwise-debilitated femininity useful and productive while at the same time tethering it to regimes of self-improvement and pleasure.[18] What Jagose then reminds us is that the dominant frameworks of the time, which are today often related to self-help via medical or extra-medical protocols, influence our desires, and that pleasure can be bound up with biopolitical control and the harvesting of (our own) potential.

The release of the newest version of the *DSM* is notable in light of our cultural reliance on codified medical discourses, and because how we define pathology has implications for how we understand what is normal (Foucault, 1973). The diagnosis of FSIAD in women is worthy of investigation because codes for race, gender, and sexuality are part of what is prescribed by the

---

18. My use of the terms *capacitate* and *debilitate* here draw on the biopolitics described by Puar (2017).

DSM, and these have particular import in a world in which sexual regulation is an exemplary tool of governance. Racially unmarked feminine receptivity is now pervasive in psychological and popular discourses, and the notion that women are disordered if they don't respond appropriately to their sexual partners' advances informs how we understand healthy femininity. Some psychologists have argued that men and women may experience sexual receptivity, triggering, or "incentive-motivation" (Brotto, 2010a, 2010b), but the female specificity of the FSIAD diagnosis suggests otherwise, discursively and via the gender-specific experimental and clinical research, practices, and treatments on which it is based and that it supports.[19] Narratives about women's fraught mind/body relations, and their proclivity to respond or receive, also lend themselves easily to corollary narratives about women's need for sexual guidance—or their essential desire to submit.

Although psychoanalytic explanations of feminine masochism are out of step with current trends, the notion of feminine submission is now naturalized and promoted through pop neuroscience and neo-evolutionary psychology. While stories about the innateness of receptivity and submissiveness for women are perpetuated and also explicitly theorized through the notion of ancestral genetic survival as espoused within evolutionary psychology, they are also perpetuated through the language of the FSIAD diagnosis and its associated practices, but not theorized. This lack of theorization is actually quite pernicious—we are left with tacit support for notions of feminine receptivity, responsiveness, and submissiveness but have no explanation for why women are like this or how this situation has come to be, as psychoanalytic explanations are actively disregarded. This is a problem with models of behaviorism more broadly, and it is arguably how they end up reiterating some of the tenets of evolutionary psychology as background theory (see Toates, 2014 for an example of this trend). The responsiveness criterion and female specificity of FSIAD suggest that these feminine tendencies are innate, or at least they suggest that describing differences in male and female desire patterns is more important than considering the etiology of those differences. Here,

---

19. At the time of this writing, MBST is still used primarily with low-desiring women. Bossio, Basson, Driscoll, Correia, and Brotto (2018) recently conducted a pilot study with men who used mindfulness for erectile disorder, and Koscis and Newbury-Helps (2016) work with couples but orient mindfulness toward relationship therapy rather than solely sexual improvement. Brotto (2018) discusses the possibility of using MBST with men, and includes a chapter on how to use mindfulness with couples (seemingly as a way for women to "take what they learn" home to their partners). But the vast majority of published studies twenty years into the twenty-first century have been conducted on individual women using mindfulness to enhance desire or alleviate genital pain, and the protocol was developed, in conjunction with Basson's circular sexual response cycle model, for use with women.

I argue, description is violent, as analyses of power, of historically oppressive relations between men and women, and of the devaluing of femininity, are left unexamined. Questions regarding why women would need to find reasons to be interested in (heterosexual) sex or to be responsive to their (male) partners outside of their own desire are not engaged with, let alone answered. Questions concerning the inequities and systems of internalized domination that might produce this unequal sexual situation are similarly ignored.

In this context, applying models of responsive desire disproportionately to women reessentializes and rebinarizes human desire, producing it once again as sexually disparate, dichotomous, and even dimorphic, and, as these models are situated on the same stage as evolutionary psychology in our current context, as neurobiological and teleological in their gender essentialism. Proponents of circular models of responsive desire for women claim to present an alternative to a masculinist psychonanalytic conception of "sex drive," but this claim rests upon an oversimplified vision of psychoanalysis. Not only is this framing of desire not in accordance with the totality of psychoanalytic and psychodynamic conceptions of desire, but it also ignores all of the psychoanalytic theorizing since Freud, from the sexual fantasmatics of Laplanche (1976), to object-relational theory in the work of Klein (2002), to Benjamin's (1988) nuanced accounts of desire as bound up with heteronormative gender relations and domination, to investigations of the imbrication of race, gender, and sexuality under colonialism and white supremacy (McClintock, 1995; Musser, 2014; Stockton, 2006; Stoler, 1995). Relational psychoanalytic accounts of intersubjectivity and mutual recognition (Benjamin, 1988) are especially useful in thinking about sexuality from a clinical perspective, but proponents of FSIAD and associated discourses do not embrace these concepts, and instead (re)emphasize sexual complementarity, which in their framing may be paradoxically antagonistic and brutal, or at the very least, conceived of as provocation/reaction, and normatively on white masculine terms (i.e., male as provoker, female as responder).

The dismissal of psychoanalytic accounts of desire by those who have paved the way to FSIAD is not only a rejection of psychodynamic accounts of one-on-one sexual interactions, it is also a denial of the broader theorizations about sex and domination that contemporary psychoanalytic and psychodynamic practices have proved so useful at accounting for. Indeed, behaviorist sexual improvement techniques (including MBST, strangely enough, as it is intended to be about nonjudgmental awareness and living in the present moment) are based on neurobiological explanations for behavior that are more rationalistic and masculinist in their very form than are many psychoanalytic or psychodynamic explanations. Mindfulness-based sex therapy appears to suggest the utility of an internalized system of (self-)domination and (self-)submission (the body dominates the mind, or should, but the mind has to train itself to get in line with this! Which is the sub and which is the dom?!), and ultimately denies or ignores sociocultural and psychodynamic explanations, proclaiming instead the importance of "taking control" of one's own thoughts and behaviors as a means to an end—that is: a (hetero/homo) normative sexual relationship in which "successful" sex is privileged. Race-analytical, feminist, relational, and object-relational psychoanalytic accounts have instead emphasized intersubjectivity, mutuality, and, simultaneously, power and trauma, and the ways in which the social and dyadic context of sexuality inform sexual experience and thus should inform treatment (the concept of treatment itself is also broadened in this field—it's not just about instituting a regimen for individual bodily attunement, but about considering social, cultural, and broadly political analyses of desire). Although the treatment protocols for FSIAD allow for some of this psychosocial/dynamic evaluation (i.e., in some psychoeducation materials there is a discussion of relationship satisfaction and partner's level of desire), the language and practical utilization of the *DSM-5* discursively produce a less dynamic system of analysis and a restrictive narrative around sex. Further, the use of MBST as a training of desire paradoxically indicates an internalized (and individualized) dominating and objectifying orientation toward one's own sexuality. Following the "brief" protocol set forth by Masters and Johnson and Helen Singer Kaplan, including the notion of bypassing deeper or remote issues deemed irrelevant to the proximate sexual concern at hand, contemporary disorder language and behaviorist interventions for women's low desire do not account for the patient's full psychic history (except as it specifically concerns the immediate reasons why she doesn't want to have sex and how she can overcome this problem), nor do they account for the social context in which men and women end up with such disparate patterns of desire, and are, in fact, *produced* as sexually different.

If receptivity, responsiveness, reactivity, lack of spontaneous interest, and in some accounts, even submissiveness are implicitly or explicitly formulated as essential feminine traits, and this assignment goes untheorized and unaddressed, then this modulation of feminine desire within the field of sexuality (particularly among women with male partners) might become a form of *husbandry*. Women who are produced as specific kinds of sexual beings live out these identities with their partners (and their partners experience them as such). Labels and experiences interact, in a feedback loop, and this process cannot be described simply in terms of "social construction." It is about the *living* of embodied hierarchies, sexual categories, and ways of being in the world, which take shape within fields of power. We modulate our sexualities through drugs, behavioral training, mindfulness, and other therapeutic interventions, in accordance with the logics of optimization and securitization, and conceptions of the health and wellness of the population, within "regimes of happiness" (Martínez-Guzmán & Lara, 2019)—all of which are presented in the form of medical and scientific expertise. In this milieu, it is easy to see how desire—the most subjective, elusive aspect of sexuality—may now be the most worthy of investment, as improper or unproductive desire might be conceived of as dangerous, or, at the very least, unhealthy and bad for society as a whole. Within the omnipresent discourses of evolutionary psychology, behavioral biology, and clinical and experimental psychology, feminine desire is produced as uniquely enigmatic and mysterious, or in need of direction. Current psychomedical discourses reinforce the purported naturalness of sexual difference, while simultaneously prescribing and deploying proper gender relations and forms of social reproduction. When desire and its peculiar feminine incarnation are framed as potential to be harvested—is husbandry on the horizon?

CHAPTER 3

Women-with-Low-Desire

Navigating and Negotiating Sexual Difference Socialization

Regina, a bisexual twenty-five-year-old white woman, tells me: "The way that we as a society talk about the way that males and females are is not necessarily true to how males and females are. That is a story that we tell ourselves, that men are more sexual creatures and have a more simplistic sexuality—and it might be self-perpetuating, too—as soon as you start telling the story, people start identifying with it." We are sitting in front of a box fan she has placed in the window of her tiny midtown Manhattan apartment, which she shares with several other people in their twenties. We have been talking for hours about her life. On the recruitment flyer for my project, brandished with a stock image of a lipstick kiss mark with the overlaying text "Not in the Mood?" I implored women with "low sexual desire" to tell me about their experiences with this, but Regina and I have been talking about a lot of other things, too. Rent in the city is expensive and it's so hot and gross in the summer. We drink ice water and we sweat, and she moves back to her unmade bed. I stay on the floor, taking notes and playing with her cat. Shedded fur sticks to my thigh; I think there is some in my eye. It isn't until at least halfway into our more than three-hour interview that Regina tells me that she also experiences pain with sex sometimes. She is frustrated that her partners don't understand why she doesn't want to do it. She wishes they would be more creative with sex—like more playful and willing to incorporate more oral stimulation. She wants it to be more fun. She is tired of doing all the work (including a brief stint with using vaginal dilators). She's not really sure if she should be dating cis men.

The conversations I had with women about their sex lives were alternately funny, intimate, heartbreaking, and stimulating. Many of them had commonalities with the one I describe above with Regina, and many participants shared similar insights about how we learn to have sex in gendered ways. In this chapter, I focus on that qualitative data and place them within the frameworks of queer feminist phenomenology (e.g., Ahmed, 2006; Grosz, 1994; Huffer, 2013) and feminist psychoanalysis (Irigaray, 1985; Kristeva, 1982; Mitchell & Rose, 1985), critical trauma studies (e.g., Malabou, 2012; Wertheimer & Casper, 2016), feminist psychiatric disability and madness studies (e.g., Donaldson, 2002; Johnson, 2010, 2013, 2015; Mollow, 2014), renewed critical investigations of neuroscience and brain/body/environment connectivity (Pitts-Taylor, 2016; E. A. Wilson, 2004, 2015), and the production of "cerebral subjectivities" (Vidal & Ortega, 2017). How might we understand the social, psychological, and biological as co-constitutive, to the point where it's impossible to disentangle them? In order to consider this, I execute multiple levels of analysis. First, I examine how feminist psychologists have responded to dominant scientific discourses, including "drive" models of sexuality and Masters and Johnson's human sexual response cycle (HSRC), illuminating how these counter-interpretations have relied on liberal and cultural feminist tropes about white cisgender femininity. Then, I examine how some low-desiring women of diverse races and ethnic backgrounds respond to both the dominant discourses (such as the HSRC) and to the feminist counter-interpretations of these discourses (including the circular sexual response models within the broader feminized responsive desire framework). Through these analyses, I analyze low-desiring participants' experiences of *sexual difference socialization*.[1] In light of the current experimental climate of research on and treatment for low desire in women, including FSIAD, with its "receptivity criterion," it is imperative to listen to what diverse women have to say about their own sexual interest, desire, and arousal—and how these link up, or don't, for them, personally. How have ideas from science and medicine made their way into women's experiences of sex? Do women think of their own sexualities in terms of "interest," "arousal," "incentives," and "motivations"? Do they feel that their own sexualities are responsive, receptive, flexible, and fluid? If so, where do they think this comes from? Or is there more to their sexual

---

1. Tolman and McClelland's (2011) notion of "sexual socialization" has a kinship here; however, rather than considering only how women are socialized into sexual scripts, I emphasize phenomenological, affective, and traumatic experiences as *productive* of specific formations of femininity—and center how women navigate medical and scientific rhetoric about sex and gender (rather than how they navigate social forces broadly).

imaginaries (Labuski, 2015), and, if so, what do these consist of? I argue that women are affected by the circulation of evolutionary, biological, and psychological ideas about white receptive femininity, sex, and desire, even as these discourses claim to make objective observations about the genders, sexualities, and desires of the human beings they interpret. My notion of sexual difference socialization does not rely on an a priori account of the biological body as sexually differentiated, and instead seeks to understand how bodies and populations are produced as masculine and feminine in relation. To this end, I elucidate how women navigate, live out, sometimes take up, and in some cases reject evolutionary and biological narratives about their own sexualities and their relationships to their sexual and romantic partners. The chapter concludes by exploring women's descriptions of the forces that have influenced their experiences of femininity, sexuality, and desire, and elucidates how women understand the relationship between their psychology and biology, or between their own minds and bodies. Here, I utilize crip theory and madness studies to consider bodyminds[2] as informed by trauma, as a corrective to the framing of minds and bodies as separate in both dominant sexual medicine discourse and in the liberal and cultural feminist counter-responses to that dominant discourse.

While evolutionary narratives of sexuality and gender are often couched in universalizing terms, it is imperative to acknowledge that these "caveman/cavewoman" sexuality narratives are actually very much historically specific (i.e., they are not only heteronormative but also cisnormative and white). However, feminist counter-responses to dominant scientific discourses also uphold certain hegemonic ideals—including the whiteness that inheres in nonintersectional and universalizing models of receptive and responsive femininity. Contemporary research on women's sexuality plays into white racial tropes that designate femininity as responsive/receptive while it ignores the ways women of color, particularly Black women, have been framed and treated (i.e., as aggressive, hypersexual, and to be experimented upon) via sexological discourse and within OB-GYN settings, historically (Fausto-Sterling, 1994; D. C. Owens, 2017; Roberts, 1997; Washington, 2006). Of course, do-it-yourself (DIY), sexual- and reproductive-focused, women-led activist movements have participated in white supremacy as well, and also in the neoliberal biopolitical management of women's bodies.[3] We must acknowledge that feminist

---

2. With the term "bodyminds," I draw on Clare (2017), who offers novel ways to consider the inextricable imbrication of minds, bodies, and the social; this framing moves us beyond traditional formulations of the psychosomatic, toward relational and often traumatic ontologies.

3. For an example of biopolitical investments within the "women's [reproductive] health movement" in the US beginning in the 1960s, see Murphy (2012).

activism and feminist psychology have both been complicit in perpetuating not only essentializing discourses that reify women's "receptive/responsive" desire but also racism and white supremacy. So this part of my story will begin with the cultural feminist turn of the 1960s, which arguably propagated all of these things, and also set the framework for the contemporary field of the "psychology of women" and its investment in white femininity. The medical, scientific, and psychological discourses I examine here are definitely cishet, bourgeois, and white, but not all of these participants are—my sample includes many women of color and not-so-feminine-identified folks who describe how they have had to navigate sexual difference deployments of all types. It is clear how even those women who do not fit into normative categories of whiteness and receptivity have to grapple with these discourses. My goal is to make space here for them to speak back.

Research on Women's Sexual Psychology in the Aftermath of Cultural Feminism

There is a long history of theorizing the constraints on women's sexuality in Western or Global North feminisms, discussions that picked up swiftly with the advent of second-wave cultural feminism in the 1960s—and that eventually made their way into the subdiscipline of institutionalized and academic psychology that came to be called "the psychology of women." As second-wave feminism and the "women's liberation movement" gained momentum through the second half of the twentieth century, scholars' and activists' critiques of the repression of female sexuality—particularly as female sexuality was constrained by compulsory heterosexuality (Rich, 1980) and by the institution of patriarchy more broadly (Rubin, 1975)—reached a fever pitch. In the mid-1970s, many feminist theorists described how domestically inclined, heterosexually oriented, and self-sacrificing women are produced *as such* within a system that negates their desire. According to Gayle Rubin (1975), "At the most general level, the social organization of sex rests upon gender, obligatory heterosexuality, and the constraint of female sexuality" (p. 40). Adrienne Rich (1980), writing around the same time, also described this system in which women are socialized to "feel that male sexual 'drive' amounts to a *right*" (p. 638), and argued that under patriarchal social relations, male power is wielded against women, who are framed as "frigid" if they don't capitulate to the institution of heterosexuality and concomitantly deny same-sex love or the possibility of "lesbian existence." Radical feminists like Andrea Dworkin and Catherine MacKinnon further inveighed against the violent institutionalization of heterosexuality at all levels of US society and especially against the production of heterosexual intercourse as specifically oriented toward not only men's pleasure, but women's annihilation. Later, as activists, Dworkin and MacKinnon held pornography accountable for duplicitously portraying women as taking pleasure in sexual scenarios that were in fact examples of patriarchal domination (Dworkin, 1987; MacKinnon, 1982). Although their earlier writing, as separate from their political lobbying against pornography, was arguably more critical of the legal and cultural institutionalization of heteronormative relations than of heterosex itself (Dymock, 2018), Dworkin and MacKinnon have been caricatured as everything that is wrong with feminism—man-hating, essentializing of sex and sexuality, and even holding a myopically pastoral and naïve view of sex as redeemable through egalitarianism. Through the 1980s and into the 1990s, all of these feminist criticisms of social relations between men and women were met with a conservative and reactionary backlash (as documented by Faludi, 1991) alongside the advent of sex-positive feminism, which celebrated the queering of gendered sexual power relations (Califia, 1994).

In the 1970s, second-wave feminism shifted toward a vision that came to be known as "cultural feminism," exemplified by the writing, in the US, of Mary Daly and Adrienne Rich (according to Alcoff, 1988). Cultural feminists viewed masculinity and femininity in essentializing, almost spiritual ways; not only did they critique patriarchal repression of women's sexuality and bodies, but they argued that women were imbued with essential *positive* feminine traits—such as cooperation, compassion, attunement, perceptiveness, empathy, sympathy, and nurturing—which were inherently better or more valuable than corresponding (and dimorphic) masculine traits. Importantly, many of those associated with this feminist strain were white women. Daly (1978/1990) went so far as to argue that women should govern men, as women are clearly superior to men due to their "essential biophilic life-loving energy" (p. 355). The whiteness of cultural feminism is key in understanding how receptivity is framed in psychology today. As Audre Lorde (1979/2015) pointed out in her "Open Letter to Mary Daly," the "feminine culture" that is most often celebrated in this moment in feminism is based in a spiritual vision shaped by and for white women, even as it appropriates Black women's culture and claims inclusivity for all women.

The self-identified feminist psychologists influenced by this cultural turn played a key role in developing theorizations of responsive sexual desire in women, as they described feminine development as essentially distinct from masculine development—thus there is a through line from this work to contemporary notions of feminine erotic plasticity (Baumeister 2000, 2004) and sexual fluidity (Diamond, 2008). These psychologists also inherited some foundational aspects of the US-based cultural feminist psychoanalysis of Nancy Chodorow (1978)—including a focus on the essential complexities of femininity, the importance and natural goodness of motherhood and mother-child relations, and a liberalism infused within pastoral framings of (the potential for) egalitarian parenting, gender relations, family-making, and sex (described by Grosz, 1990).[4] Two practical exemplars of this cultural feminism–infused approach to the study of gendered psychological development and the "psychology of women" were Jean Baker Miller and Carol Gilligan.

In 1976, Jean Baker Miller, a practicing psychiatrist at Boston University School of Medicine and later at Wellesley College, instituted her specific brand of female-focused psychology with her widely read book *Toward a New Psychology of Women*. Here, she explored the power-laden relationships between men and women, and explained how these unequal dyads of "dominants" and "subordinates" affect women's psychological development. Miller's work was indeed revolutionary for focusing on diversity in human psychological development, for taking power and inequality into account, and thus for deviating away from hegemonic models of universal and normative development that had held sway up until that time. But her research also continued a project of gender essentialism by alluding to the idea that differences between men and women were in many ways indisputable or indelible. She argued that "open knowledge about sexual matters is a pressing need, as is a redefinition of female sexuality in women's terms rather than as it is perceived by men. An important aspect of this . . . is the elimination of the role of sexual object and a greater emphasis on the connection among sexual, personal, and emotional meanings" (J. B. Miller, 1976, p. 24). She goes on to highlight emotionality, participation in the development of others, cooperation, and "everyday," "personal," and "humanity-shaping" creativity as attributes specific to female psychological development. Although Miller consistently referred to the importance of social conditioning in women's inclinations in these domains, and illuminated the feminization of empathy as it relates to psychological and embodied carework (she did not use these terms, as they were not yet in parlance), she also tended to speak of feminine proclivities in these ways as *natural*.

---

4. Andrea Long Chu (2019) has described the quintessential cultural feminist irreconcilability of *hope* and *disappointment* as the essence of all feminism, in that it encapsulates feminism's ontological impossibility—feminism is impossible insofar as it is the political project of attempting to change affects, attachments, and the structure of desire itself, to overcome disappointment in the name of hope, even with the full knowledge that gender relations can never be egalitarian, and thus that heterosex (but also all sex) can never actually be "good" in the way we want it to be (but secretly also *don't* want it to be). Here is the paradox.

Feminist psychologist Carol Gilligan also contributed to the institution of studies of women's psychological developmental as a subfield within psychology, and although she has said much about women's "resistance" to social structures that condition their sexualities and desires, she has also continued the cultural feminist project of framing women as more emotional, cooperative, and caring than men in essentialized or naturalized terms. In her 1982 book, *In a Different Voice: Psychological Theory and Women's Development*, Gilligan documented "the disparity between women's experiences and the representation of human development" (p. 1), thus critiquing the normative and universalized descriptions of growth, separation, and autonomy that individuals are expected to experience as they mature into adulthood, which characterized the post-Freudian field of developmental psychology at that time (and which Gilligan understood to be male-oriented and privileging of masculine relational styles—which were, in her view, not very relational at all). Even with an important attention to gendered power differentials, Gilligan's early work slips between a model based on social conditioning and one that makes naturalized assumptions about essential femininity—specifically women's different and seemingly superior capacity for moral reasoning and judgment. This slippage would be common to much of the feminist social psychology literature in the ensuing decades. Not only has this work in social psychology been founded upon essentializing ideas about masculinity and femininity, but it has also focused primarily on women's identity formation and psychological development at the expense of a full elaboration of the embodied and relational experiences of desire, pleasure, trauma, and power.

Contemporary critical feminist social psychologists have sought to rectify this trend (for some important examples, see Fahs, 2011; M. Fine, 1988; Gavey, 2005; McClelland, 2010; Meana, 2010; Peterson & Muehlenhard, 2007; Tolman, 1994, 2005, 2006; Tolman & McClelland, 2011; Ussher, 2011; Van Anders, 2015[5]) and, in some cases, researchers I have identified as complicit with the

---

5. Neuropsychologist Sari van Anders's research is unique in this arena. In the first decade of the twenty-first century and beyond, van Anders and colleagues have studied responsive desire from an explicitly gender-neutral perspective, focusing on state-dependent desire, contextual cues, and the effects of a variety of stimuli including solitary versus partnered sexual acts, with diverse experimental research participants, including men and queer women. Through this research, along with her "sexual configurations theory (SCT)" (2015), van Anders has worked to bring a focus on nonbinary understandings of sex, gender, and "gender/sex"; intersectionality; self-knowledge; and divergent experiences of eroticism and love, via what she calls a "sexual diversity lens," to sexological research. She promotes "dynamism rather than fixedness" (p. 1185) in research on sexuality through an explicitly queer, feminist perspective. This project is to be lauded. However, I ultimately agree with the criticisms of Subramaniam and Willey (2016), who suggest that even SCT still suffers from a certain ahistoricism of its categories of study, and that the implementation of SCT in sexological

development of the feminized responsive desire framework and FSIAD diagnosis have been involved with what may be considered more critical projects (for examples, see Brotto, Heiman, & Tolman, 2009; Graham, Sanders, Milhausen, & McBride, 2004). Much research (both quantitative and qualitative) straddles the line in terms of a cultural feminist agenda. But the vicissitudes and embodied relations of desire continue to be ignored within mainstream psychology of women, including by many of the most renowned researchers studying gender and sexuality today. In this vein, themes regarding essential femininity derived from cultural feminism have also been taken up broadly in the neo-feminist sexology research described in chapter 2 of this book, in addition to much of the feminist-branded sex therapy post–Masters and Johnson. Again, I argue that this is a direct result of the jettisoning of psychoanalysis; feminist psychologists who have eschewed psychoanalytic frames are less likely to consider desire as structural yet internal, and they ignore how trauma informs desire (in complicated and sometimes unpredictable ways). To this end, psychologists influenced by the cultural feminist turn analyze gender but not in a way that is adequate to theorizing the mimetic, iterative, and uncontrollable qualities of desire, even when they do acknowledge gender inequality.

Alongside all of these developments in the psychology of women, including the publication of the groundbreaking Hite Report (1976), which publicized (some US) women's desires for more intimacy and emotional closeness in their sex lives (and also the fact that the vast majority of women in the US do not experience coital orgasms), there was also a momentary explosion of feminist sex therapy protocols and activism oriented toward the enhancement of women's sexual pleasure. These efforts ran the gamut in terms of their orientation to the motifs of cultural feminism. Sex therapists and educators like Betty Dodson, who focused on the "liberation" of female masturbation, sometimes in group workshops (1987), and Lonnie Barbach, who referred to women who had never orgasmed as "preorgasmic" (1974) and constructed workbooks for women to enrich their sex lives on their own and with partners, arguably deviated in some ways from the cultural feminist model. This was particularly evident in their practical skills–oriented approach, in lieu of an emphasis on the essences of femininity. In *Becoming Orgasmic: A Sexual Growth Program for Women* (1976), Julia Heiman and Leslie and Joseph Lo Piccolo also articulated a program for enhancing women's sexual pleasure, based in cultivating responsiveness and receptivity. At this point in the mid-1970s, these research-

---

research would ultimately be a form of "harm reduction": "SCT will merely proliferate sexual identities (no doubt an improvement on our current world) rather than de-naturalize sexuality as such" (p. 514).

ers were still working within Masters and Johnson's four-staged, linear, unisexual response model. But their discussion of women's desire as being distinct from men's, possibly in need of triggering, and oriented toward sensuality and emotionality, was part of a project of interacting with Helen Singer Kaplan's theorization of (low) desire in women alongside the newer trends in explorations of women's "unique" psychological development posited by thinkers like Miller and Gilligan. All of this work can be considered part of a specific moment in the trajectory of compulsory sexuality as well—the idea here was that sex is healthy and orgasms are important, and women should work on optimizing their own pleasure, in specific, healthy, and, importantly, natural ways. For instance, Barbach (1980) defined the "preorgasmic" woman as one who is "unable to reliably masturbate to orgasm with her hands" (p. 59). This purism often took the form of arguments for the "naturalness" of certain ways of being sexual, and thus we can see it as a nascent form of DIY biopolitical investment in sexual difference and gendered and racialized sexual pleasure, as it was also oriented toward white women, with white women's biggest sexual concerns at the time in mind.

Many of these cultural feminist themes are still alive and well in sexology, sexual medicine, and sex therapy today. Contemporary sex therapist Gina Ogden's (2001) "four-dimensional model" of sexuality represents a certain cultural feminist hangover, particularly in her emphasis on spirituality in women's experiences of sex and desire. This is also evident in the promotion of "natural" approaches to the treatment of women's low desire (framed as superior to "unnatural" pharmaceutical approaches), for instance, in Brotto's mindfulness-based sex therapy today. And Basson's circular sexual response cycle—although developed and implemented officially only in the last twenty years or so—has been decades in the making (in addition to the use of the incentive motivation model to disproportionately describe women's sexual response). Basson's model in particular appears to have its early foundation in the cultural feminist–infused developmental theory of social psychologists like Miller, Gilligan, and others, and it was also fleshed out in the sex therapy protocols of second-wave cultural feminists. All of these strands together are aspects of the long trajectory of biopolitical and compulsory investment in (white) women's sexual pleasure, particularly as it is purported to be oriented toward receptivity, responsiveness, intimacy, and sometimes spirituality. In this vein, we might think of this network of investments as a form of what Murphy (2012) calls "protocol feminism"—a feminism "invested in the politics of technique" (p. 22), self-help, and DIY enhancement of the self, and one that often seeks to obscure its constitutive relationship with neoliberalism, racism, and hegemonic biomedical technologies. Accordingly, the therapeutic program and sexual response paradigm that has emerged at the nexus of these currents is oriented toward female sexuality as essentially responsive and receptive.

On the other side of this cultural feminist approach to sexology, sex therapy, and sexual medicine is, of course, the corporate doctors and pharmaceutical companies invested in treating women's sexual problems.[6] And since the success of Viagra in 1998, particularly, there has been much feminist activism against these trends—as the prediction of many activists was that this corporate investment would begin to focus on women (a prediction that proved correct), and that pharmaceutical treatment was, uniformly, *not* the correct path to take in treating women's sexual problems. Among the groups most keen to speak out against the medicalization of women's sexuality (Tiefer, 2001; Working Group for the New View of Women's Sexual Problems, 2002), was the New View Campaign, led by New York City–based psychologist-activist Leonore Tiefer. Tiefer became an especially vocal critic of the pharmaceutical investment in women's sexuality in the late 1990s and early 2000s, but she had been writing about her concerns with the reductionist framing of sexual dysfunctions in the medical sphere, the *DSM* as a "text of gender politics" (1995), and the "male-orientedness" of Masters and Johnson's linear four-stage human sexual response cycle (1991) since the late 1970s. Taking on a self-proclaimed "social constructionist perspective" on gender, sexuality, and the trappings of medicalized sexology, the New View's campaign took off in full force around 2000, when a working group put together a document to protest the medicalization of women's sexual problems in the soon-to-be-released *DSM-IV* (text revision). Critiques included that contextual and sociopolitical factors have not been fully addressed in the American Psychological Association's premier diagnostic manual, and that the full spectrum of reasons that women have sexual problems and low desire include many things beyond diagnosable psychomedical issues (including intimate partner violence, conflicts over money, and discrepancies between a woman's subculture or culture of origin and dominant cultural norms around sex) and thus cannot be captured in any medical diagnosis. Although Tiefer's work is rooted in a social constructionist approach and the New View's critiques forefront social inequalities and their effects on women's (low) desire, I argue

---

6. As this book interrogates the feminized responsive desire framework, I do not elaborate a longer history of how women's sexual problems have been configured and treated in Western medicine (see Kleinplatz, 2018, for an excellent review of that history), nor do I critique the pharmaceutical investment in treating women's sexual problems or the medicalization of women's sexuality (see Cacchioni, 2015; Canner, 2009, for excellent reviews of the story of how "female sexual dysfunction" came into existence, and how the pharmaceutical industry has capitalized on this diagnosis).

that Tiefer's work, taken as a whole (and the orientation of the Campaign in its full trajectory), has had an ambivalent and fraught relationship to the cultural feminism of the feminist sex therapy movements and adjacent discourses, from the 1960s' orgasmic liberation workshops through to Basson's circular sexual response cycle in parlance today. This ambivalence is particularly evident in the near-total shift to critiquing the pharmaceutical industry and its "disease-mongering" in the early 2000s, concomitant with an absence of activist resistance and targeted critique leading up to the publication of the *DSM-5* in 2013—specifically, an absent critique of the FSIAD diagnosis. I argue that the New View Campaign, although important and timely at its inception, has ultimately been complicit in the creation and institutionalization of the newest instantiation of receptive female desire within the broad feminized responsive desire framework.

What I think the cultural feminist–informed models of women's responsive desire (along with the antimedicalization/anti–FSD/anti–Big Pharma activism) miss, and what I seek to draw attention to in what follows, are the voices of women with desire problems themselves. These women have been conspicuously absent in much of the current female sexual dysfunction debates. There has certainly been some qualitative (and plenty of quantitative) research conducted on low-desiring women, including by self-identified feminist psychologists, but the question of how women feel about the discourses themselves has been less frequently asked. Instead, most psychologists of a variety of stripes seem to ask women questions, and then apply their models (i.e., models of responsive desire, incentive-motivation, intimacy-seeking, etc.) in interpreting women's answers. I have no doubt that many women describe their desire as "responsive" and that they seek "intimacy" and want their sexual experiences to be more "emotional" and "connected." But I also argue that women are *expected* to say these things, and they bring those expectations with them to clinics and laboratories. And so it seems that certain cultural feminist tendencies have become tautological here, in the "alternative" sexual response model itself; receptivity is the very heuristic framework by which women's sexualities are interpreted, and thus the notion that women are responsive is reinforced and reified, over and over again. Responsiveness has become its own hermeneutic, and gender is produced, in a certain (white hetero cis) way, recursively. Further, as is suggested by the fact that designers and facilitators of mindfulness trainings present women with data on the circular sexual response cycle and on women's subjective/genital discordance (described in Brotto, 2018 and by my participants Astrid and Kelly who have been through treatment), women also literally *learn about receptive femininity* in clinical and increasingly in extra-clinical settings (i.e., via the internet, social media, and other popular outlets). And finally, as my own data suggest, some women feel distressed about a lack of desire, but want something different—they don't necessarily feel that their experiences can be made sense of in terms of naturalized feminine responsiveness. I argue that desire cannot be reduced to stimulus/response, and that situating women's experiences of "low desire" in terms of receptivity is likely not helpful for many women—particularly when it is that very framework that constrains and produces their desire as such. And so it is through all of this that women-with-low-desire[7] is constructed as a clinical category—and as a population to be managed. I now turn to members of that population to shed light on its production.

Desire? Interest? Arousal? Linkages and Lacunae in Embodied/Psychic Sexual States

In order to gain insight into the new *DSM-5* diagnosis of FSIAD, I asked my participants about how their desire, arousal, and interest link up (or do not). Here, I am directly in conversation with the terms of the FSIAD diagnosis and with the circular sexual response cycle as it is applied to women—however, my goal was to find out more about how women feel about the *ideas* encapsulated in the diagnosis/model, and about the diagnosis/model as a presented framework for understanding female sexuality, rather than to utilize the diagnosis/model per se. Although most of the women I interviewed were not aware of the content of the newest edition of the *DSM*, they were certainly aware of scientific tropes about female receptivity, responsiveness, and flexibility; they had complex thoughts about the notion of a feminine disconnect among cognitive, emotional, and embodied states; and they were able to articulate very clearly the (important) place of desire in their own sexualities and sex lives (even as they described their desire as, at some points, "low").

Many of the women I interviewed stated that the linkage of desire, interest, and arousal is, in fact, driven by context, and that in certain specific instances, they may feel physically aroused before they "realize" they want to have sex (in keeping with the feminized responsive desire framework, including the circular sexual response cycle). But, in general, they stated that desire comes first—which challenges the idea that for most women, arousal and desire co-occur, or that arousal precedes desire. One very important aspect of desire that many

---

7. I thank Monica Casper for urging me to flesh out this notion of "women-with-low-desire" as a category and population configured via the mutual constitution of discourses of femininity, low/responsive desire, and psychosexual medicine.

participants emphasized was the need to feel truly stimulated by and attracted to a partner—but this experience could not be reduced to "incentives" to have sex. Most of the women who spoke with me said it was hard for them to get turned on physically if their desire was not already in motion. This sentiment is clearly expressed by Tiffany, who explains, "For me, it is always desire first. I have to be attracted to the person in one way or another," and by Lola, who states, "I've never been aroused and then it made someone seem more attractive to me." Sam reiterates this when I ask her to describe her problems with arousal and desire, and whether she has ever begun to experience desire for a partner after already feeling physically turned on:

> Sometimes [I have trouble getting lubricated], but if I want to [have sex], if I am into it, then no. . . . [M]ost of the time I don't have a problem getting aroused, but if I'm not super into the guy, like "Okay, I'm just going to have sex now," then I might have that problem. . . . I also feel like desire has to do with wanting something, whereas arousal seems more physical, something that is physically happening to me or my body. . . . I don't think it always has to go A then B then C, it's just that for me that feels like maybe the more natural thing.

Here, Sam makes it clear that even though she has experienced arousal preceding desire on occasion, that chronology doesn't really feel right or "natural" to her. She also expresses that arousal preceding desire might characterize most of the casual sex she has had, but that ultimately, those experiences were not satisfying:

> I think that would count for most of the one-night stands I've had, where maybe the desire is not there, then you start making out with somebody and become aroused, and then fornicate . . . but they would probably have had to be persistent.

The experience that Sam describes here explicates her view that when she feels physical arousal first, the sexual act that results is not the most pleasurable experience for her, and one that she tends to feel ambivalent about. It also usually occurs only because the (in this case, cis male) partner involved has been particularly insistent. Obviously, this does not paint a picture of the most consensual or pleasurable sexual encounter. Notably, Sam's description also challenges the standard logic that "arousal-first" desire is more common in long-term relationships, as Sam states that it is more likely to characterize her one-night stands. Regina also articulates that for her, desire tends to come first—or, at least, that she prefers it that way:

> Arousal for me usually comes after quite a bit of a lead-up, so the desire part would really have to be there first before I would ever get to a place where my body would *want* to be aroused. . . . I think of arousal as being the physical part and desire as being the social, interpersonal, psychological part. But for me I think it's a thing where the desire comes first, and then I can feel arousal.

Later, Regina describes the disconnect she sometimes feels between her physical sense of arousal and the desire to engage in sex (or to avoid it). She clarifies that the issue for her isn't finding a way to align her subjective desire with her physical arousal, it's that if she's not fully "into it," aligning them is not something she *wants* to do. This notion of preference—preferring desire to come first, rather than experiencing arousal and then engaging in sex—was reiterated by Elizabeth, who is a survivor of childhood sexual abuse (CSA) and describes a sense of dissociation in the form of depersonalization (a feeling of not being connected to her body, or of watching the sexual act occur from a disembodied perspective) during many of her sexual experiences. When I ask her how she interprets this experience of dissociation in relation to desire, arousal, and interest, she states: "I feel like it was just like my body couldn't get there if my brain couldn't."

Most of the women I interviewed said that sex doesn't really work if they are not "into it"—which implies a type of desire that can't be reduced to "motivation." The model of arousal preceding desire does not make sense for many of these women, experientially, nor do they identify with it. In fact, this model of responsive desire registered, for them, as distinctly undesirable: The idea of cognitively or rationally inducing a sense of being receptive or "in the present" (such as might be induced via mindfulness-based sex therapy, in accordance with the logic of the circular sexual response cycle) in order to tune into a physical response and thus go forward with a sex act made them uncomfortable. They expressed particular concerns about coercion and lack of consent. Annie, who is a survivor of sexual violence, explains:

> If I'm not really into it, it doesn't usually work that well; I'll have a harder time getting wet and actually aroused and excited. . . . [T]hat has happened to me before [experiencing physical arousal before desire]—but it's not really my preference. I tend to be controlling in my sexual relationships; I like to call the shots in terms of when we have sex.

Many participants similarly expressed the desire to be in control of the terms of sex, of not wanting physical arousal to dictate desire or guide a sexual experience. And notably, almost all participants stated that they did not enjoy sex nearly as much when physical arousal preceded a clear sense of desire, and that sex was much better for them when they felt a true longing, wanting, or desire for their partner. These notions of enjoyment and *preference* for a certain sequence of events (in this case, for desire first, then physical arousal) are absent in the clinical literature on women's (low) desire, even though the possibility of a preference for responsive desire is included in the MHSDD diagnosis for men (American Psychological Association, 2013). This lack of a "preference criterion" for women seems highly problematic, particularly in light of what these particular low-desiring women told me in our interviews.

Women who had experienced sexual abuse also expressed that sex is better when desire precedes physical arousal—and their experiences drive home the necessity of taking this preference seriously. Molly, for instance, expresses a similar sentiment about not enjoying sex if she is not truly interested in, desiring of, and engaged with her partner:

> A lot of times I feel very dissociated. Like my body is turned on, but my mind is not. So physically I have a reaction, like I get wet—but mentally I don't feel like I am really there. My body is showing all the signs of being turned on, but I don't *feel* turned on . . . so a lot of times I just go, "Well, I'm wet, might as well have sex," and it's okay, but it is not that much fun. But it's easier than not having sex, in my weird way of looking at things, because I have such a hard time saying no to men. . . . [E]ven with [a partner she trusts] there have been times where I have gone, in my head, "Why am I doing this?"—where I have felt really disconnected and thought, "I don't want to do this anymore" . . . and that is what started to get me really turned off, that feeling of like my body responding, when my mind is not. . . . [T]hat is a turnoff because I feel like it kind of increases the dissociative state. . . . I know that your body can respond at times, even when you are being forced to do things. . . . I don't know if that's what happened with [the man who abused her as a child], I don't remember, but sometimes I wonder if that's where some of that comes from, in terms of getting turned on physically but not feeling good about that unless my mind is incorporated.

Molly's story of disconnection, dissociation, and trauma, outlined above, is one example of why the diagnostic logic of arousal co-occurring with or preceding desire potentially amounts to a strange sanctioning of blurred consent, and perhaps even a medicalized endorsement of one partner's sexual wishes governing another's, which is potentially dangerous—particularly in that so many women have experienced abuse, rape, or some kind of sexual violence over the course of their lives (or will at some point during their lives[8]). Coercive experiences range from overt violent infractions by strangers on the street to less clearly defined situations in which consent was not adequately acquired from an intimate partner, date, acquaintance, or friend (or, instead, in which women were pressured to have sex that they "consented" to by not saying "no," but did not feel comfortable with and thus did not feel was ultimately truly consensual) (Fahs, 2011, 2016; Gavey, 2005; Peterson & Muehelenhard, 2007 have also examined this "gray area" regarding consent/nonconsent and the blurriness of everyday sexual coercion).

If some low-desiring women are keenly aware of the possibility of dissociating during sex, and feel uncomfortable with the idea of allowing their physical arousal (even if it has become "subjective arousal" insofar as they noticed it) guide a sexual experience, then it may be unethical to promote models of responsive/receptive female desire in addition to concordance-enhancing or mind/body "alignment" techniques such as MBST to them. These protocols could be interpreted (including by women themselves) as medically legitimized methods prescribed to women to induce them to overcome a mental state of not being fully "into it" and to instead follow the lead of the aroused body, or worse, an aroused partner. Although MBST has been used with low-desiring women survivors of childhood sexual abuse who are now in consensual relationships—and was deemed successful in that their genital/subjective concordance was increased post-treatment (Brotto et al., 2012)—I have serious concerns about promoting such a method to this population. One reason for my concern is that for many sexual abuse survivors, consent is not always so clear-cut, and another reason is that fully consensual relationships do not exist as entirely separate from relationships where consent is sometimes breached, including by trusted partners—these two types of relationships do not fit into neat, discrete boxes, as some psychological research on this topic would purport. Thus, Brotto et al.'s (2012) analysis of trauma is of a specifically white, cis, middle-class trauma—a trauma that is thought to be anomalous or extraordinary, that begins and ends at distinct points in time, and that can be overcome with therapy (including "brief" or focused behaviorist treatment protocols).

Cvetkovich (2003), Berlant (2011), and others have made a case for "insidious traumas" or "crisis ordinariness" and thus demonstrate the everyday experience of a range of traumas enacted against marginalized populations. This

---

8. According to RAINN (Rape, Abuse & Incest National Network) statistics: https://www.rainn.org/statistics/victims-sexual-violence

point is especially clear when considering how many cis and trans women, including women of color, poor women, queer women, and women with disabilities, are often traumatized over and over again, both in their primary relationships and structurally, out in the world (Piepzna-Samarasinha, 2018; we may also include nonbinary and gender-nonconforming folks, and many trans men here, as well). In this light, it is inadequate to relegate sexual violence, which might produce dissociation, solely to stranger rape or childhood sexual abuse. Molly's story, described above, illuminates why we should be concerned about the hypostatization of sexualized and gendered violence as exceptional. Sarah (who is not a CSA survivor) shares similar ideas, and articulates them specifically in terms of consent, when I ask her how desire, interest, and arousal are connected for her:

> It's like if I have the desire, then I am aroused; if I don't have the desire, then I am not aroused. . . . [Arousal preceding desire] *does not sound like consent*. . . . [I]t's like when I was hooking up with [kissing] this dude, thinking that maybe I didn't want to do it, but I was like, "Should I just keep doing this, and then maybe I'll get into it?" and I kept doing it . . . but I think I would not do that with sex, because for me it's like literally like it [his penis] won't enter [my vagina]! It's not gonna happen if I'm not turned on. If I have already shut it off in my brain, it's shutting off "downtown," too.

Sarah's thoughts make it clear that even women who are not survivors of childhood sexual abuse have concerns about consent and coercion in their day-to-day sex lives, and they also elucidate the quotidian milieu of sexualized violence. Most of the women I spoke with (regardless of whether or not they identified as survivors of abuse) articulated sentiments about the need for trust and safety during sex—and many shared their stories of partners introducing sexual acts or scenarios (particularly around pain and domination) during a sexual encounter when the women had not expressed interest in this, and described how they were uncomfortable with it (importantly, this was also true for women who were actively interested in or involved with subbing in BDSM, which will be explored in chapter 5). They also made it very clear that they do *not* feel that receptivity or responsiveness defines their sexuality, that they have very strong sexual desires outside of responsive physical arousal (even though they are currently experiencing or have previously experienced low desire), and that they are very much subjectively aware of their body's physiological arousal when it occurs—and sometimes actively do not desire to follow it. This is important to note, as "arousal" and "interest" are brought together in the FSIAD diagnosis and the circular sexual response cycle for women. The women I interviewed clearly distinguished desire as a unique experience, and as something not always related to their own perception of their body's vasocongestive arousal response. For them, desire is often relational, but not always responsive. And it is not simply a cognitive or rational construct; desire is not necessarily experienced as spontaneous or untriggered, but it is also not something they need a partner to "awaken" in them or something that is reactive. In fact, the women I spoke with were uncomfortable with this conceptualization of being sexually triggered by a partner, as their preference is to feel in control of—and clearly consenting to—any given sexual experience. This is particularly true when they are with cis male partners, and for women who have experienced gendered or sexual violence (and most of my participants had endured self-identified traumatic sexual experiences at some point during their lives, regardless of whether or not they identified as survivors of childhood or adult sexual abuse). Tiffany links these issues of safety and trust to her experience of being a woman in a society in which her body is regularly threatened: "I'm just trying to be a little bit more conscientious of my decisions in that regard [i.e., sexually] to protect myself." This is a sentiment that numerous other women echoed, and one that I will return to in my full discussion of violence, trauma, and desire in chapter 5.

Opening Up "Receptivity"

Many of the women I interviewed also spoke of how notions of receptivity, responsiveness, and passivity *do* fit into their sex lives—but in ways not captured by the circular sexual response cycle or the feminized responsive desire framework. Participants who had been treated in medical programs for women with genital pain and comorbid low desire had specific and cutting critiques of these types of programs and associated treatments—including the use of mindfulness-based sex therapy, or MBST, to enhance desire and subjective/genital concordance. When I ask her if the program she attended allowed her to experience any more pleasure upon sex with her male partner (the person she was married to at the time), Astrid states:

> I didn't get the sense that sexual enjoyment was any goal of this program. Not having it be impossible to be penetrated because of excruciating physical pain was *the goal*. We were taught "You have to be receptive to sexual attention, you have to be willing to receive sexual advances from your partner." Not that you should enjoy sex or that sex should be an exciting orgasmic experience or something like that—that wasn't even hinted at!

Beyond critiques of medical programs, some participants (who had not been medically treated for low desire or pain) expressed the ways they feel they have been socialized to be sexually receptive and responsive over the course of their lives. When discussing why she enjoys sex more now that she has been able to take up a more dominant position with her current partner, Valdivia tells me:

> Maybe this idea of being able to be a sexual aggressor, rather than just a *receiver* of sex, which is what I think I was indoctrinated to think that sex was supposed to be like . . . it's interesting how it might mess with your brain if you've been taught to feel that women who are delicate, and wear makeup, and do their nails, and all of these things are not sexual aggressors. But I guess that's not true! Maybe [I don't mean] aggressor, but *initiator*. . . . I come from a culture where I am supposed to be a "lady" and that implies a lot of passivity.

Here, Valdivia explains how she is able to experience herself as both femme and sexually dominant, but that being able to understand these aspects of her sexuality as compatible took a lot of work—specifically as she was raised between two cultures in which femininity and sexual dominance are sometimes posed as mutually exclusive (Valdivia identifies as Latinx and grew up in the US, and she explains how both her home culture and US culture instilled these ideas in her). Valdivia's experience also highlights the simultaneous *expectation* and *silencing* of the sexual desires of Black, Brown, and Indigenous women, and suggests that white supremacy further imperils and complicates the sexual experiences of low-desiring women of color.

Some participants spoke of receptivity, responsiveness, and passivity in our interviews, and elaborated on how these inform or do not inform their senses of their own sexuality and femininity—often in creative, unconventional, and provocative ways. Natasha outlines how what she experiences sexually could likely be medically classified as "low sexual interest/arousal" but that it might be better characterized as a type of *active passivity*:

> There is some kind of uncanny overlap between active masochistic desire and passivity . . . wanting to be tied up, and just lying there not doing anything because you're not into the experience, have a certain superficial resemblance. Which I think is complicated for me, because I do sort of like being [tied up]—I think that my instinct is a fairly passive one, and I don't know how much of that is just that I am like, "I am not that into this, you

are the one who is starting this" and how much of it is that I really actively like being in the position of having things done to me.

In this passage, Natasha points to the resemblance between the active desire to "have things done to her" and what might otherwise appear to simply be "low desire." Although she states that she is sometimes unclear about which camp she falls into, her articulation of the problem exposes that sometimes a woman's "responsiveness" does not represent a cognitive, rational, desexualized choice to engage in a sexual encounter at the behest of her own vasocongested genitals or a persistent partner, nor to maintain her long-term romantic relationship or enhance intimacy, but it can instead evidence a highly erotic, charged, and actively sexual desire to *receive,* and to agentically control the terms of that "being done to." This has much in common with discussions of queer femme receptivity, for instance as described by Cvetkovich (2003). Annie articulates a similar sentiment about her own sex life with her partner:

> My partner and I definitely have times where even if he is sort of initiating the, "Hey, I'm feeling this desire," then I'm like, "Okay, I'm into it, I'm not having this strong desire right now, but I could be into it, so okay, go ahead! Arouse me!" And then it becomes more like he initiated it but I'm still kind of like directing what's happening to get to the place where I'm aroused and then we can have sex.

Annie's statement suggests that sometimes low-desiring women might "direct" their partners to arouse them, and thus are still "calling the shots"—almost like a challenge or a playful game that becomes incorporated into the sexual landscape and subsequently becomes arousing in itself.

Many of the participants I spoke with articulated that women are socialized and learn to be receptive and responsive in a way that most men are not. In fact, "receptivity," "responsiveness," and "low desire" are in some cases the only frames available for interpreting one's own sexual, gender, and desire problems if one is a woman—hence the pertinence of the category *women-with-low-desire*. In the previous quotes from Natasha and Annie, we see how some women turn this learned responsiveness into a form of agency, however—through *active passivity* or *active receptivity*. This conceptualization of receptivity, as it specifically attends to power, seems quite different from the kind that is cultivated in desire training programs that utilize the circular sexual response cycle with low-desiring women and that incorporate mindfulness-based sex therapy within the feminized responsive desire framework.

Spontaneous Desire and "Me Time"

Throughout our interviews, it became clear that many of the women I spoke with have plenty of "untriggered" sexual desire, just not for their current partners, nor in the context of a routinized sex life that had become characteristic of many of their long-term monogamous relationships (this phenomenon is also explored by Meana, 2010; Perel, 2006, 2017; and Sims & Meana, 2010, among others). In these cases, desire becomes a special realm, "just for them," outside of the relationship. For these women, lack of interest in a specific partner does not equal "low desire" (even though many participants had come to believe that it must mean that, which is why they were talking to me). Almost all of the women I spoke with had very active fantasy lives, frequently felt attracted to strangers (often women), watched pornography and/or read erotica regularly, and thoroughly enjoyed masturbation and made time for it in their day-to-day lives. These same women still felt like something was wrong with their desires, with their bodies, with their sexualities. Although these women's desires are not necessarily spontaneous, in that they are not fully internal (as drive models would suggest), they cannot be characterized as simply responsive or receptive either. Natasha, for instance, states that she feels that her strongest desires almost categorically cannot be requited—meaning she sometimes feels that a gulf separates her desire and the fulfillment of that desire, or at least a fulfillment by her partner:

> [Desire] is sort of a wanting feeling that I really associate with *unrequitedness,* with *absence.* . . . [I]t seems like what would be nice would be to be able to bring that sense of desire into my lovely, stable, harmonious relationship . . . but it seems like there is some kind of gulf that separates them.

Corinne also expresses a sense of feeling like her desire lives in its own world, apart from her monogamous heterosexual relationship. But, like most of the other women I spoke with, she enjoys masturbating and has a very active fantasy life. She explains that she experiences the most sexual satisfaction when she is alone, because that is when she feels the freest to mobilize whatever fantasies she wishes:

> There are definitely times where I've been out doing stuff and I'm like "Oh! I know! I'm going to go home and masturbate because I *can!*" [laughing] So there is definitely that odd sort of excitement about it, I kind of enjoy doing it outside of [the relationship]. . . . [I]t's like, "You know what? It's just not

going to happen" [fulfilling sex with her partner, in this moment], so this [for her, BDSM fantasies] is what I can think about when it's "me time."

Valdivia describes a similar security in her desires during masturbation, which she has historically not always felt comfortable sharing with partners: "I masturbate a lot even when I'm dating people. I think the healthiest and longest-standing sexual relationship I've ever had is with myself, hands down." Valdivia describes how she often felt that she had to hide her self-pleasuring habits from (cis male) partners, but now that she is pursuing more "intentional," queer relationships, she feels comfortable integrating masturbation into her sex life with certain partners. Valdivia also acknowledges the role of personal fantasy in her sex life with her partner; she states that she often thinks about other people and other scenarios when having sex with her partner, and that she doesn't understand this as something that reflects negatively on their sex life (it doesn't indicate that she is unhappy). Tiffany also feels a great deal of satisfaction and directs much of her own desire into self-pleasuring, and shares Corinne's sentiment that when she is masturbating, she feels freest to explore any fantasy she wishes:

> I definitely do have those strong desires, especially when I'm alone. I let my mind wander more, whereas when you are with a certain person, you are kind of targeted into having that with them, but when I am alone and thinking my own thoughts, my mind can wander either from person to person or scenario to scenario . . . and because it's just me, there are no restraints, and I know I can make myself come, I don't have to wait on anyone else.

At the extreme end of the spectrum of "spontaneous" versus "receptive" desire, Astrid describes how her desires were actively negated in the context of medical treatment for sexual pain and low desire. At the time of treatment, she was in a relationship with a cis man, whom she was not attracted to and did not desire, but to whom she felt a responsibility to be sexually receptive. She describes how she had plenty of sexual desire for women, and regularly fantasized about them while she masturbated, but was too afraid to reveal this to the treatment program's directors or to her partner, which resulted in a complete schism between her fantasies/desires and the sex acts she actually engaged in—or, rather, desperately avoided:

> I was masturbating and stuff but I would never tell him [her partner] that, I kept that a secret . . . and to this day I can have great orgasms. My body works. To me, I'm not sexually dysfunctional, I can come, I can have great

sex, I couldn't be physically penetrated but I was still masturbating, I was fantasizing, but I couldn't say that to her [the treatment program director], so I just lied and said I wasn't interested in sex. He [her partner] was there [in some of the treatment sessions], so I told her that I wasn't interested in sex anymore, that I felt sexually dysfunctional. I was lying. But I couldn't say anything else because he was right there.

Astrid's story is particularly alarming, and it spotlights the dangers of the feminized responsive desire framework as it is taken up practically in clinical sexual medicine. Due to economic constraints, heteronormative expectations, and a variety of contextual factors, Astrid felt that she had to keep her desires (for women) hidden from her partner and the clinicians who were "treating" her—so instead, she avoided sex when she was able to, but sometimes engaged in it only at her husband's behest, and always at the expense of her own desires (which were very real and active).

What these women's comments illuminate is that the image of feminine desire that the FSIAD diagnosis and the circular sexual response cycle put forward doesn't adequately capture the lived experience of many low-desiring women's sexualities and desires. The women I interviewed don't necessarily always desire sex with their partners, and they don't always desire the kind of sex their partners want—but they are not lacking in desire, by any stretch of the imagination. These observations suggest that the FSIAD diagnosis is actually a *relational* diagnosis and thus should not be applied to individuals (categorically, women), and suggest why the "receptivity/responsiveness criterion" (and its female specificity) is clinically inappropriate and, in some cases, dangerous. It might be argued that the only people who will actually receive the FSIAD diagnosis are those women who seek it out, and who thus feel they truly have low desire and consider this lack to be a problem, but even if only a small subset of women will be treated for FSIAD, the diagnosis has a far reach and implications for all women because of the pervasiveness of the discourses that are used to support it. Under its shadow, women may pathologize themselves for not serving their partners adequately. And in the most extreme cases of medical treatment gone awry, some women might end up in treatment programs and receive a diagnosis because they feel they are not adequately meeting their partners' needs. Thus, this diagnosis and associated naturalizing discourses about feminine responsiveness and receptivity are of great concern simply because they circulate in the world, promulgating claims about women's discordant sexuality, and instantiating antiquated notions about innate sexual difference and disparate masculine and feminine desires. These discourses and regimes are also concerning because in our current self-medicating moment in late neoliberal capitalism, medical discourses are pervasive and easily accessible and thus women are regularly urged to label themselves, or, as is expressed by Astrid above, might even be coerced into this labeling and associated treatment protocols by insistent and demanding partners (or doctors).

Nurture Is for Women, Nature Is for Men: Learning Sexual Difference via Science and Medicine

Contemporary sexual medicine continues to support the notion that women's desire is organized in a fundamentally different way than is men's desire—masculinity and femininity, according to this logic, belong to incommensurable paradigms. In a sense, masculine desire is the only kind of desire that is *sexual,* per se. The association of women with the desire for intimacy, emotional closeness, and nonsexual rewards (shapeable by nurture and culture) and the concomitant association of men with a *true* sexuality (driven by nature and biology) proliferates in many guises, and still haunts sexology today—including in its feminist instantiations. This asymmetry of masculine/feminine desire is instituted in the notion of innate "female erotic plasticity" (Baumeister, 2000, 2004) and is reified and codified in the FSIAD diagnosis and supporting research, including in the near-uniform application of Basson's circular sexual response cycle to women, in the disproportionate use of MBST techniques with women, and in the continued attempt to excavate the truth of the gap between female subjective and genital arousal in experimental psychophysiological research. In relation to this broad feminized responsive desire framework, several themes emerged from my interviews that low-desiring women report grappling with: the widespread notion that penetrative sex is the only "real" sex; the idea that women have more "complex" and "emotion"-driven sexualities than men; the "obviousness" or visibility of certain body parts and cycles and how these inform experiences of the gendered body; and that feminine sexuality is associated with what one participant called the "pathologizing-healing dialectic," whereas sex itself is produced as a realm for men. All of this comes together in the summative notion that women are taught how to be "certain kinds of sexual beings"—sexual difference socialization—including through popular medical, scientific, and psychological self-help discourses (a point also noted by Gupta & Cacchioni, 2013). Many participants described these various themes adding up to a sexualized nature/nurture asymmetry, wherein masculinity becomes tethered to nature and activity, while femininity is associated with nurture and receptivity.

They stated that they often feel that they have to navigate this asymmetry in the context of their sexual relationships—which is in some cases compounded by other relational asymmetries.

Penetrative Sex as the Only "Real" Sex

One theme related to gender differences in the experience of sex was what participants and practitioners referred to as a social emphasis on the penis, including the consummation of sex being equated with men's sexual satisfaction and ultimately male orgasm, and even defining "sex" itself as penile-vaginal heterosexual intercourse. Kaye (2011) analyzes the conflation of sex with heterosexual intercourse, arguing that the naturalness of penile-vaginal intercourse is so taken for granted that "it has become the proverbial 'it' in 'doing it'" (p. 113). Gavey (2011) and Loe (2004) extend this point in their discussions of Viagra and the "coital imperative" within cisgender heterosexual relationships, and Labuski (2015) and Cacchioni (2015) also illuminate these normative themes as they relate to women's experiences of (hetero)sex and desire.

Many participants expounded upon men's expectations, stating that men themselves perpetuate the idea that "real sex" is sex that involves penile-vaginal penetration, because that is what *they* (men) desire and what they have come to expect from an "authentic" sexual encounter. Evie describes how this socialization configures men's and women's experiences of heterosexual sex—and desire for it—much differently:

> Normative sex is men getting off; it's less focused on the woman. And so I do think that our sexuality and our [men's and women's] desires are different. There's not really an emphasis on pleasing a woman, it's pleasing a man, because that's what heteronormative sex does. . . . I don't think it is biological by any means—men are probably socialized to think that that is what sex is, and that it's good for everyone, because it's good for them.

Sarah, Regina, Astrid, and Kelly—all of whom experience mild to intense intermittent pain during intercourse—described how they had suggested to cis male partners that they might incorporate nonpenetrative acts into their sexual repertoires, only to be met with protest from partners who believed that sex that did not involve penetration was somehow less "real." Regina sums up this sentiment: "I would sometimes suggest nonintercourse things, oral sex or things like that, and it seemed for my partners, that that was fine and good, but that it wasn't like 'real sex,' that it was only *half good*, for them."

The practitioners I spoke with also described this social emphasis on intercourse as antiquated and limiting. Betsy, the director of a medical center for the treatment of low female desire, describes how penile-vaginal intercourse is emphasized at the expense of other kinds of sex, a heteronormative cultural construct that makes sex less enjoyable for both men and women:

> Somehow the erection is such a central part of our Amer[ican culture]—like, the penis is what it's all about. It kills me! If you ask a person "What is sex?," they will say to you "Man puts penis inside vagina, man ejaculates, that's what sex is." Why doesn't anybody say "Man massages woman's clitoris until she has an orgasm"? Why have we decided to become so androcentric? The penis is the be-all and end-all. That's what people think when they think of men's sexuality, but it's not true! It's a very unsophisticated way of looking at men's sexuality, because men also have [problems with] desire, arousal, ability to ejaculate, premature ejaculation, delayed ejaculation. All those things are huge issues for men as well.

Here, Betsy suggests that the emphasis on the erection and penetration is harmful to men's sexuality as well as to women's sexual experiences. She explains that although the notion that men's only—or at least primary—sexual problem is erectile disorder is prevalent in our culture, men actually have multifaceted sexualities and can suffer from complex problems, just as women can. Annette, a clinical psychologist, also agrees that sex is too unilaterally focused on male performance and pleasure—which tends to be assessed through their erections:

> In the research on men there was so much focus and hype around pharmaceutical products and treatments of erectile dysfunction, that these bigger concepts about how do men define desire, how do they experience sexual excitement, were kind of left in the shadows. And most of the funding has been pharmaceutically based. And from Pharma's perspective, their primary mandate is in developing an effective medical treatment.

Annette links this phallocentric focus on the erection to the rise, proliferation, and cultural pervasiveness of Viagra. This is a sentiment that Louise and Betsy share as well, one that many of the women I interviewed suggested, and one that Mamo and Fishman (2001) and Loe (2004) also describe. It is clear that various technologies and discourses (including those produced by the pharmaceutical industry) support phallocentric views on sex, and also support the construction of penile-vaginal penetrative intercourse as authentic or "real" sex. These discourses continue to reproduce (cishet white) "men" and "women" in certain ways, and undoubtedly also negatively affect people who do not fit into those normative categories.

How Women Learn about Their "Complex" "Emotions"

Participants and practitioners also expressed that discourses about women's emotionality, relationality, responsiveness, sentimentality, complexity, moodiness, and generally complicated nature were pervasive cultural tropes, and were often internalized by women (and by men, regarding women) from a very young age. Most participants disputed these tropes' biological basis, although some did describe them in terms of innate differences. Regarding her thoughts on women's socialization into the role of being "emotional," and about the feminization of the circular sexual response cycle, Louise, a psychologist and activist, states:

> It [the circular model] sounds *girly*! It sounds feminine, emotional. For a long time the idea was that women's sexuality was more emotional and connected and related, that whole line of thinking, "fundamental gender differences." . . . I think that the [model] has a kind of stereotypic female language about "relatedness" and "connectedness" and "responsiveness" that's part of the hegemonic view of women, and I think a lot of people subscribe to that. You know, "Women are tender and sensitive because they are maternal" or whatever.

It is notable (and demonstrates a contradiction) that Louise acknowledges the contemporary feminization of the circular sexual response cycle, but still characterizes the notion that women's sexuality is "responsive" as antiquated. Amelia, who worked at a "sex-positive" sex toy store and led workshops on locating and stimulating the G-spot, among other methods of enhancing women's sexual pleasure, shares a similar sentiment about the cultural production of feminine emotionality and complexity:

> And like the fact that it [sex] is [supposedly] "emotional" [for women] is a huge piece, too. Sex is [construed as] like "biological" for men, it's like somehow more primal or something, like, "This is this technique that you use and you just like jerk a dude's dick off," you know? But with women it's like "cracking a code" and it's like "emotional" and somewhat more, something. . . . [I]t's just this *code* or like this thing that people can't *possibly* figure

out, that men can't *possibly* wrap their brains around, because it's so *hard*! [laughs sarcastically]

In this passage, Amelia, like Betsy and Louise, shares her frustrations about the way sexual difference is produced via discourses about the "primal" and "biological" nature of men's sexuality as opposed to the "complicated" and "cryptic" nature of women's sexuality. All of these practitioners, regardless of their level of involvement in normative sexual medicine versus alternative or nonmedical forms of sexual enhancement, expressed that these beliefs are a disservice to people of all genders and sexualities, and that they perpetuate a cultural focus on penile stimulation, cisnormative heterosexual intercourse as the only "real sex," and men's pleasure over women's pleasure.

Some participants expressed how these ideas about women's and men's divergent sexualities influenced their own orientations to sex—including in regard to their expectations of their partners, and even their expectations of themselves. Astrid describes how before she was able to articulate her attraction to women and claim the kind of intentional sex life she wanted to have, she also "bought into" narratives about women's sexuality as they are perpetuated through these socializing discourses, and ultimately came to believe (for a period of time earlier in her life) that she was not *supposed* to enjoy sex:

> I felt very much like I would do what he wanted, and that was like—again I feel in some ways I bought into that like "Men have sex because they want to have sex, women have sex because they want to cuddle afterwards" sort of narrative that you hear, like, or "Women are gonna have sex because we want the intimacy." . . . I just heard that from sort of, even from the media, like, "Men love sex, and women love cuddling," and so I thought, "Okay, this is normal. I give him sex and then he will cuddle with me."

Astrid was eventually able to express her very active desires for women and claim her own queer sexuality and a genderqueer/nonconforming identity, but for much of her adult life, she had a great deal of difficulty with sex, due to what she describes as an experience of being socialized into a set of very specific gendered sexual scripts and expectations for behavior, desire, and expression. Her story makes it clear that sexual difference socialization is extremely powerful, and that the beliefs it produces are profound, psychic, embodied, and, ultimately, very difficult to overcome. Unfortunately, being treated in a medical setting for sexual pain and low desire did not help her either, and, in fact, iatrogenically harmed her and made her situation worse.

Visibility, "Obviousness," and Phenomenological Experiences of the Gendered Body

Another important aspect of sexual difference socialization includes coming to experience parts of the body and bodily processes as gendered—including through an evolutionary or biological lens that is white and hetero-/cisnormative. Phenomenological writing on "[cis] female body experience" (Young, 2005), productions of sexual difference (Butler, 1993; Grosz, 1994; Irigaray, 1985), and heterosexual and queer "orientations" toward (or away from) other bodies that are gendered and raced (Ahmed 2006, 2007) are all of import here. I draw on this work, focusing on how medical discourses about sexual difference come to influence individuals' psychic and affective experiences of themselves as members of—in this case, feminized—populations. Embodied experience is social and relational (Merleau Ponty, 1962/1995; Oliver, 2001), and this phenomenological coding of the world is productive of forms of bodily difference (de Beauvoir, 1952/1989; Weheliye, 2014).

The practitioners I spoke with had much to say about gendered bodily coding and subsequent phenomenological and psychosocial experiences that result from this coding, but they were more likely than low-desiring participants to characterize these differences in biological terms. Betsy discusses the "obviousness" of erections and what they imply about differences in male and female sexuality and sexual dysfunction, again considering the impact of Viagra:

> People think Viagra because it's on television, and because erection is sort of a dramatic, something you can *see*, whereas desire isn't something you see, which for women, again, arousal isn't something you can see, orgasm, you know, everything seems to be more visible in a man. Erection is more visible. Ejaculation is more visible. Orgasm is more visible. . . . I think it is more situated, but given that, *I still think that women are slightly more complicated.*

In our interview, Betsy further alludes to how erections become evidence of masculine desire, spontaneity, and activity, while premenstrual syndrome or PMS and menstruation become instantiations of feminine complexity, moodiness, and cyclical ambivalence. These bodily coding schemas are fraught for the women I interviewed; women are often aware of the fact that they have internalized these essentializing notions, and move quickly between espousing their beliefs in these notions as the "truth of biology" and rejecting them as hierarchizing social scripts with no real or natural basis. But, regardless of how much these women identified with or rejected these coded parts and processes, they ultimately described how deeply they felt the impact of these systems of meaning—in their bodyminds and behaviors, which were indelibly marked by these schemas. Sexual difference socialization is thus enacted in part through gendered conceptions of arousal, which is understood to be more easily detectable in men, versus "hormonal cycles," which are purported to be more easily detectable in women. This comparison of the *visible* or *obvious* provides an interesting entrée into a phenomenological explanation for how men get coded as more desiring via their (potentially) visible erections, whereas women get coded as more complicated via their (potentially) visible menstrual cycles—and also how gendered individuals code themselves accordingly. That these phenomena happen on completely different time scales perhaps further solidifies notions of male spontaneity and female receptivity (men's desire is cast as immediate, pressing, and positive, whereas women's desire is framed as slow, cyclical, and negative—and more often oriented to reproduction). The notion of what is visible, and what this visibility means, is something that came up over and over again in the interviews. In this vein, Zola illustrates her fraught feelings about divergences in male and female embodiment and experience:

> I think it is different, just because of the differences between us [men and women]. We go through different things, our cycles are different . . . [and] the monthly hormonal influxes do not help! But I am very sure men experience some type of "menstruation" inside of themselves, because there's no other way to explain some of the hissy fits my ex-husband used to throw [laughter]. . . . [I]t's just that all of their stuff is internalized. . . . [I]t is very hard as a woman to keep these things inside, it takes a lot of strength to keep your stuff suppressed.

What Zola relates here is a very complex imbrication of social, psychological, and embodied experience that she describes as different for men and women. It is clear that she believes some of these differences between men and women are purely "biological," but she also espouses a phenomenological explanation for divergent embodied experiences, based in socialization and lived experience of the coded body. Interestingly, she also reverses the sexual difference logic that emphasizes the externality and visibility of male erection-as-desire, for instance, by focusing on men's "internalized" or "suppressed" emotions. Lisa expands this notion of the experience of sexual difference based on bodily coding:

I think there is something to say for emotional cycles in men that I am curious about and I don't think is studied enough, because men aren't having their periods or ovulating—my [female] roommate and I would sometimes have these moments where we would be like, "I don't know, everything just seemed really hard today, and I burst into tears!" and I'd be like, "Didn't you say you are about to get your period?" And she'd be like, "Oh yeah!" [laughter] or it would happen exactly in reverse. My male roommate was like, "I kind of wish that I got my period because I wish I could justify my crazy cycles according to something beyond my control! I wish I had something to blame it on because I'm also feeling that way but it's not as obviously hormonal!" So I think that men don't get credit for having emotional cycles, but they obviously do.

These statements about the visibility of body parts and bodily functions are provocative, because they suggest that psychosocial and phenomenological experiences of the body and its processes—which are always marked and coded, and always experienced in relation to other bodies and their processes—are not innate or unchangeable, but are simultaneously very *real*. Thus, the lived experience of gender is absolutely biological, in that it is part and parcel of embodied awareness, but it is not essential, innate, originary, a priori, or presocial. This is something that the participants I interviewed tended to agree upon.

Femininity and the "Pathologizing-Healing Dialectic": How Sex Is Produced as a Realm for Men

Many participants described their belief that despite the narratives about gender and sexuality that are put forward through visibility discourses, men do, in fact, have psychological problems related to sexuality—their issues simply don't get labeled or pathologized in the same way that women's do. According to the individuals I spoke with, it's almost easier for women to acknowledge their issues with low desire and other psychosexual problems because of expectations about femininity as "complicated." Participants articulated that these conceptualizations have a negative effect on men's sexuality, in that it becomes performance-driven, goal-oriented, and that any issues that they have are characterized as purely physiological—which puts a lot of pressure on men to maintain their erections, and their (heteronormative) desire (see also Murray, 2019, for more on this theme). This is an inversion of the phenomenology described in the last section; here, women have an easier time seeking out treatment for low desire because "it's obvious" that they ought to do so.

Annie refers to this gendered system as the "pathologizing-healing dialectic" when she describes a cis male friend of hers with low desire who has had a difficult time "coming out" as having these issues or seeking treatment, because of expectations about masculinity:

> I don't see him going to a doctor or getting really into the sort of like "pathologizing-healing dialectic" like women do. But I feel like he does [have similar issues]—if he were a woman in a [sexual] relationship, he would have some sexual difficulty.... [L]ike, I could see him getting—in a relationship context—if he was the woman?!—it would probably get labeled that way [as low desire or sexual dysfunction].

Taja expresses a similar view of the gendered nature of self-medicalization, which might be described as part of this "pathologizing-healing dialectic" or the feminized trajectory of seeking out diagnoses that one can then attempt to treat. When I ask her if she thinks there are gender differences in the sexual issues that people commonly experience, Taja states:

> Men are just as obsessed as women are, the difference is that they do not medicalize it.... [T]hey are worried about it, but it is different than the way I am worried about it somehow.... I'm all concerned about it being some deep *psychological* dysfunction... [but] I don't think men are worried about some big psychological problem. They're like, "Oh, it must be a physical problem."... [M]en just aren't as in touch with their emotions, I think they aren't *trained* to be in touch with their emotions, so they are not trained to assume that it *is* emotions.

Many participants echoed similar ideas about the "pathologizing-healing dialectic" and self-medicalization as something that women are more likely to experience and engage in than men. Elizabeth, Corinne, Lisa, Tiffany, Rose, and Valdivia all expressed the notion that it is "easier" for women to identify low desire and other psychosexual issues, whereas it is easier and more acceptable for men to stick with the narrative that their problems are purely physical. They also shared their beliefs that these gender differences are produced—including a generally "less complicated" orientation to sex for men, in spite of pressures to perform—through sexual difference socialization processes. Gendered phenomenological experiences of embodied states indicate different expectations for men and women around sexual concerns and dysfunction—and come to be experienced and lived in correspondingly different ways. Through these processes, sex is produced as a realm for men, that participants felt women are excluded from—or at least a realm wherein their roles are constructed very differently.

Lola describes this phenomenon of the masculinizing of sex itself as something that hinders women from asking for—and getting—what they want sexually: "I feel like dudes can just be like, they can say that they *need* sex, whereas I'm not comfortable articulating that." She explains this in terms of women being socialized to not pursue their own sexual desires, or not to even understand sex as something they have a stake in. Elaine supports this notion: "I feel like men are really told that any level of pursuit or enthusiasm [in sex] is okay for them. And I think it just makes it less complicated for them." Penelope reiterates this sentiment about sex being "less complicated" for men:

> I think in general it is easier for men to just perform the act of sex and feel really amazing physically and have no emotional connection to their partner; I think it is much harder for women to do that . . . and in terms of just the level of desire, I guess it's connected because you [men] are encouraged to go out there and desire lots of women, or you [women] are encouraged to be with one person. . . . [T]hat would contribute to the level of desire and also the connecting emotionally to your sexual partner, because if you are just supposed to be with one person, *that's your person,* but if you are supposed to be with lots of people, why should it matter how you feel towards them, I guess?

Generally, participants stated that sex is produced as the domain of men—or that it is culturally constructed and coded as such, through media representations, in popular medical and scientific narratives, and through other discourses that they learned about at early ages from their families, from religious institutions, and at school. In this context, women are understood to have a different domain that they are expected to tend to and that is important to them—one that is characterized by emotionality, intimacy, domesticity, and caretaking. Or, alternatively, they are framed as having a different orientation to or role within the sexual landscape, but that it is not a place to cultivate their own fantasies, desires, or intense sexual feelings. Instead, women are socialized to experience sex as something they should engage in and even enjoy primarily as a service—a framing that ignores women's own subjectivities as sexual beings or that produces women as very specific kinds of sexual beings, always in relation to men.

How Women Are Socialized to Be "Certain Kinds of Sexual Beings"

Many participants described how they have come to experience themselves as "certain kinds of sexual beings." This production and pursuant experience of femininity is a crucial aspect of sexual difference socialization—which, in some cases, happens at the hands of the very clinicians who are in charge of helping women to get in touch with their own sexualities. Astrid illuminates her experience with being "coerced" into a "certain kind of femininity" through her participation in the treatment program. To her, it represented this messaging taken to an extreme, coercion legitimated through science and medicine: "But in terms of sexual function, I can't even imagine going back to those freakshows, because I feel like they were telling me that I needed to work through my 'sexual dysfunction issues' to become *a certain kind of sexual being.*" When discussing sexual development with Elaine, she states:

> I think that [biology] relates more to men, and I think for women it's more sort of social and psychological, these issues of desire, and for men, it's more sort of biological and medical, they are less affected—maybe not less affected—but affected differently by the social and psychological factors. . . . [I]t [socialization] tends not to suppress [men's] desire in the same way that it does for women.

Elaine's framing here is intriguing; she suggests that men's sexual issues—including men's physiological and phenomenological experiences of these issues—are *produced* as "medical" or "biological." According to Elaine, it's almost as though sexuality is *allowed* to be "biological" for men, whereas women are socialized into their own complex and emotional experiences of sex, which are ultimately more "social" and "psychological." Elaine describes a very complicated and nuanced view of the material-discursive production and concomitant embodied experience of sexual difference, including of gendered sexual disorders and dysfunctions.

Throughout the interviews, participants expressed a certain ambivalence and cynicism around questions of "biology" versus "socialization"—the notion that even if men's and women's sexualities are ultimately more similar than they are different, even if we "start out the same" (in Marianne's words), the dominant narrative that masculinity and femininity are dimorphic persists, and that difference is ultimately lived out among real people in the world, and becomes a force in itself. Regina sums up this sentiment:

> I generally do not like explaining things by like a male-female dualism, but I don't know? I perceive them [her ex-boyfriends] as having very high sex drives. . . . [I]t's not that they didn't have those [psychological/emotional] issues, but maybe their awareness didn't match the level of awareness I was giving to my own issues. . . . [W]e definitely have the stereotype of men as being much more quick to be aroused, you hear of teenage boys having an erection when they don't want to and *even grown men not being able to control that thing*! I could not imagine a world in which that happened to me . . . but the way that we as a society talk about the way that males are and the way that females are is not necessarily true to how males and females are. I believe that that is a story that we tell ourselves, that men are more sexual creatures and have a more simplistic sexuality—and it also might be self-perpetuating, too, as soon as you start telling the story, people start identifying with it.

In this rich quote, with which I also began this chapter, Regina elucidates feedback loops among our bodies, psyches, relationships, discourses, and the world around us. She also returns to the notion that women are more inclined than are men to self-pathologize or self-medicalize (the feminized "pathologizing-healing dialectic") and that sex is produced as a realm "for men." She articulates the notion that it is difficult to disentangle different forces (the "physical," "social," and "personal") as discrete phenomena; so, as much as biological forces may produce a certain type of embodied experience, the stories that we tell ourselves and each other about biology have specific embodied and psychic effects as well. If this is the case, then how useful is measuring the gap between the subjective and physiological, as is endeavored in psychophysiological plethysmographic research? What do gendered narratives of sexual concordance and discordance offer us? What do these experimental measurements, for instance, of the disconnect between the "subjective" and the "physiological," actually offer us?

Embodied Feedback Loops among the Biological, Psychological, and Social

Discordance (between genital arousal and subjective desire) is a key frame within twenty-first-century sex research on women. I argue that the way it has been pervasively disseminated and deployed is damaging to women, and that it perpetuates the notion of specifically feminine sexual responsiveness or receptivity. However, notions of concordance and discordance, or of mind/body connections and disconnects, are worth exploring phenomenologically—particularly in the context of trauma-related dissociation and women's experiences of their bodies "shutting down" during certain sexual experiences. In this last section, I focus on trauma and the special questions that trauma raises for theories of mind/body relations, intersubjectivity, and the social. Insofar as they provide frameworks for understanding a certain process of feminization that is embodied but not essential, critical disability studies, feminist psychiatric disability and madness studies, critical trauma studies, and asexuality studies offer us a better way to understand how bodies and minds link up (or don't) than the cultural feminism–informed psychological paradigms I began this chapter by describing. They also provide alternatives to the more rigid and essentializing technologies associated with the feminized responsive desire framework that I have analyzed in this book so far—including those that use behavioristic protocols as a means to an end.

In her 2018 sexual self-help book, Brotto describes the different ways that female discordance can manifest. In a chapter wherein she discusses "how mindfulness works" (i.e., by promoting concordance, or aligning the body and mind), she makes it clear that women's biological tendency toward easily activated and powerful physiological arousal, including when a woman does not subjectively feel turned on, should never be used as evidence of the fact that she secretly "wanted it"—specifically citing cases of sexual violence, wherein the fact that a woman became lubricated or even had an orgasm does not indicate anything about her desire. Brotto deplores this notion, stating that "a woman's self-report of how she feels is the ultimate reporter of her experience and the only way that consent can be given" (p. 139).[9] I have often wondered why—if a woman's word is the only thing that matters—so many contemporary sex researchers continue to explore female discordance, why research that quite literally probes this gap has exploded so much in the first two decades of the twenty-first century, and why it continues to be the gold standard in sexual science and medicine today. More importantly here, though, I am interested in how clinicians and researchers frame other types of discordance and concordance (and why they are less likely to attend to these). In this same section of Brotto's popular book, she describes how mind/body discordance "can happen in the other direction, too"—when one feels turned on but "the body says 'No!'" (p. 139). To illustrate this example of

---

9. This is also mentioned in a toolkit available on the #debunkingdesire social media campaign's website (https://1dodfd67-9812-43f7-a73f-9bc624a65f9a.filesusr.com/ugd/1f8b67_96 7a13a8f5374d17bcbc839861a9e509.pdf), wherein the importance of consent is highlighted after a discussion of Basson's circular or "arousal-first" sexual response cycle and its applicability to women's desire enhancement.

what she calls "reverse discordance," Brotto describes how many women who have had pelvic surgeries (for instance, following gynecologic cancer) might feel turned on mentally but lack sensation in their bodies. While this "reverse discordance" is hypothesized as an example of another type of discordance some women might experience, it is also broadly understood to be a much less likely scenario in sexually "healthy" women—rapid and intense genital arousal without subjective desire to match is what is instead regularly documented in almost all of the published studies of female discordance (i.e., women experience free-flowing physiological arousal even if they can't detect it subjectively; according to "the preparation hypothesis," they can be physically ready to go at pretty much any moment but are less likely to report subjective mental desire to match).[10] "Reverse discordance" in women is thus an anomaly within the scientific lexicon, and this is borne out in the fact that it is significantly less frequently studied (specifically in regard to women who have not undergone pelvic surgeries).

While "reverse discordance" may be one interesting counterpoint to the overarching logic of feminine responsiveness and easy genital arousal, my research suggests that there are others; bodies, psychologies, and the social link up in all kinds of complex ways. One way is when the body shuts down because the mind does not want something, a very different type of *concordance*, which shores up a taboo topic in contemporary psychology and sexology: the unconscious. Yet we need not enact a full psychoanalytic discussion of the unconscious here in order to analyze embodied subjectivity in this vein. Some of my participants describe how their bodies enact things almost on their behalf, and thus they force us to grapple not only with the notion of the unconscious but also with that of hysteria. As Labuski (2015) noted with her participants with vulvodynia, an enactment of hysteria in the context of trauma—whether physical, psychological, or both (and it generally is both)—is simultaneously produced via raced, classed, gendered, and sexualized codes *and* experienced viscerally at the level of the body. Reckoning with hysteria

---

10. Lalumière, et al. (2020) explain what they see as the practical utility of disseminating knowledge about "the preparation hypothesis" (that women's easy lubricative and vasocongestive response is an adaptive mechanism evolved in prehistoric environments to protect the vagina against injury during sexual assault)—the idea is that having a scientific theory in place for why women become physiologically aroused even when they are being sexually assaulted may help destigmatize women's automatic genital response and can be used in the vein of forensic evidence and education with police and in the courts or criminal justice system. Following Chivers (2005), they also suggest that knowing that other women also became physiologically aroused when they were raped may be reassuring to some survivors. It is one thing to tell women this fact; it is another to provide an explanation for it rooted in evolutionary psychology. And of course, we would not need this type of forensic education regarding a theory of cave-rape if we didn't automatically distrust sexual assault charges made by women.

here may offer a crip (McRuer, 2006), cripistemological (Johnson & McRuer, 2014), or crip*hys*temological (Mollow, 2014) standpoint through which we might make sense of embodied experiences that bring populations together, thus theorizing both hysterical subjectivities and hysterical populations.

In 2014, Johnson and McRuer posited "cripistemologies" as a way of thinking through how a "crip" (McRuer, 2006) standpoint is a place from which to theorize, a way to make sense of disability and debility as both culturally coded and viscerally experienced in the world. This work has moved us away from thinking of disabilities as purely medical *or* as socially constructed—but instead, as political, relational, and always embodied (Kafer, 2013). In the same journal issue in which "cripistemologies" was introduced, Mollow (2014) described hysteria from this standpoint, arguing for an embodied perspective on hysterical subjectivity that takes pain and trauma into account. My participants offer a cripistemological intervention—the low-desiring feminized (and often traumatized) subject may now be a revolutionary figure who offers a new way of thinking about race, class, gender, sexuality, minds, bodies, desire, and dysfunction. The low-desiring woman as a potential FSIAD diagnosee exposes the limits of the "social" and "biological"—she has been socialized via sexual difference discourses and is produced as such within them; however, she is always at risk of failing at femininity. Some may experience this failure as liberating in its sabotage, some as a painful condition that requires treatment—but for many of us, it will always be both.

Several of the women I spoke with had experienced sexual abuse or some type of gendered or sexualized violence at some point during their lives. They were clear that regardless of any other biological or social factors, this fact alone had deeply influenced their experiences of sex, and the substance of and ability to pursue their own desires. They spoke of a variety of ways that they believe their brains have been affected by trauma, and then additionally by the types of drugs they've used to treat those conditions. Molly, who is a survivor of sexual abuse and who now helps other women who have experienced sexual violence, discusses her own embodied experience of trauma:

> There are times where I will have a very physical reaction, or feel something physical, but I'm not able to say, "Okay, I feel this because he did this specific thing to me." . . . [I]t's frustrating to not be able to say, "I know that this happened, and I know that that happened and that that other thing happened." . . . [A]nd then certain weird things can trigger it, trigger sort of a flashback. . . . [I]t's like the stuff that I can't deal with in my head comes out in my body.

Annie also shares how her experience with sexual abuse as a child has deeply influenced her embodied responses to sex today, focusing specifically on how she believes her neurocircuitry has been affected by trauma and then by taking selective serotonin reuptake inhibitors (SSRIs) to alleviate her symptoms:

> A situation that might elicit a kind of "fight" response for me would elicit a kind of like "hiding" or "fleeing" response in someone else, or vice versa, and I would say that's common and kind of the underlying biological piece of having a post-traumatic stress disorder [PTSD] diagnosis. So that's the starting point for it, and then enter the medication to treat that, in addition to the fight-or-flight thing influencing my interactions with sexual partners; the medication [an SSRI] adds this other layer of then having difficulty with orgasms, maybe having less sexual desire, and having frustration and tension around control over sex and having orgasms.

Here, Annie highlights the iatrogenic perpetuation of her low desire through her own experience of treatment for PTSD; the drug of choice for women with depression and anxiety (including women who experience these because of trauma) is often an SSRI. SSRIs are known for their sexual side effects, including a general lowering of libido and anorgasmia. Annie describes how being abused affected her neurochemistry and "fight-or-flight response," which led her to take an SSRI to treat this condition, which subsequently negatively affects her sex life and desire, which then affects her relationship with her own body and her relationships with partners. Annie has a particularly nuanced and complex analysis of this feedback loop of embodied-social interaction, which she believes is common to the way many low-desiring women experience sex. It exemplifies the thoughtful and deeply intricate ways the women I interviewed think about the interactions among social events (including traumas), personal psychology, and embodied states.

Some of the participants who experience pain upon penetration concomitant with their lowered desire had similarly sophisticated analyses of how trauma has affected their bodies and sexualities. Sarah discussed how her chronic pain condition, which is not specifically vaginal but which does make penetration uncomfortable for her, has deeply affected her desire to have sex (or rather, to avoid it)—with men, particularly. She explains how her body has become so accustomed to experiencing pain that she almost automatically "shuts down," often before the experience has even begun, in anticipation. Regina, who experiences pain upon penetration, describes a similar phenomenon:

> I went to a physical therapist, she gave me these dildo-looking things—you go up in size to stretch and things like that and I did find that if I used that the day before, or a couple of hours before I was going to have sex, then that did help things. . . . [T]hen we [she and her partner] kind of made it part of our thing, that I would do this, or maybe take a bath to relax things . . . but this all gets to be very mechanical—it is not the playful spontaneous sex that is fun and enjoyable, it starts to be like, "Okay, how can we get it so that Regina's vagina does not revolt?" Like every time we had sex I had all these *chores* to do in order to be able to have sex.

This notion of her body "revolting" against penetration is one that other participants with genital pain expressed. Maya, who has not been diagnosed with dyspareunia or vulvodynia, but who has begun to experience more intense vaginal pain in the context of her marriage, describes her thoughts on the etiology of the problem:

> It was always a little bit painful, but now it is just excruciatingly painful and I think it is because I am totally not into it. . . . I think I turn it off because it is one thing to be aroused, and another to know that the arousal will go through a complete process and you will end up having sex, and I don't want to be aroused only to have pain. . . . I have totally told myself that I don't want to do this anymore, and because of that, my body is devising ways of making it easier for me to *prove* that I cannot do it.

Both Kelly and Astrid, who have been diagnosed with vulvodynia and who completed a treatment program to help alleviate their physical pain and simultaneously treat their low desire, shared similar sentiments about the possibility of a psychophysiological materialization of their trauma and lack of desire as physical pain. Kelly discusses her experience with treatment:

> KELLY: We all had pain *and* low desire. . . . [W]hich came first? I don't know.
> ALYSON: Do you have any speculations in your own situation around which came first?
> KELLY: At first I thought it was just the pain that came first and the low desire was a by-product of it, because naturally you don't want to do something that hurts, but looking back, the guy I was with definitely was not the right person for me in a lot of ways, so part of it may have been not really wanting to have sex with him.

Astrid's story is particularly alarming, as she describes her body as literally waging war against a way of being sexual that she could simply no longer tolerate:

> I think my body stepped in where my mind wasn't willing to step in or was incapable of stepping in at the time and said, "This isn't right, I don't want to be submitted to this practice of being receptive to this kind of abusive treatment, this heteronormative—" . . . I really believe that my body just said "No!" and sort of drew a line in the sand. . . . [T]his "disorder"—it changed everything for me, it made it impossible for me to continue to engage in this very dysfunctional relationship where I traded sex for security at the expense of my own identity and my own politics. . . . I feel like my nonconsensual sex turned from only an emotionally painful sex into also a physically painful sex and that that became a physically *impossible* sex over time, to the point where I was no longer able to engage in that abusive, nonconsensual sex, just because my body made it impossible. . . . [B]ut [in the treatment program], we were told, "It's because you're in pain that you developed this uninterest in sex"—rather than the other way around.

These women's stories provide a sobering counternarrative to the tales evolutionary psychology, FSIAD, and the feminized circular sexual response cycle tell about the embodied "truth" of female desire. Rather than the female lubrication-swelling response being an indication of a woman's evolved physical proclivity to become aroused, instead we have evidence of the body shutting down as a form of embodied revolt or resistance. As we have moved away from psychosomatic medicine and into the terrain of neurologically based differences with "organic" etiologies and essentialized attributes, these narratives may seem atavistic, anachronistic, or anathema. They certainly feel out of place in our current neoliberal technoscientific moment, characterized as it is by neurocognitive behaviorist framings. But these accounts raise the question of the psychosomatic, they hearken back to Freud's hysterics and neurotics, to Anna O., to Dora, and to psychoanalytic conceptualizations that might have previously been framed as frigidity, hysteria, or peculiarly feminine neuroses. But these phenomena, experiences, processes, and practices might also be interpreted as subconscious or unconscious political acts, forms of revolt or resistance, and reclamations of bodies and identities that have been colonized and oppressed (Bordo, 1993 Cixous & Clément, 1975/1986). With this in mind, might we consider certain enactments of low desire among the feminized, and their physiological manifestations, as potentially political, subversive, or even as insurrectionary?

CHAPTER 4

Embodied Invisible Labor, Sexual Carework

The Cultural Logic and Affective Valorization of Responsive Female Desire

In 2014, Los Angeles psychotherapist Lori Gottlieb published an article in the *New York Times* titled "Does a More Equal Marriage Mean Less Sex?" This article reported on a study conducted on the relationship between household division of labor and sex frequency among heterosexual couples, and concluded that the less "gender differentiation" between two parties in a romantic partnership, the lower the frequency and quality of sex they will have. Gottlieb's take is only one of the most recent to proclaim that egalitarianism in romantic relationships, particularly among heterosexual couples, dampens desire (see Roiphe, 2012 for another example, which I will examine in chapter 5). The standard logic is that feminism has had an unfortunate side effect; women might feel more equal to their partners in all kinds of ways nowadays, but that equality was only acquired at the expense of their desire—and a hot sex life. At the same time, the concern that women still describe doing more of the most traditionally feminine domestic duties—including some that are sexual, sensual, and affective—is easily rendered passé in a purportedly postfeminist climate. In light of the popularity of media accounts and research suggesting an inverse relationship between gender egalitarianism and exciting sex, and alongside the feminized responsive desire framework that I have outlined in this book thus far (which includes the circular sexual response cycle, the new female sexual interest/arousal disorder [FSIAD] diagnosis, myriad reports of female genital/subjective discordance, and biopolitical regimes such as mindfulness-based sex therapy [MBST] to cultivate women's desire), it is imperative to consider the persistent feminization of sexual, sensual, and caring work, including within the often-gendered terrain of romantic and marital partnerships. How does performing this work affect women's desire and experiences of sex? How do medicalized and extramedical protocols for feminine sexual responsiveness and receptivity influence, frame, and delimit women's experiences of providing care? In the twenty-first century, do we see new demands for relational caretaking in light of these protocols? If so, what do they consist of?

In this chapter, I analyze the gendered configurations of intimacy and sexuality that remain hidden beneath popular accounts of "lackluster" and "unsexy" egalitarianism, linking them to more traditional forms of carework and also to biopolitical self-care regimes under late capitalism. Extending analyses of the social organization of care more broadly, my data from low-desiring women suggest that many intimate relationships—particularly wherein there are gendered desire discrepancies between partners—involve what I call "sexual carework." With this concept, I am in dialogue with Hochschild's analysis of "emotional labor" and "feeling rules" (Hochschild, 1985; Hochschild & Machung, 1989); for Hochschild, emotions are social, performed for others, and people of different (race, gender, class, and other) statuses are expected to perform them in different ways. More so than Hochschild, however, I find Weeks's (2011) attention to the naturalization, feminization, and racialization of socially reproductive care via the idealization of the nuclear family most useful. It is also imperative to examine carework's colonialist, racist, and classist contours in terms of how these affect women of color, immigrant women, and poor women, across national borders (Collins, 1998; Francisco-Menchavez, 2018; Hondagneu-Sotelo, 2002; Kang, 2010; MacDonald, 2015; Parreñas, 2002; Wingfield, 2015). Other recent conceptualizations focus on the care that women with low desire and sexual pain perform (Braksmajer, 2017; Cacchioni, 2007, 2015; Labuski, 2014, 2015). I add to these analyses by placing "sexual carework" within a broader medicalized frame of female receptivity and responsiveness, and by attending to the biopolitical invectives that result, in terms of mandates to care for the self. This type of analysis of feminized sexual carework helps to shed light on the relational production of women's "low desire," as examining medical, scientific, and popular discourses that revolve around the broader feminized responsive desire framework illuminates the deployment of women's low desire and helps to clarify the work this configuration of receptive femininity performs at a cultural level.

There are two different formulations of *work* underwriting my analysis here. The first form of labor is in line with the typical work of liberal capitalism, in which a woman services her partner (including, in some cases, by putting on a certain kind of affective performance, often within the context of a power imbalance). Cacchioni's (2015) conceptualization of women with low desire and pain who perform sexualized "labors of love," and Braksmajer's (2017) analysis of sexualized care as a form of obligatory compliance that women with dyspareunia must navigate, are both situated within this formulation. Similarly, Labuski (2015) also describes the relational and embodied work that women with vulvodynia execute as part of a regime of intimate care and both sexual orientation and gender identity protection. All of these theorists focus on heteronormative expectations for sexual service that women engage in for the benefit of their (often cis male) partners. My own conceptualization of sexual carework, in regard to this form of labor, has much in common with these framings.

The other aspect of sexual carework I describe in this chapter is an example of Foucauldian governmentality (2000) and a form of biopolitical (1978, 2003) labor under neoliberal capitalism—it is the labor that a woman directs *inward*, to make herself more enjoyable, appealing, or optimal to others, but that also includes an expectation that she will do this labor *to and for herself*. This type betrays the mandates of neoliberalism (including its sexual imperatives), in which femininity itself is understood along an axis of debility and capacitation (Puar, 2011, 2017), and in which self-care, self-optimization, and pleasure itself become work. Not only do the low-desiring women I interviewed describe laboring in this second, self-optimizing or biopolitical way, but this theme emerges in medical, scientific, therapeutic, and consumer discourses—including in the feminized responsive desire framework described throughout this book. The logic of self-optimization as compulsory has been theorized at length (Ahmed, 2010; Berlant, 2011; McRuer, 2006), as have its sexual components (Barounis, 2019; Gupta, 2011, 2015; Gupta & Cacchioni, 2013; Milks & Cerankowski, 2014; Przybylo, 2013). But my analysis makes clear that there are specifically gendered facets of this labor that can be examined as particularly relevant in the case of women-with-low-desire—members of a population who are expected to work on themselves and conjure up a desire for the sake of their lovers, themselves, and even the nation, the public, and the population or species body. If sexuality is compulsory, it must also be a type of work. Under this model, those who cannot work are thus debilitated; they *ought* to work on themselves, or allow themselves to be worked upon, with an eye toward their own (in this case, gendered and sexual) capacitation.

The heart of this chapter, then, is to add this deeper biopolitical theorization of sexual care; consider how this type of service operates over the life-span for many women and how they are socialized into it; and to analyze sexualized, sensualized, and affective forms of gendered neoliberal citizenship—a form of what Cossman (2007) refers to as "sexual citizenship." In this vein, Cacchioni (2015) describes three different aspects of what she calls "sex work"[1]—"discipline work," "performance work," and "avoidance work." Both "performance work" and "discipline work" involve self-improvement strategies that develop one's "sexual capital" (p. 85) and thus have implications for governmentality. I am in conversation with Cacchioni's framing but take this Foucauldian analysis a step further, via two moves—(1) I consider sexual carework as a mode of compulsory self-optimization or self-care (as a form of anatomopolitics) as elucidated above. And (2) I analyze it as a mode of population production (as a form of biopolitics)—those who perform care in this way are produced as part of a responsive, receptive, feminized population. So, in addition to qualitative analyses of low-desiring women's narratives of pressure to provide sexualized care, and the gendered logic of receptivity they describe learning at young ages, I also illuminate discursive productions of femininity as receptive, reproductive, valorizable,[2] and always ready to labor—including as these are found in psychomedical discourses and popular accounts. This is necessary, as the feminized responsive desire framework does not only impact women who are formally diagnosed with desire troubles or sexual pain; its impact, in fact, goes much further—as it has been taken up in alternative health and wellness circles, other popular self-help accounts, and under the guise of sex positivity and feminism. Here, the logic of receptivity contours the logic of care.

In analyzing these two forms of labor, I engage with a revised Marxist feminist critique of heterosexuality, social reproduction, and gender relations under capitalism, specifically framing it alongside contemporary cultural narratives about the purportedly negative effects of gender equality, and bringing the medical and scientific discursive logic of feminine receptivity to the forefront. Building on the scholarship of pioneering theorists of gendered carework, the social organization of care, and the undervalued labor of women, particularly women of color, in global production and social reproduction more broadly, I argue that intimate relationships themselves involve

---

1. Cacchioni's (2015) notion of "sex work" is not to be confused with paid sex work—sex work proper—that involves providing sexual services in exchange for money. Her terminology is drawn from Duncombe and Marsden (1996), who use the term *sex work* to describe unpaid sexual labor in long-term relationships. I dislike this term, as I understand sex work to be a paid service that requires a separate analysis in terms of precarity, vulnerability, and economic justice for sex workers. I will discuss sex work proper briefly later in the chapter and explain what it does and does not have in common with the concept I develop here: sexual carework.

2. Here, I mean *valorizable* in the Marxist sense—simply, to make valuable or profitable.

sexual carework. Primarily, this duty falls upon women in heterosexual dyads to maintain harmony in their relationships by using their bodies to provide certain kinds of sex, at certain times, and in certain ways, to their male partners—but this socialization process begins early and thus extends beyond heterosexual monogamy. Women are, of course, socialized to be sexual caretakers—their role in sexualized social reproduction is not naturally given. Yet, women who labor in this way are not simply victims of false consciousness or ideological dupes. As Cacchioni (2015), Labuski (2015), and Braksmajer (2017) also found, low-desiring (and sexually pained) women's sexual care is often very much considered, concerted, methodical, creative, and strategic, and it is something that many of the women I interviewed ultimately derive pleasure from—albeit not necessarily orgasmic pleasure of the type that is generally associated with sex and sexual desire.

Let me be clear: Not all gendered and sexualized work is the same. Paid sex work is not the same as sexual carework in the service of others, which is not the same as the work of self-optimization. Different groups of women are targeted to perform and are affected differently by doing these types of work. As Grant (2014) and Mac and Smith (2018) articulate, the work that sex workers perform should never be conflated with carework, nor should the sex worker's experience be made to stand in for the "experience of all women"—"for this person, sex work *may* be sex—but it is also *work*, in a world that allows no alternative" (Mac & Smith, 2018, p. 39). However, we may also fruitfully consider the ways that sex work is devalued precisely because it is interpreted within frames of gendered and racialized care and essentialized and naturalized feminine responsiveness. Similarly, paid nonsexual domestic and caring work is also gendered and racialized, and performed disproportionately by women of color, immigrants, and poor women working under heteropatriarchal cisnormative white supremacist capitalism (Collins, 1998; Weeks, 2011).

Outside of paid sex work and paid nonsexual domestic and caring work, the medicalized logic of feminine receptivity that informs unpaid sexual carework also impacts marginalized low-desiring women disproportionately—and so there is a paradox here. This is because while the work of self-care or self-optimization, with its biopolitical implications, works within a white, middle-class, hetero-/cisfeminine logic, as does the feminized responsive desire framework writ large, the day-to-day banal work of care—including sexual carework as a form of social reproduction—often falls disproportionately upon low-desiring women of color, poor women, Indigenous women, immigrant women, women with disabilities, and trans women (more so than middle-class, able-bodied, cishet white women). So, while the medicalized logic of feminine receptivity targets all women, it does not affect all women in the same way. I will attend to this tension between who the logic targets, and who is affected most in the day-to-day experience, throughout the analysis but especially at the end of this chapter.

Social Reproduction, Receptivity, and Feminized Labor

Today, *carework* is a common term among social scientists and conveys the type of work done, usually by women, in the home or other domestic realms (DeVault, 1991; Hochschild, 1997; Hochschild & Machung, 1989). Carework encapsulates housework, sexual reproduction, and child and elder care, and some feminist scholars have argued for a sexualized component as well, beyond sexual reproduction per se, but in terms of the provision of sexual pleasure. In order to fully elaborate the relationship among sexual carework, other forms of gendered carework, and social reproduction, it is crucial to look at the Marxist history of these concepts. Marx (1990) only briefly mentions the processes involved in what he refers to as *reproduction* (sometimes called *social reproduction*)—or the notion that in order for the worker to be productive, to effectively produce saleable commodities, he (and importantly, it is a "he" in Marx's formulation) also requires the maintenance and reproduction of his body, his labor power. For Marx, social reproduction is the process by which the worker, in a capitalist economic system, is cared for— generally within the home—so that he may continue to work. Marx (1990) states: "Just as on the first day of his appearance on the world's stage, man must still consume every day, before and while he produces" (p. 272). But what happens before, during, and after production is a crucial aspect of work that Marx largely neglected, and a lacuna in his analysis that has been roundly critiqued by materialist, Marxist, and autonomist feminist scholars for many decades (for examples, see Dalla Costa & James, 1972; Federici, 2004, 2012; Fortunati, 1995; Mies, 2010). These critiques reached a fever pitch in the 1970s after the publication of Friedan's *The Feminine Mystique* (1963), and with the International Wages for Housework Campaign (WfH), which drew attention to the unpaid work women do to sustain the family (and the capitalist wage relation) within the larger political economic system.

The International Wages for Housework campaign, a global social movement that grew out of the autonomous Marxist tradition in Italy in the early 1970s, had a deceptively simple core tenet: Women's domestic work ought to be paid. The Wages for Housework critiques primarily focused on the unpaid work women do to supplement and sustain the family within the larger political economic system; the type of work usually considered part of the social reproductive economy and that creates an environment sustainable for the (male) worker to go out and earn the real "family wage" included cooking, cleaning, childcare, shopping, and other quotidian duties. Importantly, these activists took up this framework not because they actually wanted housewives to make money for their duties, but rather to draw attention to the insidious and methodical way capitalism exploits a certain type of work, naturalizing it as feminine, disguising its racialization, and as such, not treating it as work at all. WfH activists believed that illuminating this fact would highlight for the working class how they have been held apart and hierarchized by this sexual division of labor, and suggested that it would ultimately create a space for women to refuse this work while simultaneously refusing to partake in the capitalist system of exploitation, which would result in the fracturing and ultimate collapse of capitalism (see Weeks, 2011 for a full analysis of this goal of the refusal of work in WfH's platform).

The emotional, affective, and embodied labor involved in providing a "happy home," clearly crucial to any worker's sustenance, is an integral aspect of social reproduction. Von Werlhof (1988) argues, regarding women, and particularly women of color, who are colonized and designated as "nature" under capitalism: "The labor of these people is therefore pronounced to be non-labor, to be biology: their labor-power—their ability to work—appears as a natural resource, and their products as akin to a natural deposit" (p. 97). S. James (2012) writes that women have always "service[d] those who are daily destroyed by working for wages and who need to be daily renewed" (p. 93). Federici (2012) extends von Werlhof's analysis of the naturalization of women's work and James's notion of women being at the "disposal" of men, framing the work that women perform in intimate settings as something that has been "transformed into a natural attribute of our female physique and personality, an internal need, an aspiration, supposedly coming from the depths of our female character" (p. 16). She goes on to explain how women are socialized into this role: "From the earliest days of your life, you are trained to be docile, subservient, dependent, and most importantly, to sacrifice yourself and get pleasure from it. If you don't like it, it is your problem, your failure, your guilt, and your abnormality" (p. 17). Federici also describes how multifaceted the labor performed by women in intimate settings is, as they are expected to service the male worker "physically, emotionally, and sexually" (p. 17). In a provocative essay entitled "Why Sexuality Is Work" (originally published in 1975), she comments on the reasons for women's particular experience within the "schizophrenic character of sexual relations" under capitalism:

[Women suffer most] not only because we arrive at the end of the day with more work and more worries on our shoulders, but additionally because we have the responsibility of making the sexual experience pleasurable for the man. This is why women are usually less sexually responsive than men. Sex is work for us, it is a duty. The duty to please is so built into our sexuality that we have learned to get pleasure out of giving pleasure, out of getting men aroused and excited. (Federici, 2012, p. 24).

Even with the recent rise of the #MeToo movement, this particular analysis may seem outdated. After all, even as a certain kind of (white liberal) feminism has been mainstreamed, we continue to live in a highly individualistic neoliberal moment, in which sexuality has purportedly been liberated, and is celebrated as something that everyone should naturally have the right to enjoy. We are all aware of the number of women who have joined the workforce; of the "equality" with which women can now access the public sphere; of the rising number of countries around the world, including the US, that have legalized gay marriage; and of the supposed tolerance of queer sexualities, as evidenced in media portrayals and other public discourses in the Global North. But what remains salient about Federici's and others' analyses cited above—particularly for my current project—is the attention they focus on the simultaneous biologizing and feminizing of care, and of feminine sexual receptivity. This is important in light of new trends in scientific sex research and sexual medicine (and their popular depictions), through which sexuality is configured in terms of essential gender difference, and through which masculine and feminine behaviors, desires, and expressions continue to be discursively produced and essentialized, in new and ever more insidious guises—what Preciado (2013) might call a form of *technogender* or what Repo (2016) would consider a disciplinary and normalizing deployment.

With the rise of childless straight white couples today—especially among those who identify as middle class in the US—carework is now increasingly framed as a less pivotal or useful category of analysis. According to many popular and social scientific accounts (Gottlieb, 2014; Kornrich, Brines, & Leupp, 2012), the "new" family dyads are egalitarian, with each member of a couple or reproductive unit (regardless of that couple's sexual orientation) contributing to the earned income and sharing in the housework. Not only should this be critiqued as a white middle-class framing that purports to be neutral, it also conflicts with the findings from my data with low-desiring women. The women I interviewed for this study suggest that there is still an invisible and gendered element to the social reproduction of a home and a family—specifically when the home consists of a cis male and cis female partner—and that the division of labor is not so egalitarian. According to my participants, this embodied invisible labor involves sexual carework—an aspect of sexualized social reproduction and also an aspect of sexual difference socialization (as defined in chapter 3)—in the form of embodied and energetic sustenance that the female or feminine partner most often provides to the male or masculine partner. My participants described long histories of providing sexualized or other forms of affective caring labor over the course of their lives—and many of them described learning early on that their mothers had also provided it to their fathers, or that other women in their lives provided it to the men in theirs. They also described a hegemonic cultural (and scientifically instantiated) ideology that supports the notion that the feminization of this care is "natural."

In our contemporary moment, the relegation of the housewife to an alienated domestic enclosure, an undisputedly gendered division of housework, and a rigid romantic relationship that necessarily involves childrearing or that involves a male-identified and a female-identified partner, are no longer assumed nor expected when it comes to cohabitation, family, and home. Much has changed since the inception of the International Wages for Housework campaign, but it is also the case that many cis women still do find themselves in monogamous, long-term partnerships with cis men, and that this type of family or some variation of it, of this core economic and reproductive unit, is the norm—or, alternatively, it is a normatively raced, classed, and heterosexualized ideal that many folks aspire to (or are pushed to aspire to). However, boundaries between work and leisure must increasingly be reconfigured (DeVault, 1991), not only due to the "second shift" that many women describe taking on (Hochschild, 1997; Hochschild & Machung, 1989) but also because what it means to work is being reconfigured—work must now be understood in terms of affect, performance, biopower, and other circulations that extend beyond the workplace, and that cannot be relegated to the "public sphere," but that are absolutely social (Clough, 2007; Foucault, 2003; Hardt & Negri, 2000, 2004). In light of this reality, it is necessary to (re)explore the gendered configurations of embodied labor that still circulate within intimate settings and the effects these configurations have on women's sexuality. As these prototypes have cultural sway and maintain a hegemonic persistence, they have import for gender-nonconforming and trans folks and for queer sexualities and relationships, as well as for hetero- and homonormative cis partnerships.

Beyond the gendering of production and reproduction historically, we must also consider how these (productive and reproductive) categories of labor are increasingly collapsed under neoliberal imperatives toward self-branding, self-appreciation, and self-valorization (Feher, 2009, 2018), and also how desire itself is reified under regimes that deploy sexuality, quantify and schematize behaviors and expressions, and put sexuality to work—ideologically and materially (Floyd, 2009). These schemas of optimization, and the simultaneous way in which they encourage self-modulation (anatomo-politics) and population production (biopolitics) (Foucault, 1978, 2000, 2003), are examples of how we might understand work in contemporary biopolitical terms. Taking up this type of analysis, Ruído (2011) argues that contemporary work must be reconfigured not only in light of social reproduction, but in regard to affective economies, performances, and circuits of pleasure and desire:

> Defining work and its limits in abstract terms at the present time, where the times and locations of production become blurred and extended, is not an easy task. However, experiencing its consequences on our bodies seems to be less complicated, especially if we consider a definition of work that goes beyond the economistic view (whether neoclassical or Marxist) and, especially, if we understand our sustainment of a daily life and our daily incorporation of personalities and social actions as spaces and (re)productive efforts. Everything that tires, that occupies, that disciplines and stresses our body, but also everything that constructs it, that takes care of it, that gives it pleasure and maintains it, is *work*.

These nuanced accounts of work provide an entrée into my own intervention, as they bring together autonomist/Marxist feminist and biopolitical analyses. Work is relational and social, it is something we learn and experience phenomenologically and psychically, and it is written on our bodies and into our intimate relations with others. It can feel like a violation or a chore; it might be gendered, raced, or otherwise forced upon us through powerful discourses; it can be pleasurable, or we may feel like we are failing at it (and, importantly, these experiences can all occur at the same time). This unique intertwining of coercion, pleasure, failure, and desire might be particularly descriptive for those who are socialized—and sexualized—into receptive femininity, and so I will now explore sexual carework through participants', clinicians', and other healers' and educators' narratives about these processes. It must be acknowledged that the low-desiring participants in this study inevitably experience sex as more of a "chore" than do women who have never experienced low sexual desire. But, these low-desiring women's narratives, while not generalizable to all women, still reveal something important about what feminized sexual carework looks and feels like, because in a circumstance of low desire, the work cannot be ignored. Thus, it's not so much that these women are an exception to the rule, but rather that they throw into sharp relief the extent to which women more broadly are expected to approach sex as carework. Their stories also shed light on a certain spectrum of ambivalence: For these women, performing care sometimes felt pleasurable, yet at other times, it felt deeply coercive, and like it must be refused.

Feminine Socialization and Sexual Carework

The participants that I interviewed grappled with the heavy burden of the intimate labor that they know falls on their backs as individuals in the category of women-with-low-desire. For some, the specifically feminized indoctrination into this work—the way that it involves a necessary power imbalance, a mandate to please someone else, and in some cases an imperative to excavate and bring forth their own pleasure (or at least a performance of that pleasure)—was striking. Rather than solely providing pleasure in the form of servicing their partners' bodies or providing their own bodies as a service, some of my participants spoke of how they work to produce an experience that feels "authentic," and described a socialization into this type of socially reproductive work beginning at an early age.

Early Experiences with Embodied Invisible Labor: "Giving Daddy Five Kisses a Day"

Feeling as though they had to perform affective, embodied acts of labor from very young ages, specifically for their fathers, other male relatives, or family friends, was a common theme among participants. They contrasted this to the experiences of their male siblings, whom they believe were not expected to perform in the same way. Rose, a straight, thirty-three-year-old Black woman, describes this type of experience while we sit across from each other at my kitchen table. Rose's parents divorced when she was very young, and she only saw her father once or twice a year after that, as he lived in another country. But when he did visit, she was expected to "give him kisses" and perform for him in other ways that felt disorienting to her, even at the time:

> He would say, "I miss you so much, I love you so much, you have to give me five kisses a day!" And I would like negotiate with him. I'd be like, "No, I'll give you three kisses today, I don't want to give you five!" because I didn't like it, I didn't like being physical, hugging him . . . because I didn't really know him. . . . [I]t's funny, because he was a cool guy, he was fine, he used

to like to cook a lot, he always wanted to do fun things, so I thought he was a cool guy, but we just didn't have that *relationship* . . . and I think you go along with it out of guilt, because you're like, "Well, he's my dad, he's *supposed* to do that."

Rose elucidates the ambivalence she felt for her father, and also the ambivalent and transient place he had in her life. She only saw him once a year, but when she did see him, she was expected to be physically affectionate with him. Researchers and writers of color have documented the ways in which the burden of various types of emotional labor falls disproportionately on women of color (Collins, 1990, 1998; Lorde, 1984/2007; Piepzna-Samarasinha, 2018), but much of the contemporary research has focused on how that burden is enacted in the workplace, for instance through racist double standards regarding "body labor" and "feeling rules" (Kang, 2010; Wingfield, 2015). Collins's (2004) seminal work on sexual violence enacted against Black women has opened up a space to consider how this coercion takes many forms, and my own research suggests how the intimate, sensual labor that women of color are expected to perform from young ages may also feel coercive to them—especially when they identify as low in desire and are also regularly exposed to other forms of gendered and racialized structural violence.

Although this theme may resonate particularly for Black women with low desire (including as they experience coercion and intimate transgressions at the hands of white people), other low-desiring women of color and white women I interviewed also described experiences with early expectations for emotional, sensual, and embodied forms of labor. Across racial backgrounds, low-desiring participants articulated a similar dissonance that Rose describes—their fathers were emotionally unavailable and distant, yet these young women were still expected to be physically affectionate with them when they were around. This tension was something that many participants did not know what to do with; they described being "too young" to simply say no to physical affection they did not want to provide. They felt uncomfortable being physical with men they were not close to, including their own fathers, but at the same time, did not experience the request for physicality as an outright violation. This is part of the murky terrain that young women find themselves in at early ages regarding expectations of their bodies and the provision of physical expressions of care and love. Many participants who described experiences like those of Rose were not victims of child sexual abuse or molestation (Rose was not either), and in some cases, they expressed this ambivalence even if their parents were not divorced—even if their fathers were "around," they did not feel particularly close to them, yet were expected to perform affectively and physically for them. This fraught experience is crucial to analyze, as it occupies a space just to the side of what we would normally deem sexually inappropriate.

Participants also described learning about sexual caretaking at young ages, often from their mothers, who felt it was a duty they had to perform for their husbands and boyfriends. Maya describes learning about sexual carework from her mother early in life. Maya's mother told her that she did not enjoy sex, and that it was something that wives "just do" for their husbands, like a chore. She describes how her mother made it clear, when Maya was very young, that sex was never going to be something that she would enjoy, because most women just don't enjoy sex: "My mom made that very evident, that that was her experience, that *it was something that men liked to do; women don't like to do it.*" Jill also describes her experience with learning a woman's role in invisible sexual labor from her mother and illuminates her own experience of providing care for a father whom she felt conflicted about. Jill's mother told her how she never wanted to have sex with her own husband, Jill's father, and how she regretted that she had never had the chance to experiment sexually. Jill states that she thinks that this lack of sexual experimentation negatively influenced her mother's desire, and speculates that her mother "passed that trait on" to her:

> I don't know if that's why [I have low desire].... I think that maybe she just didn't have orgasms with my dad, and that's why she never wanted to have sex.... [S]he told me that she just never wanted him, she never wanted to be with him sexually.... I don't know if that affects me somehow.

Like Jill, Taja describes a complicated circumstance in which she not only learned about sexual caretaking from her mother, but also feels that she inherited some of her mother's experience of sexual trauma (even though Taja herself does not identify as a childhood sexual abuse survivor):

> I have trouble getting aroused all the time. I've pinpointed it as being about dissociation ... but I think it's also related to my mother's sexual trauma as a child. She was sexually abused, and I have had several shrinks tell me that I "think" [i.e., her body "thinks"] that I was abused, but it is purely that I absorbed all of this [trauma] from my mother. She imprinted on me in such a distinct way.... [S]he told me that men were not safe, she told me that I was never safe, she was always yelling my name, terrified that something had happened to me—she is a very anxious woman—I just inherited all of it.

Later in our interview, Taja describes how she had to balance this constant anxiety with a conflicting sense of being responsible for men's feelings and experiences, including sexually, which ultimately made extra work for her in her present-day life. It is important to recognize that these women do not identify as CSA survivors and all of them come from purportedly "intact" families and homes. Rose is the only one whose parents are divorced. These are women who learned unhappy lessons early on about relationships between men and women, and they describe how many of their expectations in this regard—which they learned from their fathers' persistence and/or their mothers' warnings—were borne out in their relationships with men as they progressed through life. Rather than pathologizing these specific parents as teaching their children antiquated or coercive lessons about sex, we might instead consider the framework within which little girls come to know themselves as affective providers and, ironically, as caretakers—for adult men—at such young ages, and in which at least some mothers teach their female children to guard their bodies, to protect themselves, and to consider "the sexual" as a realm that will never be fully theirs to inhabit.

"Men Only Want One Thing"

The low-desiring women I spoke with expressed their beliefs that dominant Western cultural expectations regarding men's and women's sexuality—or gendered assumptions about who sex is for, how it should be done, and why these ways are "natural"—are still rampant today. These participants—like Jill, Maya, and Taja cited in the previous section—stated that they learned at early ages that sex was not "for them," or at least, not for them to *enjoy*. They expressed that they had learned—not only from parents and caretakers but also in their schools, from their peers, and through media accounts and representations (including representations of scientific and medical research)—that, as women, their roles in sex would necessarily be fraught and ambivalent. They described conflicting messages around being encouraged to be sexy, voluptuous, and enticing, while at the same time being expected to guard against the advances of men—who "only want one thing." For these women, it is difficult to navigate this terrain and to find a place for one's own desire. Valdivia describes feeling confused about what her role in sex was to be as a young woman, as she was taught that women don't enjoy sex, but only "trade" it:

> I think we are taught to mask our sexuality, or to look at sex as something that you trade. You trade sex for respect or for dignity or for class position-

> ing or security. Sex is the price you pay to have someone who's going to respect you or be with you for the rest of your life. And [this idea has] never been able to account for the person that I am, which is someone who wants to be like, "You're hot, and hopefully you respect me ... that would be nice if you respected me, but ... you're hot!" ... [S]o my cultural education on sex has not only been extremely unscientific, oppressive, *but it's taken out desire,* it's taken sexuality out of the equation, it acknowledges sex as this thing that you have to keep safe because "men only want one thing from you." ... [T]hat's how I was raised, "men only want one thing" ... but it's like, "What if I want that thing, too? What if I only want that one thing? Then what?!"

In this statement, Valdivia highlights the notion that sex is constructed—through discourse and embodied learning and experience—as a realm for men, and a space that women are generally excluded from, unless they are playing a very specific role within the barter system. This notion rearticulates the tenets of the feminized responsive desire framework in which femininity operates in accordance with its own receptive logic—a logic in which women's desire is never a driving force on its own, and never sexual, per se. But Valdivia's narrative also makes it clear that she very much desires sex, and that she does not feel comfortable trading it in a system in which men are purported to "only want one thing." She does not desire sex on these terms, but she *does* experience a great deal of sexual desire. Her experience challenges the logic of medicalized feminine receptivity. Later in the interview, I ask Valdivia if she experiences desire in her current relationship (with a female partner), in light of her experience of self-identified low desire throughout her life. She is able to characterize her sexuality more clearly and explain how she thinks that cultural narratives about women serving men are perpetuated through sexual difference socialization processes (see chapter 3 of this book for more on this), and how they have affected her own sense of guilt and resentment around sex:

> I hate it when I feel like it's something I have to do. No one is forcing me, thankfully, but it's more like I have this internal thing that's like, "Well, you *should* have sex." ... I hate that. I try to be really cognizant of it, like "Why? Why should I?" But it's like, "It's been five days, your partner is going to feel bad." ... [L]uckily I date someone who doesn't take it personally. She'll be like, "I want you to touch me" and I'll be like, "I'm not feeling very sexy right now, sorry" and we'll cuddle, but I feel that's something I've never had before, the ability to be like, "Sorry, I just don't feel sexual." ... [I]n the past I've never felt able to say that because usually, specifically with guys, it would make me feel like I would lose their interest. Or because I'm negotiating sex

in exchange for your respect or your love, if I don't give you sex, then why would you stick around? So it's a nice thing that when I'm not feeling sexual, I get to negotiate that now.

Valdivia describes the internalized pressure she has always felt to have sex, even when she didn't want to or wasn't feeling "sexy," but states that she always succumbed out of fear of losing a partner's love or attention. This was a common theme expressed by many participants. Valdivia is currently dating a woman and feels that some of this pressure has been removed, but importantly, even in her current queer relationship, she hasn't been able to fully shake this narrative about women's roles in sexual carework—it is clear that a certain barter logic also extends beyond heterosexual relationships. She links it to being raised in a culture in which women are taught to "mask their sexuality" (she was raised in a Latinx American household but also states that she adopted potent ideas about sexuality in a hegemonic white US context) and also to admonitions she heard about sex from the woman who raised her, her primary caretaker, growing up:

> My primary female caretaker taught me to never depend on men because she was abandoned by her husband, and her way of surviving was to completely *forgo* men. . . . [T]he way she raised me was like, "You need to get an education, you need to work, don't depend on anyone, especially men!" It was this independent mentality tied in with like "because men only want one thing from you."

In this last passage, Valdivia expresses how she was taught to protect herself from men, and to live as independently as she can, as a mode of survival. Other participants, including Maya, describe how many young women are raised to believe this, often by mothers or other female caretakers who are framed as having had a different experience when they were coming of age, during a time when some women still had no choice but to be housewives, or were tied to men because of economic dependence. However, it is clear that the economic vulnerability of being a white housewife is very different from the financial precarity experienced by many women of color who have always had to work. The specific admonitions of Valdivia's caretaker (an immigrant woman of color) might offer a unique reading of how the "men only want one thing" logic operates differently for immigrant women, women of color, and poor women, or those from working-class backgrounds—with a focus on independence and self-sufficiency. This is consistent with Nelson, Cardemil, and Adeoye (2016) who illuminate how women of color are often socialized to be "strong" and "independent" in the face of widespread racism and sexism—and it is a theme that has been put forward by many women of color feminist theorists for decades (for one example, see Moraga & Anzaldúa, 2015, especially the essay "La Prieta" by Anzaldúa).

When I asked the participants about their current sex lives, most did not tell a story of complete liberation from some of the very pitfalls that Valdivia's caretaker described to her. It is also important to note that although Valdivia does not identify as a survivor of sexual abuse, she does experience regular harassment and verbal assault. Most of the women I spoke with had experienced some type of sexual abuse, assault, or other violent experiences at some point in their lives. This gendered violence—which spans a spectrum from quotidian microaggressions in the form of harassment, catcalling, and inappropriate touching to more extreme sexual violations, including child molestation and incest (described, for instance, by Fahs, 2016)—is clearly a variable that is correlated with "low desire," but it is unfortunately and shortsightedly a variable that is not often cited in mainstream clinical and experimental psychological literature on gender differences in sexual response.

"Doing It Anyway"

The women I spoke with for this study described how sometimes they would go through with sexual acts—including penetrative penile-vaginal intercourse—even when they did not want to (i.e., when they did not want to as a result of their own sexual desire for their partner). They cited many different reasons for this. As Valdivia alludes to in the passage above, a common reason is simply that they feel they *should,* that they are expected as women to perform sexually, and that they have known their whole lives that this expectation falls upon them. This is consistent with the findings of Cacchioni (2015), Labuski (2015), and Braksmajer (2017). Many low-desiring women initially had no explanation for why they engaged in sex even when they did not want to, many explained that they simply felt they "couldn't say no," and many did it for their partner's benefit or for "the good of the relationship." Importantly, these phenomena (and many of the reasons women report having sex) are also described by Basson (2000, 2001b, 2002) in the design of her circular sexual response cycle, further solidified in the receptivity criterion in the FSIAD diagnosis and in the feminized responsive desire framework more broadly. To restate one of the main premises of this book: While Basson and other sex researchers who study women's responsive desire usefully note this tendency that women have to engage in sex as a duty to the relationship, they do not critique it. Instead, they too often leave this discussion in the realm of the descriptive, and because of the presumed objectivity of contemporary sexual medicine and technoscientific explorations of sex more broadly, that description becomes a truth (women's desire is inherently more responsive than men's) and eventually a prescription (women ought to be responsive, and this is how they can enhance their receptivity). So, while this service orientation to sex may be true of many women—and I agree with Basson and others that it is—I want to consider *why* some women have this orientation to sex so as to explicitly denaturalize it, and to consider where it comes from, why it is not necessarily good for women, and how we can rethink treatments for low desire in light of it. In the absence of this rethinking, I argue that *description is violence*. The stories of the women in this chapter bring home the gravity of the need to rethink the feminized responsive desire framework, and they illustrate how the mandate of feminine receptivity is particularly pernicious when it is codified in purportedly "apolitical," "atheoretical" medical and scientific discourse.

On this point, when I ask Sadie if her partners had ever experienced her low desire, interest, or arousal as a problem, she tells me: "I don't think they ever noticed. Meaning that I was having sex with them [anyway] . . . they thought everything was all good." Annie similarly states:

> There have been times that I kind of just did it to please my partner, and I feel like there have been times where they have been able to get off and be okay with it and I'm just kind of like, "Aah, I'm not really that into this . . ." And it's a little distressing sometimes, you know, having sex when you're not really super into it. . . . [T]here have been times that are sort of like in that middle space . . . where I sort of just dissociate a little bit, and I'm just like, "Okay, this is happening, and that's fine, and great, and . . . it's done."

Here, Annie's story throws into critical relief the assumptions of the circular sexual response cycle and the incentive-motivation model as these are embedded in the FSIAD diagnosis as part of the feminized responsive desire framework. At least in some cases, when women are in that receptive, responsive, "middle space" of "sexual neutrality" (in which they are said to be easily swayed into being sexual by a partner—if they are sexually functional as women, that is), they never do get to a place of full-on desire, arousal, or enjoyment (as the circular sexual response cycle would suggest). In some cases, they may continue to participate in an act simply because they have already started, and they feel like it would take too much energy to stop. This is the ugly side of feminized responsive desire—wherein these response models do not make sense for some low-desiring women, and become, instead, a prescription for coercion (or, at the very least, a prescription for mediocre and service-oriented sex). Rather than rocking the boat, or disrupting the moment, many of the women I spoke with dissociate and continue to "go through the motions." Rose gives an example of what this might look like:

> The problem is, I have sex when I don't want to. The guy that I dated last year, at one point I said, "Why is it that we automatically have sex like every time we hang out?" And I think it totally caught him off guard and he was like, "Well if you don't want to, we don't have to . . ." but I had also been on certain occasions like, I did not really want to—he had a friend over once who was sleeping in the living room, and I was like, "I don't really want to have sex right now because your friend is in the living room," but he like kept pushing it and I just kind of went along with it.

And Molly, a survivor of childhood sexual abuse, makes the problem particularly clear. She describes how she sometimes has sex with men to make them happy, to placate them, or because she is afraid that if she says no their "feelings will be hurt." She links this inability to tell her partners what she wants (or doesn't want) to her experience of sexual trauma, and describes certain present-day experiences as a form of retraumatization. When I ask her if any of her partners have experienced her low desire as a problem, she tells me a story about her experience of performing sexualized labor when she was working at the beach one summer:

> I don't think so, because even when I have no desire, I still have sex with them. I have never said no to sex. So I'm sure from their perspective it's not really an issue. . . . [T]here was this one time, when I was younger, I was hooking up with this really hot guy, we went down to the beach and had sex, and he came, and I did not, and then I gave him a blow job and he came again, and I still had not come, and he was like, "Oh thanks, I really needed that!" and he was done, and that was it. And he was like, "So, should I walk you back to your house?" and I was just like, "What?!" . . . [B]ut there is somehow this idea that women exist to service their needs, and our needs don't even register a lot of the time. . . . I felt like, "Wow, I am just a stress reliever for you! Thanks!" [laughs sarcastically]

Molly paints a complicated picture of the sexual terrain in which mutuality, consent, desire, and pleasure must be navigated—or, in which they are not always adequately navigated—at each and every sexual encounter. Unfortunately, what she suggests is that the intersubjective context of sexual relations is sometimes not given adequate attention, and rather than mutuality being actualized, one person functions to serve another's needs. It is important to recognize that this is not a clearly coercive situation; it is not the case that these low-desiring women are being actively violated or abused, but rather, that long-held assumptions—and traumas—have become so deeply ingrained that some of these women are left feeling voiceless, unimportant within, and ultimately detached, disconnected, and dissociated from certain sexual experiences.

Many of the women I spoke with did not feel voiceless, though, and clearly articulated why they chose to have sex, in spite of their lack of desire. Some participants described this in terms of feeling like they wanted to make their partners happy, or because performing this work was their responsibility. DeVault (1991) highlights how other forms of gendered carework, including food preparation and provision, are perceived as a responsibility that women feel they have (often to their cis male partners, and to their families). The notions that much of this gendered labor is paradoxically invisible yet highly necessary to the functioning of a cisheteropatriarchal white supremacist capitalist society, and that it is naturalized as feminine, are similar themes in DeVault's work on women's caretaking and in my own conceptualizations of sexual carework here (and its concerted, thoughtful, and intellectual enactment on the part of the feminized laborers). It is important to note that all of this work also indirectly results in surplus value, and thus services capital. Jill explicates this perspective of performing sexually because she feels it is her feminine responsibility, but one that she chooses to enact only for specific partners:

> It was like a chore for me, to have sex, and I was staying at his apartment a lot and I was just thinking, "I would rather be at my place with my computer, with my book, or hanging out with my friends rather than hanging out with him," so I decided that I can live without him as a boyfriend. . . . [B]ut I was in a relationship with one guy, a very successful guy, but I never told him "I don't want to have sex tonight" because he did a lot of things for me, he bought me a lot of stuff, we were traveling, we did a lot of cool things, and I thought, "Well he's doing so much stuff for me, I could definitely have sex with him and not reject him, even though I don't want to [have sex]" . . . like a favor. And it worked for some period. . . . I did not enjoy myself that much, but I was like, "It's only fifteen minutes, it's only twenty minutes, half an hour, and then that's it!" and he's happy, and then he makes me feel happy. . . . [B]ut with just *regular* guys, I would rather say, "No, I just don't want to."

In this statement, Jill articulates how sexual carework is something she sometimes provides, but only to very special (in this case, "successful") men, to partners that she cares about, and whom she really wants to make happy. This experience is complicated for her by the fact that—at least in the situation she describes above—some of these special men also provide for her financially. Her comments are reminiscent of Valdivia's thoughts on women trading sex for security, respect, and class positioning, although her perspective on this is not a critical one. Regarding feeling like she needs to have sex to make her husband happy, Penelope states:

> I instigate it sometimes, but sometimes it's just because I feel like, "God, we haven't had sex in a while, I feel like we need to, so I need to instigate this."
> ... I think for him it is not that satisfying because it doesn't last that long but I'm like, "Okay, good, you came."

Penelope makes it clear that it is not just her husband's expectations of her, but also social expectations that compel her to have sex with him: the feeling that it's "been too long—we *should* have sex." Penelope's statement is in line with Valdivia's thoughts on her responsibility in terms of sexual frequency to her partner, articulated above. Corinne states that she feels the need to fulfill "her end of the bargain" in her marriage, and Elaine likewise describes her sense of sexual responsibility to her husband, linking it to her religious identity and beliefs:

> If I can just get interested *enough,* then he can kind of just do it, and that doesn't sound very nice but on some level I do feel—and this is going to sound negative but it's not—or at least not in my sort of world view—that I do have an *obligation* to provide my husband with a certain amount of sexual satisfaction, I believe that is part of my sort of Christian worldview and I don't think that's demeaning. I just think that's part of the agreement. And if I can just—it comes to the point where my feeling is, "If I can just get interested *enough* . . ." then we can have a sexual experience, and it's not too fraught, it's not *horribly* uncomfortable. . . . [B]ut that's the thing that I really have the trouble with . . . just raising that interest sufficiently to sort of go through with it.

Penelope, Elaine, Corinne, and Maya all describe feeling pressures to have sex—either to fulfill their "wifely duties," to make their partners happy, or because of more abstract reasons such as societal expectations placed on women to please men, or in line with the notion that "that's what happy couples do." These normative conceptions about sexual frequency and quality—or injunctions or imperatives to have great sex and lots of orgasms—is something many participants discussed. But what is striking about the four women mentioned above is that although they express experiencing low desire with their partners, and feel like they have to really push themselves to get "interested enough to go through with it," they also describe having an abundance of intense, free-flowing, and even spontaneous sexual desire in other contexts and moments in their lives and/or for other people. These women's stories also illustrate my concerns regarding nonconsent and the feminized responsive desire framework, and suggest that tuning into the aroused body and tapping into "responsive desire" is not the answer for many women with low desire. But these narratives also raise the question: If the problem is interpersonal and structural rather than individual and medical, how can it be fixed?

"Faking It" and Affective Performances of Pleasure

Many of the women I spoke with explained how they labor affectively to perform a certain kind of sexual pleasure for their partners. Rather than just providing pleasure in the form of servicing their partners' bodies, they instead talk about how they work to produce an experience that feels authentic. According to them, this notion of authenticity is crucial to successful sex, yet it is an experience that can be difficult to create, particularly in light of conflicting ideas about women's roles in sex (the familiar virgin/whore dichotomy outlined initially by Freud). My analysis of "faking it" here resonates with Duncombe and Marsden's (1996) theorization of "deep acting," Cacchioni's (2015) extension of this into what she calls "performance work," and Fahs's (2011) description of how women use their bodies and voices to make the role more "convincing." Molly states that she does her best to "play the part":

> ALYSON: So when you're having sex with these men, sometimes maybe you're doing it just because you are not saying no?
> MOLLY: Yes, and secretly planning my Christmas shopping list in my head! [laughter]
> ALYSON: Are you acting like you are into it?
> MOLLY: Yeah, sometimes. I'm so worried about them feeling bad, that a lot of times I think I just go along with it.... I definitely don't just *lay* there, doing the 1950s housewife kind of thing. [i.e., she performs an experience of sexual pleasure]

Some participants who described performing pleasure for the benefit of their partners also characterized their agreement to engage in sex with their partners at all as a performative act of reassurance involving considerable embodied and affective labor. Regina describes sex with some of her long-term partners as a constant source of conflict, in large part because for her, intercourse tended to be painful, and doing it was something she avoided. She explains how this ambivalent situation became particularly problematic with one partner after an alleged episode in which she cheated on him at the beginning of the relationship (in her view, they were not yet officially together and thus it wasn't cheating), and then she felt like she had to constantly "make it up to him" or "reassure him"—including by having sex with him when she didn't want to:

> I wouldn't want to [have sex], so I would never initiate it, and then I would go along with it sometimes, and then feel bad and not want to, so then try to make it be a little bit longer before I *gave in* the next time. I remember having a conversation with [him] like, "You have no idea what it's like to feel like not wanting to sleep with someone but feeling like you have to and doing it anyways. How can we even be having this conversation when you have no idea what that feels like?!"

Maya expresses a similar sentiment regarding feeling like she has to reassure her husband that she loves him by having sex with him, even though she generally does not enjoy the act itself and also finds intercourse painful. She laments the lack of passion in her sex life with her husband but feels conflicted, because she also deeply cares for him, and wants to make him happy. She articulates how part of the "marital contract" includes not only having sex when she doesn't want to, but doing it in a way that makes it seems like she does, in fact, enjoy it—via an affective performance of pleasure:

> Apparently, the other night I let out an exasperated sigh, and he was destroyed! This poor man, I feel for him, he is not unattractive, he's not uncaring, he is a wonderful human being, but I cannot bring myself to be interested! I feel bad and that's why I often have sex just to be like, "Oh, poor guy, let me make him feel like I love him," but oftentimes I really do just feel like, "Oh god, really?! It is 10:30, I am tired!" And it's not just me *pretending* to be tired—sex requires *mental* energy, too! It's like, "What am I doing, how do I please this person, am I acting like I care?" In order to coexist—and we do love each other—so to make that work better, I feel like it is one of the things I have to get myself to accept. Because it is part of the bargain.

For Maya, this performance of pleasure and her experience of the embodied and affective carework that she provides are very fraught. She feels ambivalent about the role she plays in her marriage. On the one hand, she loves her husband and honestly does want to make him happy—that is something that she desires. She also desires to hold up "her end of the bargain"—she feels that she agreed to be sexually intimate with her husband for life and wants to fulfill that agreement. But she also feels that there is an imbalance in the relationship because she does not derive pleasure from the type of sex her husband wants to have:

> If there is no physical pleasure, there is no incentive to do it, it's all one-sided, I'm not getting—why would I go through the motions, if I'm not having pleasure? I really despise this idea of marriage as a sexual contract, you just do it and you fake it, and that's part of life as well as baking cookies.... [S]o if there's nothing in it for me, I don't like this idea of me always *giving* just to please him.

Comparing the above two passages illuminates Maya's ambivalence—as much as she loves her husband and is thus willing to care for him sexually, she also can't help but feel resentful toward him at times, as she feels the deal is so "one-sided." Labuski (2015) also found that women who experience pain with intercourse still had sex with their partners—with mixed affects. Sometimes they engaged in intercourse to solidify their feminine heterosexual identities (and counter the idea that they weren't "real" women—also described by Ayling & Ussher, 2008 and Kaler, 2006) or to please a partner—but they often resented their partners while doing so. This theme of a deeply rooted psychic and embodied ambivalence around sex is a common theme in my research with low-desiring women, as in Labuski's work with women who experienced sexual pain, including vulvodynia, and it also appears in Cacchioni's (2015) analysis of the conflicted place that women who feel compelled to have sex in spite of pain—who "stick it out" (p. 88)—find themselves in.

Valdivia discusses "faking it" as well, and explains how women are caught in a double bind regarding their affective sexual performances. She explains how women are "demonized" for faking it (orgasm), but are simultaneously and paradoxically *expected* to perform pleasure:

> People really demonize women who fake it. They put you in a place where you are like "dishonest," you are a bad person. There was a time where mainstream media talked a lot about faking it, and I remember it really touching a part of me, because I was like, "*I* fake it . . ." And I didn't fake it because I

was trying to deceive anyone, I think I faked it because I thought something was wrong with me . . . because I couldn't get off.

Valdivia explains here how she also faked it because she felt abnormal for not enjoying sex more—in this case, penile-vaginal intercourse with cis men. She states that she performed in this way not only to please her partners, but because she thought that she should be experiencing that same kind of pleasure herself.[3] She goes on to explain how she eventually learned that other types of sex with different partners would offer her more pleasure, and this allowed to her to stop feeling compelled to fake it:

> I feel like sometimes we treat people who fake it in an unfair way. I think we are told that all you need is a dick, and then the dick is in you and you have this really incredible communion with this person, and you sigh a lot, and then some kind of music happens, and then you come together! Or at least that's what movies have told me . . . but that's what movies *tell* you! And that's what I thought was going to happen. . . . [I]t was either that, or like [it is in] really bad porn. . . . I thought that one of those two things was going to happen for me, and neither happened!

In this quote, Valdivia explains that she "faked it" because she thought something was wrong with her for not having orgasms from the kind of penetrative heterosexual sex she had experienced up to that point with cis male partners. She explains that she always thought that she should be able to enjoy sex in the same way that her male partners did, because of portrayals of sex in movies and porn—the main type of "sex education" most participants say they received (especially those who grew up in the US). It wasn't until she determined that *sex takes work* in order to be enjoyable that she was able to really "get off" and finally be in a place to stop faking it—which she had done for so long in the hope that something would ultimately fall into place and allow sex to become pleasurable for her (the way it appears to be in movies and pornography). What does it mean that the solution to low desire is to realize that sex

---

3. Jagose (2013) describes the "counterdisciplinary" potential of fake orgasm as "an innovative sexual practice that makes available a mode of feminine self-production in a constrained field of possibility" (p. 196). I find this interpretation provocative in that it challenges the normative impulse to "authentic" sexual experience and reveals disciplinary aspects, particularly within the broader field of cis/heterosexuality. But for the participants in this study who "faked it," even though fake orgasm may have operated as a practice of self-production and thus offered a certain kind of control or agency, it was contoured by their deep disappointment with heterosex (at least in their lives at the time of the interviews). They seemed to have less (cruel) optimism about heterosexuality than Jagose might expect, then.

takes work? How might we understand this type of work as being far different from sexual carework as it has been described thus far? And if mindfulness-based sex therapy also constitutes a type of sexual carework, how and why has this work become so feminized and individualized?

Other women discuss what happens when it is impossible to fake it, including the deleterious effects this impossibility can have on a relationship. Zola describes how, when she was depressed, she could not muster the affect that her husband ultimately seemed to need her to mobilize when they had sex:

> ZOLA: He would complain all the time and I would just be like, "If you want to have sex, go find somebody to have sex with!" and he would be like, "I don't want to have sex with anybody else, I want to have sex with you!" And I'd be like, "Well, I don't want to have sex. I am not feeling it. I'll do it if you want me to do it, but I just don't feel like it," and he would be like, "I want you to be into it, I don't want you to just feel obligated because you are my wife," and I would be like, "Well, that's how I feel. I don't want to touch you, I don't want to be touched, but I will sit through it, I will let you do whatever you are going to do so you can get your rocks off, and I can go to sleep, or finish my day, or do whatever it is . . ." and so that used to be a big problem for him.
> ALYSON: When you would have sex, did he know that you were not into it?
> ZOLA: Oh yeah.
> ALYSON: But he would do it anyway?
> ZOLA: Yes, we would have sex anyway.

All of these stories suggest that both women and men are led to believe that sex should be "easy," that it should come naturally, that it should not require any time or work or effort, and that somehow, all of this magic will happen from penile-vaginal intercourse alone (this is consistent with many of Tiefer's critiques, for instance in Tiefer, 1995). What these low-desiring women describe is all the (ideally mutual and reciprocal) time and work and effort it actually takes to make this event happen, and how they feel that the labor is, in practice, often one-sided; they perform and tend to the occasion, whereas they feel that their (cis male) partners often do not put in as much effort. Importantly, the sexual landscape these women illuminate is not something that is the effect of "natural kinds" of desire; it cannot be reduced to the interplay between an innate biological male drive to have sex and an innate biological female drive to care or be empathetic—or, in line with the feminized responsive desire framework, to be receptive. Instead, what is being described is an aspect of sexual difference socialization (discussed in chapter 3), in which women have been taught to play a certain role and take up a certain share of the work, whereas men are generally taught to have expectations regarding their own pleasure and that these expectations will be met.

Feminized Sexual Carework beyond the Bedroom

Masculinity requires its own type of labor in terms of performance (Murray, 2019), but here, I want to put forward the notion that sex requiring work is a given, that it is (or should be) obvious, and I want to focus specifically on the feminized side of this sexual division of labor. According to Penelope: "We [women] are not taught to go out and get a bunch of men, we are taught to attract them and do things that make us attractive to them, we are taught to love and take care of them." This eloquent statement sums up the feminization of sexual carework that these low-desiring women experience. Penelope's statement also suggests that sexual carework, the invisible embodied labor that is also always affective and performative, often extends to the entire relationship, family, and home, for women. The participants that I interviewed often grappled actively with the heavy burden of the intimate labor that they know falls on their backs as feminine subjects. On this point, Ava states:

> In my relationships, I'm very much a caretaker, I buy people meals, I buy them presents, if they're sick I make them soup. In my past relationships that's put me at a disadvantage. . . . I've always been really submissive in my sexual and personal life—whereas in my public life, like in school and with friends, I'm very loud, people know me as kind of assertive, I'm a bitch, I say what's on my mind, and I stand up for what I believe in, so there are these two very different sides of me depending on whether I'm in an intimate relationship with someone or if I'm not.

In this passage, Ava explains how she enjoys caring for her partners, but also feels like she has to keep her guard up, lest she be taken advantage of by men who expect her to perform sexual and relational carework out of obligation, or to play a certain role to accommodate them. Elaine also discusses the work that she does for her husband (and plans to do in the future) within the context of their sexual relationship, but in this account, it doesn't concern his sexual pleasure, specifically. In her case, having children will be part of the (reproductive) responsibility she enacts to care for her husband, an obviously feminized form of care:

I am ambivalent [about having kids], but my husband really wants to, and so we're negotiating that terrain right now, but realistically we will have them in the next year and a half to two years. . . . [H]e comes from a family of four children and all of his aunts and uncles have multiple—it's just a big—it's important to him.

Ava, Elaine, and other participants describe their intimate relationship to cultural narratives about women's responsibility to engage in carework, and the ways in which it is sexualized but also extends to other domestic duties within families and households. This work has been *responsibilized* (Cossman, 2007; Murphy, 2012) in a managerial sense—the burden of intimate maintenance is pushed on to women, who become sexual, sensual, and affective managers of the home. As this work is also part of social reproduction (and sexual reproduction, in Elaine's case), it is useful to consider all of these different forms of work as part of a kind of feminized affective labor—around which the women I interviewed felt much ambivalence. This affective labor can also be linked to the feminized responsive desire framework: If women are consistently framed as responsive and receptive, it makes sense that they would feel ambivalence around providing care. There is a paradox here, as a type of *activity* is mandated within this *receptivity*—feminine responsiveness becomes work in itself that is both naturalized and prescribed. Women are expected to open up in an active way, a way that entails work, and thus a deep ambivalence runs through the experience of performing feminized affective labors—from sexual carework to other forms of social reproduction—as these fit within the essentialized logic of feminine responsiveness.

Carework as Coercion

In the most extreme and troubling cases of women performing sexual carework in domestic relationships, low-desiring women have sex because their partners materially and economically support them, because their partners are coercing them, or because they feel they have no choice but to have sex. Astrid explains how she felt compelled to sexually perform for her ex-husband, because she was so young when they were married, and because she was completely dependent on him:

> I had sex because he wanted to have sex. That was it. From the very beginning of our relationship . . . sex was what I did to make myself useful, or like worthy of that [his economic support], I guess? Because we did get together

when I was so young, and I like moved in with him while I was still in high school and stuff. . . . [A]nd yeah, I guess, I felt like sex was kind of like—sex was something that I did as a trade-off for benefits I got in our relationship, like he paid our rent, he paid for our groceries, things I did in return were I made him dinner and I let him fuck me. Like, that was my role, you know? So yeah, like when I became sexually nonviable [because of sexual pain], I had to deal with it, right? Like, I mean, there was no alternative to that. *I wasn't of any use if I couldn't have sex.*

In this quote, the fraught terrain around consent and coercion that many participants describe becomes disturbingly stark. Although Astrid's example is not representative of the type of sexual carework most of the women I spoke with performed on a regular basis, it is still a deeply disconcerting example of how this type of care sometimes manifests as particularly coercive and violent—specifically within a system in which women are configured as naturally or essentially receptive and responsive, and in which men are configured as "only wanting one thing" in a way and to a degree that is beyond their control.

The Biopolitics of Sexual Carework: Medicine, Science, Therapy, Capital

One way sexual carework protocols become feminized in the present day is through medical and scientific discourses that perpetuate notions of female sexual responsiveness, receptivity, flexibility, and fluidity. This is specifically apparent in some of the contemporary clinical and experimental psychology research, diagnoses, and treatment protocols that I analyzed in chapters 1, 2, and 3. The medicalization and feminization of receptivity—including the widespread notions that women "just don't really like sex" or that they are "hard to get off"—are questioned by some of the clinicians I interviewed and also by low-desiring women themselves. Betsy, the director of a holistic clinic that treats women with low desire, tells me that many doctors (doctors who are not associated with her clinic) seem to expect women to "grin and bear it" when they have pain or discomfort during intercourse—a common problem among the low-desiring women I interviewed:

[At the medical center, we would tell women:] "We're going to put you on the following medications to see if we can get your body in better shape, and we're going to see you in a month or two. . . . [O]nce we feel like your body is a little bit more responsive, then we'll say, 'Okay, now we want you to try these sensate focus exercises, we want to schedule sex with you and your husband, we want to introduce specific sexual activities.'" If you try to introduce those sex therapy activities when a woman's body is not ready for that, that's just like, it's so enraging, when the woman says, "I don't have any desire!" and the doctor says, "Oh, just do it!" like "Take one for the team!"

Betsy expresses her frustration over this type of treatment model, which she describes as antiquated and misogynistic, but which she says is unfortunately still prevalent in sexual medicine. For instance, pop therapist Michele Weiner-Davis made the case that low-desiring women should "just do it"—have sex for the sake of their marriages—in her 2003 best seller *The Sex-Starved Marriage*. In making this argument for what she calls "Nike sex," she cites Basson's circular sexual response cycle as a way for women to achieve this, and as a reason why it should be easy for women to do this (a point also noted by Cacchioni, 2015). The fact that this mentality is still alive and well is further instantiated by Astrid, who experiences pain on penetration along with low desire and who previously sought medical treatment (at the behest of her partner) to help her deal with these issues:

> One of the gynecologists I saw literally said, "Put this anesthetic cream on a cotton ball and put it into your vagina ten minutes before you have sex so then you don't feel it," and I was like, "Um, but what's the point of sex then?" and he was like, "Well, what do you mean?" He just didn't understand how that was weird, to like numb all feeling before you have sex!

The women I spoke with who had been treated in medical therapeutic programs for sexual pain and low desire had many specific critiques of this type of program and associated treatments—including those that were arguably oriented toward enhancing female receptivity and responsiveness. Kelly, who had been enrolled in one of these treatment programs, expresses similar concerns around the medical treatment of vaginal pain, and questions for whom the remedies are actually designed:

> KELLY: It was kind of weird—because it wasn't supposed to have anything to do with sexuality, it was just like, "When you are reading your book, put this thing in" [here, she is referring to a vaginal dilator], just to kind of get your vagina used to having something in there. . . . [I]t was awkward and strange.
> ALYSON: Did they ever actually say, "This is so that you can continue to have sex with your boyfriend?"

KELLY: Not outright. But . . . that's sort of where it was going. . . . [T]he only reason I could think of is so that I would still be able to have [penetrative] sex *even though I didn't want to.*

All of these examples show how women experiencing low desire and pain—specifically if it interferes with their ability to be penetrated—becomes framed as *a problem for men* within dominant medical and therapeutic paradigms. Similar to the findings of Kaler (2006) and Labuski (2015), my research suggests that, in certain medical treatment programs, women are taught how to use their bodies for sexualized service. And here is where the older (liberal capitalist) form of work and the newer (biopolitical) form bleed into each other—in both instances, the work is about heteronormativity and service, but the newer version is also about the purported *self*-care benefits of experiencing this type of responsive femininity (i.e., service to oneself, partner, family, and even the broader population in the name of "therapy"). In this way, more traditional heteronormative medical frameworks provide the foundation for the biopolitics of sexual carework. At the time of their enrollment in the program, neither Kelly nor Astrid was interested in having penetrative intercourse with their male partners. Yet, in the program, it was always assumed that part of their treatment for low desire would include maintaining the ability to engage in heterosexual penile-vaginal intercourse—and both Kelly and Astrid stated that no clinician ever asked them how they identified sexually or if, how, or with whom they liked to have sex.

It is not only within clinical medicine and therapy that these imperatives to feminine receptivity and their linkage to sexual carework surface; these norms circulate in alternative healing and educational spaces as well. In fact, in a "biomedical" (Clarke et al., 2003) milieu, wherein medicalization becomes neoliberal *self*-medicalization and enhancement, these alternative wellness spaces are where we see the biopolitics of feminized sexual carework really take shape. I interviewed a small number of women who worked in sex toy stores that sold products and also held workshops designed to enhance desire and sexual pleasure. Amelia describes what it was like to work in such a space, and how she felt about leading workshops:

AMELIA: I didn't realize that the content of the workshops that I would be leading would be all male-centered. I had an understanding of [the store] that I think was something different.
ALYSON: But why were those the ones you would be teaching?
AMELIA: Because those were the ones that were repeated with the most frequency. They were the ones that brought in the money. We had work-

shops about BDSM bondage rope-tying stuff but we'd get five people, whereas "How to Please Your Man" and "How to Give a Blow Job" routinely sold out. There was another one called "How to Please Your Woman" and we *never* sold out of that one [laughing].... I thought the workshops I was going to be teaching were going to be for women—'cuz that's what I thought [the store]'s modus operandi was, that's what I thought the store was *about* ... but it wasn't necessarily—not because [the store] philosophically isn't about that but because that's not what *sold.*

Amelia describes how even at a purportedly sex-positive, feminist sex toy store, women still took up the bulk of the work of making sex pleasurable—for themselves *and* their partners—whereas heterosexual cis men routinely did not take such an interest. Notably, the workshop leaders themselves were also most often femme-identified, nonbinary, or genderqueer, so the educational labor was also less likely to be performed by cishet men. Here, the relationship between sexual production and consumption is worth examining in its own right.[4]

Linking this heterosexual imperative (Gavey, 2005; Loe, 2004) with feminine receptivity under protocols of capacitation (Puar, 2017) and within regimes of sexual citizenship (Cossman, 2007), it is also illustrative to analyze some of the data I gathered from Celeste, a yogic, tantric, meditation-based, and spiritual healer who focused on sexual enhancement techniques designed to increase desire and pleasure, primarily for women. Celeste expressed particularly strong views of the plight of women's sexuality in our current moment. She explained to me that women's desires are being dampened by too much work outside of the home, and too much alienation from their innate feminine sexual energy. In Celeste's view,

Men evolve and grow spiritually and emotionally by ordeal, by going out into battle. Women grow by being adored. Women need to be worshipped.... [W]hen the woman is happy, the whole *household* is happy. When the woman is *not* happy, in a household with family, with kids, if the woman is bitter and resentful and dried up and stressed out, *everybody* suffers! When the woman is soft and open, and enjoying life, everybody feels that around her! That's what I always say to the women in my training—that is *women's work.* Forget about whether or not it's supposed to be women in the kitchen

---

4. Comella (2017) elaborates the capitalist tensions involved in running a sex-positive feminist business, and similarly speaks to the difficulty of navigating the heterosexist demand involved in programming.

or whatever—it's women's work to be sensual and to be in love with life, and then everybody benefits from that! . . . So that is what my work is, it's helping women to realize how high the stakes are. This is not just about, "Oh, reclaim a great sexual relationship"—this is your *life!* This is the life of the *planet!* The same thing that is happening to us, it's happening to the planet, we are burning it up!!!

Here, Celeste links the gendered provision of sexual carework to women's sensual nature and natural receptivity and makes a case for the feminine duty to provide not only a comfortable home but a type of cosmic equilibrium. She goes on to state: "Women are so stressed and pulled in every direction, we have no time to be voluptuous. And I mean that in the sense of just voluptuous, soft and pleasurable, and loving life. *That's the woman's job.*"

It is imperative to highlight Celeste's words here next to the words of participants who spoke in the previous section about the carework they perform "beyond the bedroom," in their relationships more broadly, and to interrogate the feminization of this relational work. Celeste's framing of the feminine responsibility to not only be sexually receptive but to be "voluptuous," "soft," and "pleasurable," and implicitly to be sensual, empathetic, responsive to others, and nurturing—while making this entire production appear carefree and natural—clearly resonates with many of the women I spoke with. But many of these low-desiring women did not see carework—sexual or otherwise—as a naturally ordained feminine duty, and it was something they felt much ambivalence around (even when it involved caring for people they loved).

Celeste describes this feminine sexual responsibility in terms of maintaining a certain kind of energy, sensuality, voluptuousness, and capaciousness—something that women in our contemporary society have lost because they do not have time to be "in love with life." When I ask Celeste to describe how this energy imbalance affects women and their families, she explains: "Really, what that translates into is that we don't get to indulge in those feminine pleasures anymore. Those are the societal pressures, and that's what I meant when I said that *it's up to women to be that way.* Because men *biologically* won't indulge in that." Here, again, Celeste encourages us to consider that women's capacity to be so nurturing is founded in an innate biological drive to conviviality, and further prescribes the feminine duty or responsibility to not only sexually satisfy one's partner but to sexually satisfy one*self*—"to love life"—in order to provide a happy home, to create a welcoming and hospitable environment in a relationship and for one's family, and, potentially, to save the planet. Celeste thus illuminates a different kind of sexual carework—a type of work that is the product of biopolitical imperatives under neoliberalism; her narrative spells out the mandate toward pleasure, or the work of self-care, self-optimization, self-capacitation, and ultimately of self-valorization, in bluntly gendered terms. If we link this back to the way carework was discussed earlier in the chapter in regard to race and class, locating it within white supremacist and colonialist capitalism, and also consider its cultural feminist underpinnings within contemporary feminist psychology today (discussed in chapter 3), it is easy to see how this biopolitical framework will affect different populations very differently. Which women will be able to *afford* to optimize? Which will be accepted into the valorized fold? Which will be excluded based on race, class, nationality, disability, or their status as genderqueer, nonconforming, or trans, before they even get to the capacitation/debility threshold? Who will be expected to labor in the older service-oriented way, while simultaneously still being held to the standards of self-optimization under a regime of "voluptuous" femininity?

Capacitating Femininity

Sexual carework, as part of an embodied and affective system of invisible labor performed within intimate settings, including the home, is a complex enactment. The low-desiring women I spoke with were well aware of the "stakes" of reclaiming their "natural" feminine energy—the receptive responsibility that has been prescribed to them through scientific and psychomedical discourses, sex therapy, popular culture and media accounts, and now via alternative, holistic, and "Eastern" medicine, or yogic and tantric healing protocols. Narratives and expectations about how great sex can be—or should be—inform women's desires to engage in sexual acts just as much as "wanting to get off" (or to get someone else off) affects their desires to engage. And it is unsurprising that some women, particularly the low-desiring participants I interviewed, feel that the sexual labor dynamics in their own households or intimate relationships are fraught and one-sided (this might be especially unsurprising when those relationships are with cis men, for all of the reasons I have outlined above). Narratives about women's inherent drive to be sensual, the feminized requirement to produce an embodied and affective ambiance in a sexual relationship, and the notion that women have a responsibility to be responsive and receptive are found in diverse discourses and domains in our contemporary world—even when there is so much apparent sexual freedom. This circulation itself undoubtedly influences women's desire—or lack thereof.

In light of the turn in queer and biopolitical theory to reexamine bodies as information (Clough, 2007, 2018; Terranova, 2004), which make up populations produced and managed through (self-)governing modalities and citizenship regimes, it is imperative to continue to consider how the "old" categories of gender, sexuality, race, and labor are reinvented in a neoliberal context. It is important for queer theorists, feminists, critical theorists of race, and disability scholars and activists to consider the biopolitical productions, structures of regulatory control, and possibilities for transgression within these regimes that are characterized by a sexual imperative to pleasure, but gendered and racialized affective labor must be attended to as well—as there is a very specific version of white receptive feminine pleasure mandated in the biopolitical carework protocol I identify. This feminine pleasure is part of an apparatus in which participation in sex becomes bound up with sexual citizenship. In this context, female sexual refusal becomes not only a barrier to full citizenship, but refusing feminine subjects (or even *potentially* refusing feminine subjects) run the risk of being posited as intransigent, as debilitated, of being counted as "killjoys" (Ahmed, 2010), or as a population to be worked upon, to be made more productive, more capacitated, more capacious—always already asymptotically closer to seamless self-governability, self-appreciation, and self-valorization. This feminine capaciousness (and here, I am not only talking about sexual receptivity but about feminine hospitality more broadly) has a special relationship to the biopolitical mandate of sexual optimization, as feminine receptivity is an essential aspect of neoliberal governance strategies of rejuvenation and reinvigoration—not only of the feminized subject, but of the larger populations to which she is held responsible. The receptive feminine citizen will not only rejuvenate and reinvigorate herself, according to these mandates, it is her duty to rejuvenate and reinvigorate the world. As the words of my participants—first and foremost, Celeste—and these accompanying biomedical, therapeutic, and popular discourses suggest, feminine receptivity offers the promise of unification, of harmony, of solidification—of the (cishet romantic) relationship, the (nuclear) family, the (bourgeois) community, and the socius or species body at large. Thus, the woman who refuses receptivity is herein produced as not only an enemy of mankind—she is an enemy of The State. She is an enemy of humanity itself, of democracy, freedom, and progress. Here, feminine capacity/debility take on a specific tenor and weight, and they expand and extend well beyond the bedroom. This particular white-hetero-cis-gendered version of the sexual imperative also shores up the specter of that old liberal concept, what Marxist feminists call social reproduction, or the unpaid labor of care, of pleasure, of happiness—both the mandate to please others and the mandate to please oneself—which are so invaluable to capital today. If neoliberalism has indeed collapsed the space between private and public, spirit and market, reproduction and production, as Feher (2009, 2018) suggests—so that we are all self-governing nodes within ever-productive populations—what can we say about this mandate to sexual receptivity and its white, bourgeois, hetero, and cis gendered prescriptions? Further: What regimes of capacitation do we have in store for us as we trudge forward through late capitalism? What new forms of husbandry are on the horizon as we move into a moment in which various sexual and nonsexual desires and pleasures are prescribed and proscribed, according to affective delimiting within populations, but also sharply in "real live" sexual scenes?

During the course of our time together, Astrid revealed to me that after finishing the treatment program for low-desiring women with sexual pain, she finally left her husband, started having sex with women, and embraced a queer and genderqueer/nonconforming identity. Within a paradigm that explicitly links feminine competence with receptive and responsive sexuality and sensuality, Astrid's story may be one example of the potential of queer failure (Halberstam, 2011; Hoskin & Taylor, 2019). Avowed *in*competence, in the form of feminine refusal, may be one of the most subversive strategies in a neoliberal workplace in which our sexualities are increasingly optimized and our bodies are made more and more capacious. Further, if we consider the spectrum of ambivalence, from pleasure to refusal, that structures experiences of feminized affective labor and sexual carework, it is possible to see how Astrid is not such an outlier, at least not among the population of women-with-low-desire. While refusal of this work may be one avenue for sabotage, a type of (direct) work action, it is imperative to remember the ways in which different populations are treated differently when such boundaries are transgressed. So: While refusal may be the only option for some, it is also a dangerous option for many. Given this, the best form of resistance may be to sabotage *together*.

CHAPTER 5

Reclaiming Receptivity

Parasexual Pleasure in the Face of Compulsory and Feminized Trauma

> I think that experience of being fucked and feeling like a technology of a penis, like a vehicle or vessel, is a very common experience for women who have sex with men . . . but submission is also something I'm drawn to [that isn't unique to me]. . . . [I]t can be really hot if it's with someone you trust and who wants to make you happy sexually. . . . I've realized that lots of women have that experience and I think it's tied in really closely with bondage and that it's about some kind of "soul-shattering" thing or something [laughs]. . . . I do find sex soul-shattering whether it's good or bad, because if it's bad it's shattering in one way, and if it's good it's kind of shattering in a different way, because I feel really vulnerable and open. . . . [I]t's kind of too much . . . and I haven't trusted men my whole life. I really haven't trusted men my whole life, that is very true. (Mallory, thirty-two years old, white, bi/queer)

A few years ago, when I was conducting interviews for this project, one of my participants asked me if anyone was going to interview me for the study. At first, I was taken aback. I identified as a very sexual person, as someone who did *not* have "low desire." But, pretty quickly, I realized that I've had all of the same issues that most of the women in this study describe—including many times wherein I didn't feel sexual at all. Like many of the participants who have been introduced throughout this book, I had primarily but not exclusively dated cis men up to that point in my life. I had at one point identified as straight. I had come to eventually identify as a queer femme,[1] but I had been socialized into thinking about sex in very cisnormative and heternormative ways (including in regard to my absent—at times—desire). I had a very whitewashed view of sexual difference and feminine receptivity. I had also alternately internalized and rejected discourses about the way women *are* sexually. I had performed sexual and sensual carework, including from a young age. I had experienced violent sexual experiences, some of which I didn't label or understand as violent at the time, and I lived with what could only be described as some kind of trauma. Sometimes I dissociated during sex. But I was also becoming more and more interested in BDSM, and particularly in being submissive in these scenarios—including in some cases with men. I literally laughed out loud when I realized I had not seen myself in this project in this way. And the "reverse interview" commenced a couple weeks later. Like all of the other interviews, it felt a bit like a verbal account of my "sexual biography" or what one participant called a "queer intake" (as opposed to a more conventional psychomedical intake). I didn't transcribe that interview for a very, very long time. And when I did, it made me cry.

This chapter examines the nuances of desire and fulfillment as they are framed within women's own narratives, focusing specifically on their experiences of receptivity, submission, consent versus coercion, and sexual intentionality. Participants, like me, articulated how sexual enjoyment is complicated for them by concerns around trust and safety, due to the widespread experience of sexual violence that is disproportionately afflicted against women and femmes. During the course of our interviews, the women I spoke with elaborated a variety of desires and fantasies that had not been met, specifically by the cis male partners they had over the course of their lives. They described a multitude of reasons why these fantasies had not been fulfilled—including a lack of trust, safety, and intimacy in their relationships, which these women would require in order for fantasies to be acted out. Many spoke of fantasies involving BDSM, and they had diverse desires about their own roles within these power/play scenarios and disparate ideas about what they most wanted from different partners in regard to the enactment and exertion of power. At first glance, it may seem that there is something paradoxical about the place

---

1. Long before I began this project, a friend referred to my gender as "andro-femme." I found this term quite fitting and as this project has progressed, I have embraced it even more, and come into a more nonbinary identity. It is unclear whether or not this experience is related to conducting this research, but of course doing this work has affected me in all kinds of ways, and so my shifting experience of my own gender subjectivity toward a nonbinary femme-of-center identity is at least a worthwhile autobiographical and reflexive sidenote.

of power in fantasy here, and indeed, almost all women spoke of how they required a safe environment to explore certain fantasies, particularly those involving BDSM. At the same time, though, they explained how too much comfort could "ruin" the fantasy, in some cases was associated with routinization and boredom, and was thus framed, in those cases, as unappealing. Their accounts suggest a delicate balance at work between taboo and trust, novelty and comfort, and subversion and safety, often held in a complex state of tension. Upon further analysis, it is apparent that most of the women I interviewed actually did not experience this tension as a paradox, though; the key to upholding safety while also allowing sexual taboos to be explored involved carefully implementing an environment of trust, intentionality, and consent. In fact, it seemed as though *consent was produced in the context of trust* (rather than trust being produced in the context of consent). Creating this environment and ambiance takes care and work—something many participants felt their (particularly cis male) partners did not readily contribute.

The women I interviewed had many ideas for the best ways to alleviate their low desire, and almost all had strong critiques of what they identified as conflicting and ambivalent social expectations for women, double standards for men's and women's sexual behavior and desire, and the problems that people inevitably encounter when they "learn how to have sex" from watching pornography—as they claimed was the case for many people. In general, participants seemed to have lots of desire, contrary to even their own self-characterizations as "low-desiring." Through our discussions, in fact, many women identified this self-diagnosing trend and revised their initial self-diagnosis, stating instead that they do, in fact, experience sexual desire, just not for the type of sex they are *expected* to have, and, in some cases, not for the type of sex that their partners want to have with them. This phenomenon evidences how the hermeneutics of "low female desire"—and now the "naturalness" for women of "receptive/responsive desire"—are really the only frames of reference women have available to interpret their experiences if they don't like the sex they are having. The feminized responsive desire framework thus dictates how women register—and *interpret*—their own sexual complaints, including when these complaints are actually about gender relations or gender itself (for instance, the receptive femininity that has been forced upon them). Here, we have another example of how the category and population—*women-with-low-desire*—is produced and lived out by those who are socialized into femininity.

Participants also identified many nonsexual desires, which seem to border on the sexual in a larger sense, and which, in fact, push the boundaries of and urge us to question what the sexual may or may not incorporate (Kleinplatz, 2006). This experience of pursuing nonsexual desires via sex is not to be confused with the "non-sexual rewards," "incentives," and "motivating factors" described in Basson's (2000, 2001b) circular sexual response cycle, however; instead, the nonsexual desires I describe might be associated more with Kleinplatz's (2006) "lessons from the edge"—including "unconventional" intimacy, self-knowledge, delving deep into experiences of trauma and power, provoking intensity and intensification of sensations, and playing with affect regulation, more broadly. In thinking about "motivations" in this new way, we might also consider psychoanalytic and queer investigations of sex that are similarly nonpastoral, nonredemptive, and certainly not romantic, for instance in the vein of what Cvetkovich (1995, 1998, 2003) describes regarding butch/femme sexualities, including active or agentic femme receptivity and butch untouchability, and also in terms of Bersani's (1986, 1987) self-shattering or disintegration via sex as "anticommunal, antiegalitarian, antinurturing, and antiloving" (Bersani, 1987, p. 195) (specifically, for Bersani, this is experienced via the "humiliation" of receptive anal sex). Some low-desiring women in this study describe experiencing submission during BDSM encounters as a form of meditation (LaMorgese, 2016) and/or as therapeutic (Lindemann, 2011), a notion that I argue opens up a radical potential for a form of *para*sexuality—a set of subversive and queer practices, sometimes associated with BDSM, that is beyond or beside the sexual as it is currently configured in contemporary psychomedical discourse. To this end, BDSM reveals possibilities that are very different from those associated with mindfulness-based sex therapy (MBST), as BDSM, unlike MBST, forefronts a full engagement with all of the psychic and social structures of desire, including with trauma, taboo, and power relations, more broadly. Research from psychoanalysis and cultural studies that considers the phenomenology of the Freudian death drive (Bersani, 1986, 1987; Brothers, 2008; Cvetkovich, 1995, 1998, 2003; Hart, 1998), in addition to BDSM-positive sex therapy (Moser & Kleinplatz, 2006; Rogak & Connor, 2018), asexuality studies (Milks & Cerankowski, 2014), and queer theory and phenomenology that engage with negative affects such as shame and abjection (Kristeva, 1982; Ngai, 2005)—especially those that attend to racial inflections within biopolitics and formulations of desire more broadly (McClintock, 1995; Musser, 2014; Nash, 2014; Stockton, 2006; Stoler, 1995)—can all help us rethink feminine responsiveness and receptivity as *active* or *agentic,* outside of the power vacuum of contemporary sexological discourse (which includes the feminized responsive desire framework), and without the trappings of essentialized femininity inherent in today's mainstream psychology of women as it is informed by the white cultural feminism of the 1960s (and white liberal feminism, today). I argue that it is possible to interpret femme receptivity as agentic without idealizing, romanticizing, or pastoralizing it, and without assuming that power relations in sex can somehow be recuperated or recast as pure or egalitarian. Instead, my data suggest that justice-seeking and radical care need not negate sexual domination and submission, and that parasexuality might inform and be informed by nuanced conceptions of asexuality beyond normative discourses of sexual rights, health, intimacy, eroticism, and ability/capacity (see the essays in Milks & Cerankowski, 2014, and specifically for this project, Kim, 2014 in that volume, for nuanced and sophisticated analyses of asexuality with which my concept of parasexuality finds much common ground).

Questions of trauma, power, and agency were raised again and again in these interviews, and it is my project in this chapter to tease apart these complicated themes around the sexual experience of the low-desiring women with whom I spoke. One of the most important conclusions derived from my qualitative analysis is that the medical and scientific discourses I analyze—including the feminized responsive desire framework as it includes the new female-specific low desire diagnosis (FSIAD) in the *DSM-5*, plethysmographic research on female subjective/genital discordance, the circular sexual response cycle, and biopolitical training protocols such as mindfulness-based sex therapy—simultaneously both *require* and *erase* women's and femmes' disproportionate experience of trauma. These discourses thus perpetuate institutionalized sexual and gender-based violence, including iatrogenic violence within the medical and scientific sphere itself. I will elaborate on this important theme and describe how it emerged at greater length in the conclusion chapter of this book.

Popular Depictions of Feminine Sexuality: Receptivity, Submission, Masochism

In the first decade of the twenty-first century, much popular journalism focused on the problem of women's low desire. But popular work has also taken up the themes of feminine responsive desire (Basson, 2000, 2001b), sexual fluidity (Diamond, 2005, 2008), and erotic plasticity (Baumeister, 2000, 2004). Most recently, popular writers (some of whom are also clinicians and academics) with the intention of reaching broader audiences in the vein of self-help, have deployed these scientific findings to make arguments for women's disproportionate experience of responsive/receptive desire (Brotto, 2018; Nagoski, 2015), women's potentially hardwired tendency toward insatiable lust (Bergner, 2013b), and the surprisingly common experience of female infidelity (apparently also driven by insatiable lust) (Martin, 2018). Women, in these popular works, have even been described as "super freaks" (Martin, 2018, p. 45) with "anarchic arousal" (Bergner, 2013b, p. 5). In this interesting turn, we see a simultaneous eschewing of some of the core tenets of evolutionary psychology (such as the idea that women's truest drive is toward motherhood), combined with the maintaining of other core tenets (such as naturalizations of female subjective/genital discordance via "the preparation hypothesis," or the notion that as an evolutionary adaptation, women are biologically "prepared for anything"—including rape—in the words of sex researchers Suschinsky & Lalumière [2011]; as a reminder from previous chapters, this has been offered as an explanation for why women become genitally vasocongested and lubricated by literally any stimuli deemed "sexually relevant," including, infamously, bonobo sex). All of this emphasis on feminine sexual anarchy then appears as receptivity in a new guise—and the old virgin/whore dichotomy is dressed up in some nice new clothes.

As we have seen, much of the clinical and experimental literature on the subject over the past two or more decades has continued to paint a picture of women as more complex than men when it comes to sex and sexuality. The notion that women's sexuality is not only complicated and complex but also receptive, responsive, and even submissive remains a mainstay in contemporary popular interpretations of sexual medicine. And the theme of responsiveness easily lends itself to notions of inherent masochism or submissive tendencies, even as this sits uneasily next to new trends that frame female desire as lascivious, hedonic, and salacious. It is via the truism of female genital/subjective discordance that both arguments—unbridled female concupiscence, on the one hand, and the more demure feminine responsiveness and receptivity, on the other hand—are maintained. As I have argued in previous chapters, the purported disconnect or gap between women's minds and bodies has been instrumentalized—it is literally made useful or *put to work* in these discourses. The mind/body gap is ripe for exploration and excavation, and it is overdetermined—it can be and has been made to suggest a number of different things about women and femininity.

Importantly, the instrumental work of the gap is evident in arguments that ultimately link female discordance, prurience, and hardwired desire for submission. For example, in a series of blog posts for *Psychology Today* (2012a, 2012b, 2012c), clinical psychologist Leon Seltzer describes how, even as it may seem "mystifying" " how a woman's mind and body, sexually speaking, can be at war with one another," (2012c) this conflict is evolutionarily pragmatic.[2] Regarding women's biologically ordained attraction to "alpha males" who exhibit "status, confidence, and competence," in addition to being "distant, brutal, and untamed," Seltzer states: "Male authority, or ascendance, is what most women appear hard-wired to be susceptible to, as well as willing to *submit* to" (2012b, italics in original post). He goes on to discuss popular interpretations of Meredith Chivers's plethysmographic research and claims that women's innate subjective/genital discordance may be evolutionarily pragmatic, but that it also leads to a lot of confusion for both women and the men who want to have sex with them. This is because women are programmed with two conflicting drives: one to submit sexually to men, and one to be choosy with their mates. Their long-term and short-term "mating" impulses are thus essentially in conflict. Through discourses like Seltzer's, the naturalization of female genital/subjective discordance becomes quickly and easily correlated with biologically adaptive and neurologically ingrained feminine submission. Further, a feminized mind/body disconnect and women's unconscious desires to be dominated are rhetorically linked. And this essentialization of feminine dissociation, naturalization of female submission, and concomitant neglect of gendered sociocultural violence is particularly problematic in light of uncritical discussions of the best-selling status and warm reception of women-targeted submission fiction such as *Fifty Shades of Grey* (E. L. James, 2011)[3]—which has recently been criticized not on account of its portrayal of women's submission, but for its romanticized heteronormativity and lack of a real discussion of consent (Downing, 2007, 2013; Dymock, 2012, 2013).

As mentioned previously, evolutionary neuropsychologists Ogas and Gaddam (2011) (who Seltzer cites heavily in the above blog posts) have also made a link between the feminine mind/body disconnect and women's unconscious desire to sexually submit to male domination:

---

2. As a related facet of the aforementioned "preparation hypothesis," female discordance is said to serve another adaptive purpose; it is in the best interest of the fitness of the human race if women don't know when they are turned on physically, because if they were aware of this, they might be less selective with their mates and thus have genetically inferior offspring (see Buss, 1994, for more on this evolutionary psychology hypothesis).

3. There is nothing inherently sexist or misogynistic about portraying women's sexual submission as enjoyable in a fictional work; my concern instead is with the placement of this type of prolific fiction next to increasingly popular neuroscience-based and evolutionary psychology-informed studies that suggest that women are submissive by *nature*—and particularly when an adequate conversation around sexual ethics, consent, and communication is sorely lacking in the contemporary public sphere.

Study after study has demonstrated the erotic appeal of male dominance. Women prefer the voices of dominant men, the scent of dominant men, the movement and gait of dominant men, and the facial features of dominant men.... [S]cientists believe that the ventrolateral prefrontal cortex may be responsible for processing cues indicating social status or dominance, and it appears that *almost all female brains are susceptible to dominating cues*. (p. 96; italics added)

These researchers make the case that women have a "primordial" urge to be dominated, and quote Chivers, who speculates that female coercion fantasies are about "the wish to be beyond will, beyond thought . . . to be all in the midbrain" (p. 115). What Chivers says here sounds plausible enough, but the authors then go on to extrapolate, "In such fantasies, it often seems like something is going on other than the mere desire to be irresistible" (p. 116), and describe an exemplary hypothetical/anecdotal woman who abashedly likes "the rough stuff"—pornography in which a woman is being violently coerced or exploited by a forceful man—but is too ashamed to tell her husband about her rape fantasies. According to Ogas and Gaddam, this innate masochistic feminine desire must be rooted in the deepest recesses of the "unconscious subcortex," in the hypothalamus and the midbrain.

Importantly, these discourses about female discordance and feminine masochistic hardwiring often take shape as a reaction formation to modern-day feminism. As in chapter 4, in the contemporary context in which female sexuality is framed, there is a tendency to highlight the purported problems that egalitarianism within romantic relationships presents, specifically for cisheterosexual couples—and particularly when it comes to their sex lives. A 2012 *Newsweek* cover article titled "Working Women's Fantasies" by Katie Roiphe is one example of a cultural fixation with women's low desire as a problem resulting from "too much political correctness"—particularly following the popularity of *Fifty Shades of Grey* (E. L. James, 2011) and other forms of what Roiphe and others refer to as "mommy porn" (depictions that almost always involve women as "bottoms" or "submissives" in BDSM scenarios). Roiphe (2012) states:

It is perhaps inconvenient for feminism that the erotic imagination does not submit to politics, or even changing demographic realities; it doesn't . . . peruse feminist blogs in its spare time; it doesn't remember the hard work and dedication of the suffragettes and assorted other picket-sign wavers. The incandescent fantasy of being dominated or overcome by a man shows no sign of vanishing with equal pay for equal work, and may in fact gain in intensity and take new, inventive—or in the case of *Fifty Shades of Grey*, not so inventive—forms.

Similarly, Jan Moir (2012) questions: "Is this sudden and widespread female thirst for bondage and sadomasochistic sexual fantasy a sign that, tired of the struggle for equality, women want to take refuge in being bossed around in the bedroom by a man?" The main themes in these hot takes in the wake of *Fifty Shades of Grey* appear to be: (1) Women are overworked, (2) Their lives are too much like those of men, and (3) They want to "surrender to" and "be seduced" by men—this will put them back in touch with their essential receptive or responsive desire. When these interpretations that operate under the sign of *anti*feminism are placed alongside clinical and scientific research that reifies female discordance and "arousal-first" desire (and their popular interpretations), it is not difficult to see how we end up with a naturalization of not only female receptivity, but feminine submission. And when examined critically, these depictions don't seem so different from early psychoanalytic conceptions of feminine masochism (the same ones that contemporary psychologists and sexologists have gone to such great lengths to distance themselves from). It is worth questioning why Roiphe, for instance, seems to want to claim that the fact of women participating in BDSM and the experience of female submission are somehow "unfeminist," while simultaneously leaving readers with an empty or facile analysis regarding if, how, and why women are drawn to submission. I am not arguing that (some, perhaps many?) women are *not* drawn to submission (my data and my own experience suggest that some, particularly those with low desire, are drawn to it); instead, I argue that this reality is not incompatible with a feminist analysis, and that we need not assume some natural or biological basis for this phenomenon in order to understand it. Essentializing female submission does us more harm than good, as it negates other, more complex and nuanced explanations (i.e., those that are sociological, psychoanalytic, and otherwise rooted in analyses of power, trauma, and racialized, gendered, and sexualized violence).

Furthermore, there is an irony here: Contemporary medical and scientific discourses of female *receptivity* and *responsiveness* are often posited as feminist (insofar as they are framed as part of more female-friendly sexual response models), while there is a simultaneous eschewing of the *ills* of feminism within popularized evolutionary accounts of feminine *submission*. This is a strange concoction, indeed, and one that demonstrates how useless the language of "feminism" has become in medicine, science, and popular instantiations when it comes to expectations and prescriptions for women's sexuality. A consideration of the range of ways in which self-identified feminist scholars and activists (from radical "sex-negative" feminists to third-wave "sex-positive" feminists) since the 1970s have framed sexual relations, including relations wherein women submit sexually, complicates things even further. My point here is not to claim that there is a proper feminist analysis of feminine receptivity, responsiveness, submission, or masochism; instead, I seek to emphasize how these terms have come to have very different valences. I also want to illuminate what their very different inflections tell us about our cultural obsession with the truth of female desire. In what follows, I interrogate this cultural obsession with naturalized gendered sexual power relations, especially as it exists alongside a simultaneous refusal to responsibly analyze or theorize race, class, gender, and other differences in this domain.

Feminism and BDSM: Social Debates about Sexual Power Relations

In addition to considering current trends in popular, clinical, and scientific discourses about women's sexuality and how these might affect women today, it is necessary to examine historical debates around female sexuality, pleasure, and trauma from within the realms of critical feminist response. Explicit enactments of power in sex, particularly as these occur between cis men and cis women, have been the subject of much feminist contention. Radical feminism of the 1970s into the 1980s has been broadly associated with the strong critique of not only pornography but also of BDSM, and of heterosexual intercourse itself.[4] The essays published in *Against Sadomasochism: A Radical Feminist Analysis* (Linden, 1983) represent the way this critique has largely been taken up by those within the "anti-pornography" or "anti-SM" tradition. As Hart (1998) identifies, these critiques have tended to rely on "analogical thinking" (p. 84) in which BDSM—particularly scenarios in which women are dominated by men (or by other women, which devolved into its own fraught debate)—is framed as akin to atrocities as diverse as the Holocaust and the Jonestown massacre in their duping effects on naïve victims.

---

4. Although Bersani (1987) argued that Dworkin and MacKinnon were guilty of framing receptivity during penetrative sex (for Bersani, an inherently violent and unrecuperable act, which is exactly what gives it the transformative potential for self-shattering) as potentially redeemable outside of heteropatriarchy, I instead associate that type of redemption and pastoralism with cultural feminism (discussed in chapter 3), including with models of the "psychology of women" developed in the '70s and '80s through today. In this reading of Dworkin and MacKinnon as actually more proto-queer and exemplary of the "antisocial" or "negative" turn in queer theory, I am indebted to Alex Dymock's excellent essay on this topic (2018) and to the work of Anne Cvetkovich (2003). Andrea Long Chu's (2019) discussions of the "impossibility of feminism" here are also invaluable.

This conservative strand of radical feminism has argued that women being sexually dominated (or doing the dominating) is never safe, never consensual, and certainly never feminist. However, a disparate tendency emerged in the late 1970s and early 1980s to counter this notion. Some feminists associated with this "pro-BDSM," "pro-sex," or "sex-positive" feminist movement have argued that BDSM is actually safer and *more* consensual than so-called vanilla sex because it involves explicitly negotiating power relations, rather than assuming that the best or most natural sex does not involve eroticizing power or sexual hierarchies (and thus ignoring the damaging potential of these hierarchies and power relations, particularly under heteropatriarchy). This trend also questioned the idea that there can ever be *any* type of sex that does not involve the negotiation of power (Langdridge, 2011). Many writers associated with this trend frame BDSM as liberating (for some examples, see Califia, 1994; Hollibaugh, 2000; Rubin, 1984), and some argue that it is specifically a form of liberation from, or that it can provide a way to master or transform, sexual trauma (this notion is found particularly in the work of feminist and queer theorists such as Hart and Cvetkovich who have taken up the work of author Dorothy Allison on her experience of incest and her subsequent emergence into lesbianism and BDSM subcultures).

This notion of mastery over trauma via masochism, self-destruction, or self-shattering can be traced through various strains of psychoanalysis and critical theory, including in the works of Freud, Battaile, and Deleuze. It can also be attributed in its practical, contemporary form (i.e., in BDSM as therapeutic practice) to the early formulations of Heinz Kohut, as described more recently by Doris Brothers (1997). BDSM is understood by some contemporary practitioners as liberating, and communities have formed around this notion, but the limits or uses of BDSM in this vein have also been raised and questioned in the works of contemporary critical, poststructuralist, and queer theorists (Bersani, 1987; Cvetkovich, 2003; Halberstam, 2011; Hart, 1998), who have tended to be less interested in arguing for BDSM's liberating (*or* oppressive) potential and who have been more interested in how questioning the "truth" of BDSM has become a battleground upon which wars over sexuality are waged in public discourse—including within the feminist "sex wars" of the '70s and '80s. Further, some theorists have looked to the political economy, social structuring, and biopolitics of BDSM scenes and communities (Weiss, 2011) thus helping to further remove BDSM from debates over "morality."

Feminist contestations over BDSM have also been compared to other debates around embodiment and women's agency. For instance, Pitts-Taylor (2003) documents the pathologization of women's body modification in many medical and wider cultural discourses, which occurs alongside its celebration by many of those in the alternative communities who practice this type of self-inscription of their own bodies. Pitts-Taylor (2003) describes how many of those who practice body modification see it as a form of self-mastery, a way to gain and exhibit control over their own bodies, and notes that some of these individuals are the survivors of previous traumatic experiences, including sexual abuse. Questions of bodily ownership, integrity, and control are critically raised in relation to these practices, and those who take a Foucauldian or poststructuralist feminist stance tend to critique the binary in which women are produced as (and reduced to) "dupes of culture" *or* "rational actors" within this framework (Pitts-Taylor, 2007). Instead, these feminists look to the larger power structures through which self-inscription and sexual submission are discursively framed. In this vein, asexuality studies scholars (Barounis, 2019; Kim, 2014; Milks & Cerankowski, 2014) have also challenged these dichotomies by making (compulsory) sexuality itself the object of scrutiny, and raising questions around power, consent, desire, and embodiment outside of and beyond the sexual. I will return to these themes at various points throughout the remainder of this chapter, but I go now to the stories participants told me about their own sex lives, including how and why desire is lacking (or has been lacking at some point) within them, in light of these larger questions around receptivity, responsiveness, discordance, dissociation, submission, domination, violence, power, and trauma.

Taboo, Trauma, and Trust

The historical relationship between feminism and BDSM—particularly of women submitting in these scenarios—is not an easy or comfortable relationship. It has been suggested that the desire to bottom or submit is linked to sexual trauma (at least as one possible avenue)—as a way to regain control over not only specific traumatizing experiences but also the daily and more "insidious traumas" (Cvetkovich, 2003) that women endure against their bodies and psyches (including via street harassment, objectification, sexual coercion by intimate partners or acquaintances, and "date rape"). Gendered violence runs the gamut from these more casual, everyday violations and microaggressions (which many women may understand as normal) to more clear and obvious forms of sexual violence, including child sexual abuse and "stranger rape." Valdivia describes the everyday, quotidian, almost banal experience of gendered violence, and explains how she experiences this as a perpetual potential threat, as a constant nagging at her body and psyche, and as a pervasive ambiance of insistent inquiry as to whether or not she will give consent—concomitant with a felt disregard for her answer. She frames this *foreclosure of consent* as a deep, constitutive aspect of her own experience of femininity, and something that she learned and has lived from a very young age:

> One of my first sexual experiences was when I was thirteen, my first French kiss, it was a super big deal, this intrusion of bodies, there was a tongue involved, there was groping involved, and it was sexual, it was definitely sexual, even if it wasn't called that. And I remember that this person didn't *ask* me. . . . [T]hat's the thing, consent has only made its way into my life very recently . . . and consent is a thing that is so nebulous, it is frightening to me how nebulous it is. . . . I can't find anything sexier than consent at this point, but that French kiss began a long career of *nonconsent*.

In light of Valdivia's comments, it is also important to note that some survivors of sexual abuse describe providing a service—not only to their abusers, but to a society that relies on imagery and narratives of "valid," "authentic," and "exceptional" sexual abuse in order to excuse everyday, mundane, and casual aggressions toward women and others who are feminized.[5] As long as we have "legitimate" victims of child and sexual abuse, who have suffered at the hands of the "authentic" criminals who are pathological and ill, individuals who enact violence all the time in more insidious and mundane ways can be absolved (and the pervasive phenomenon itself can be absolved). Here, we have an affective economy in which one type of violence is authenticated, and is thus made to excuse other types. This system—as it promulgates a narrative of child sexual abuse and "stranger rape" as idiosyncratic occurrences primarily perpetuated by the pathological, deviant, and "mentally ill"[6]—simultaneously exotifies and fetishizes these more obvious violences, making it appear as though they don't happen every day, all the time, and are actually part of the quotidian landscape of many women's lives (and, importantly, part of a spectrum of gendered violence—a spectrum in which instances at one end are not necessarily considered violent at all, and, in some cases, are even considered natural). Fahs (2016) has made a similar argument regarding this

---

5. I use the term *women* in this chapter, again as it is mainly about participants, who, at the time of the interviews, identified as such. However, I am clear on the fact that this experience extends well beyond cis and trans women, and that many non-binary, gender-nonconforming, genderqueer, and AFAB folks also experience this violence disproportionately. Part of my argument here is that this violence is *feminized,* even if those who experience it do not always identify as women or femmes.

6. It is also important to note the overt ableism demonstrated in assigning the perpetration of sexual violence specifically to those who are "mentally ill."

hypostatization of sexual and gendered violence, stating: "Categories of *rape* and *sex offending* obscure the pervasive qualities of perpetration and victimhood in the culture at large. . . . [T]he 'rape victim' and 'sex offender' become categories of 'otherness'—often seen as *outside the norm* and *outside of ourselves*—that blur and erase the many different ways sexual violence disrupts, traumatizes, and circulates within women's lives" (p. 62).

Importantly, much data suggests that gendered and sexualized violence is experienced disproportionately by women and femmes of color—and that this is particularly true for Black women and femmes (Green, 2017; Human Rights Campaign, 2019). Over the last several decades, Black feminist researchers have examined the precarity of women of color and of Black women, specifically, in regard to sexualized microaggressions within longer histories of culturally legitimized assault and abuse. According to Collins (1990), Black women have not only been disproportionately violated through "physical assault during slavery, domestic abuse, incest, and sexual coercion," but ongoing "violence against black women tends to be legitimated and therefore condoned while the same acts visited on other groups may remain nonlegitimated and nonexcusable" (p. 177). In light of the work of Black feminists and other feminists of color who write on the racialization of sexual violence and carework (described in chapter 4), alongside research on the whiteness of sexual difference as it is embedded in colonialist science and early gynecological practices through to today (described in the introduction to this book), the experiences described by the low-desiring women of color in the present study are especially important to pay close attention to. I highlight their accounts below.

Given the widespread normalization of these types of violence, linking the experience of sexual trauma to the desire to submit in a BDSM scenario (and juxtaposing them, as I do in this chapter) feels extremely taboo. It seems possible that this is because the only explanations we have come to imagine to be at our disposal for women's enjoyment of submission are conservatively psychoanalytic (which many self-identified feminists shy away from) or are reductively biological in nature (which most feminists—hopefully—abhor). But if we are able to conceive of a social phenomenology which attends to how power relations are lived out and embodied, more than just as gestures, but not as monolithic instantiations of a uniquely feminine repetition-compulsion (which ends up sounding just as essentializing as neurobiological explanations for women's hardwired desire to submit), we may be able to make more space for individual desire, even as we acknowledge that individuals are part of populations that are, at least in part, produced through common experiences of trauma.

For the participants in this study, there is certainly a delicate balance between owning the experience of being subjected to power (i.e., being sexually dominated) and feeling retraumatized. Most of the women I interviewed—even those who describe being turned on by submission—have experienced situations where being dominated has gone awry, and they describe their anxiety around getting into a situation where this might happen again. Other participants reject being dominated by men on principle, even if they think it might turn them on, because of their experiences with violence at the hands of men in the past. Rose illustrates this notion of a scene of sexual domination not being executed with care, and of ultimately feeling nonconsensual:

> I had one very bad sexual moment with this guy I was dating, sex started to get rough, but there was one night when it got really rough, and I just kept saying, "Stop it, what are you doing?!" But he just kind of kept going and afterward, I was like, "What the . . . ?!" . . . [H]e was kind of choking me a little, and I was right at the edge of the bed, so I kind of felt like I was gonna fall off the bed, and sometimes he would smack my butt, and sometimes it was playful, but it was starting to become painful, not fun, really. . . . [B]ut it was more like the choking part, it was like, "He's like really getting off on this, me feeling like I can't breathe and like I'm going to fall off the bed!" It was just weird . . . but the thing is—you never know what men are going to do . . . especially if you've been with guys who slap or choke you.

Rose had previously expressed how she likes being dominated sexually, so I ask her what makes a sexual experience of submission feel safer for her, what makes a positive experience different from the one she describes above. She explains that feeling like she and her partner are "on the same page" and that boundaries have been communicated clearly are crucial aspects of fostering an environment in which rough play feels like a turn-on rather than a violation. She goes on to describe how a lack of communication tends to breed the cultural misconception that *all* women "like it rough" and thus that men should simply "go for it" when they are having sex with women:

> I think he thinks there are women out there who really enjoy that kind of thing [nonconsensual rough play], and I guess he thought I was that person. . . . I can totally see someone else [whom he was having sex with] thinking, "Oh yeah, I am *supposed* to like this" and not saying anything . . . because no one else is going to say, "Yeah, that's weird, that's wrong, it's disrespectful, it probably didn't turn you on, it probably didn't feel good!"

Here, Rose is not talking about rough play, in general, as disrespectful; what she describes as disrespectful are the widespread notions that consent and intentionality are not necessary. Later, she communicates her belief that part of fomenting a healthy and respectful sexual relationship means actually taking the time to find out what your partner desires, what gives her pleasure, what turns her on. This complicated view of domination and submission exposes the complexities and vicissitudes of a desire-trauma matrix—this is rocky terrain to navigate, and there is clearly not a recipe (psychoanalytic, neurobiological, or otherwise) that can explain who will enjoy what kind of power play and role within that schema. But, taking the material and cultural situation of women into account (i.e., under racist, ableist, cisheteropatriarchy), and considering social variables and the population-producing experience of repeated and feminized trauma, are clearly important when considering patterns around desire for submission versus domination and the ways in which these play out along gendered lines.

Most of the low-desiring women I spoke with had experienced sexual and/or gendered violence at some point in their lives. Several had experienced sexual molestation or abuse at very early ages, but many had not experienced childhood sexual abuse (CSA), per se. Almost all of the women I spoke with described the larger milieu in which their sexualities had developed as traumatizing, however, and they described how heteronormative expectations tied to male aggression are often deployed to excuse violence against and harassment of women, and of women's bodies being violated in a variety of ways in everyday life and spaces. Sexual incursions could also happen closer to home, and many women described having sex with cis male partners with whom they did not feel they had particularly intentional sex lives. This illustrates the blurry terrain of consent versus coercion and of intentionality versus haphazardness within mundane, banal forms of sexual intimacy—a realm that we do not generally associate with trauma, unless it results from more "extreme," "exceptional," and thus *identifiable* forms of domestic or intimate partner violence. Regina sums up this sentiment about the murkiness of consent/coercion within intimate relationships when I ask her if any sexual experience happened to her in her life that she thinks may have contributed to her low desire:

> I don't think so, other than the history of having not wanted to have sex with my partner but doing it anyway, on just kind of a daily level . . . and certainly "consenting" the entire time, but doing so very reluctantly.

Regina's statement makes it clear that what happens in the bedroom is not as far from what happens in a dark alley as people might like to think, and it also hearkens to the types of insidious trauma described by Cvetkovich (2003) and the notion that bad and even traumatizing sex can still be technically consensual. Evie extends this idea to street harassment and other forms of violence that women endure in non-intimate spaces:

> I think that what happens is because these things are so normalized in our culture but not acknowledged—like the attacks, constant hollering [on the street, out in the world], the fact that one in three women get raped in their lives, these statistics, women are subject to sexual violence whether it is physical or emotional in nature—but at the same time our society refuses to acknowledge it as a real problem and so it's not "cool" to talk about being a rape victim, like things get really "heavy." And it is very serious, but it becomes this thing where people don't feel comfortable talking about it in everyday life even though it is part of our everyday life. And by not living in a society where people feel comfortable talking about it, you kind of have to hide it. And since sexuality is already a shameful thing, it gets channeled into that, and it becomes a somewhat shameful thing.

Evie's statement elucidates the insidiousness of sexual violence and resulting traumas, which are muted in women's sex lives and intimate partnerships. She also notes that the silence around what happens to women's bodies becomes tethered to the notion that it's not "cool" to talk about these serious issues, that it's too "heavy," and that women should "lighten up." Many participants articulated similar thoughts, and some of them also expressed this notion of voicelessness in terms of silence and dissociation during actual sex acts, or with regard to speaking about the traumas they have endured over the course of their lives. Many women described feeling voiceless not only in cultural representations and conversations about violence against women but also in their intimate relationships, including while having sex. This theme is expressed by Elizabeth, who experienced sexual abuse as a child:

> I find it very hard to speak up for myself when it comes to sex. . . . [I]t's harder than fighting with my landlord! I can fight with my landlord like it's nobody's business, but I don't feel like—or I feel like I have that option [to say "no" to sex] but I have watched myself not take it in sexual situations.

Many other participants expressed similar notions, including Molly, Tiffany, Penelope, Evie, Sadie, Taja, Rose, and Jill—to mention only a few. These women also associated it with the sentiment Evie expressed about the everyday cultural silencing of women's stories about violence, and lamented that women don't "communicate" enough—with their partners and with each other—about their sex lives, including the traumatic aspects. Sadie articulates this idea:

> I think a lot of women don't communicate, we are not taught to be up-front about that . . . [and] that's when I get these insights about other women's experiences that maybe we are not talking about—it's like, "Oh man, are we all just doing this fucking missionary position shit?!" You know? Has anyone ever said, "Hey, it can be different than this!"?

This multifaceted notion of voicelessness is a crucial aspect of sexual difference socialization. Participants elucidated how women are socialized to shut up about sex—including about infractions against their bodies. These women's descriptions of their experiences of sexual violence and trauma—or even more mundane, banal descriptions of the obscurity around consent/coercion that they have experienced in their everyday lives and sexual relationships—shed much light on why women express the need to feel safe, comfortable, and trusting in order to be able to truly "lose themselves" in a sexual experience.

For many of the women I spoke with, being dominated was a fantasy primarily because they so rarely felt comfortable or safe enough to play with the boundaries of domination/submission (in this light, it makes sense that so many of these low-desiring participants were drawn to BDSM!). They spoke of the intentionality that was required to make the fantasy work and not have the enactment disappoint, nor go too far. In a sense, then, the fantasy is actually a fantasy about *consent itself*—consent is fetishized precisely because it is so exceptional. And again, for the women I interviewed, it seems that trust engenders consent, rather than vice versa—*trust* is the foundation upon which good sex is enacted, and *consent* is no longer the key term.[7] For example, Ava had very clear reservations regarding the limits of her own submission and the reasons for those limits. When I ask her what she wants from a partner who is dominating her, she tells me:

> I have this fantasy that—if I am a sub, and this person is really attracted to me and really cares about me, then when he is in total power—let's say I'm tied up and I have a blindfold on—then if he really cares about me—even

---

7. As the notion of "consent" is so bogged down with legal and liberal valences, I argue that the focus on "trust" that emerged in my data instead offers a helpful corrective. See E. A. Owens (2019) for more on the problems with consent as contract, wherein the equal standing of "consenting" parties is always a liberal fantasy.

though I'm totally at his will—he will put my desire above whatever else it is that he would want to do to me, whether it's to penetrate me or choke me or pull my hair or whatever it is that someone would want to do to someone all tied up and vulnerable—but if I was in a position of complete vulnerability and someone just wanted to make me feel good? That's like the ultimate test of whether or not you really care about someone.

What Ava describes here is a performance of trust and safety. If someone is in a position of total power, total control, and they still want to please her, and do what she wants them to do, then for Ava, that is the ultimate enactment of trust and respect, and, potentially, an enactment of a certain kind of (not necessarily romantic) love. It is certainly a form of care. Many of the women I spoke with described similarly wanting the dominant partner (for most of the participants in these interviews, a cis man) to know what they (the sub) want and to follow those intuited guidelines during the encounter. They explained that it would obviously defy the whole purpose of the BDSM scenario if they—the submissive partner—told the dominant partner exactly what they wanted him to do; for these women, there is something very real about wanting the dominant partner to perceive what they want in terms of domination, and to be able to trust that person to not overstep their boundaries, but instead, to push them in just the right ways. Submission here is bound up with a paradoxical sense of being in control. Ava goes on to describe a situation in which BDSM play did go too far. Like Rose, she enjoys submitting sexually, but she only feels comfortable realizing that fantasy when the relationship is established as safe, consensual, and intentional, and with a partner who is trustworthy. She describes a relationship where that was not the case:

> In [a past] relationship, he knew that I wanted him to dominate me, but sometimes he was too rough. . . . [S]o instead of feeling like I could trust him and have a positive rough sex experience, I would feel even more objectified and more crappy. So that was a case of him indulging in what I wanted but not doing it right. . . . I've wanted to be blindfolded and tied up and it's not that a person wouldn't do that for me, it's that I've never been with someone I trusted enough to share that with. . . . I often find myself not sharing fantasies that I feel like have a high potential of not being carried out in the right way.

Molly, a childhood sexual abuse survivor, is involved in a long-term BDSM relationship with a sexual partner she trusts completely. Importantly, this partner is not someone with whom she is involved in a traditional, monogamous, or domestic relationship—but she also does not describe their relationship as "purely sexual." She shares similar thoughts to Ava on the requirement of safety and the power/control of submission:

> The responsibility of the dom I see is fulfilling the sub's desires, [it's about] making them feel comfortable, making them feel good about relinquishing control, because if they don't, then it doesn't work.... [W]hen I am the sub I can just be relaxed about it, and trust that he is going to run the whole show.... I feel a very strong connection to him, and we are very intimate, but just in a different way, I guess. I trust him completely, which allows us to do things that I cannot do with other people, and one of the things that I like about it—having so many issues with sex—is that when I'm with him, because he's in charge, I don't have to think about things, I don't have to get caught up in my head and worry about stuff.... [W]hen I'm with other guys I'm always trying to make them happy; with him I don't have to do that.

Molly describes how her intimate BDSM relationship provides her with more safety and security than relationships with men she tries to date and have sex with in a more "conventional" manner. Although her relationship to the institutionalization of submission is not representative of most of the other women I spoke with (she is involved with a defined BDSM subculture, whereas most participants were not), her particular example sheds much light on the relationships among trust, safety, comfort, intentionality, and sexual submission. Interestingly, and importantly, her experience of the pleasure of submission with her trusted dom is something that is often lacking in her more traditional heterosexual relationships, where power is at play, and is often gendered, but is less likely to be formally negotiated or even discussed at all.

In a world in which trauma and violence are so often sexualized and feminized, there is something clearly comforting about taking control of that power imbalance in an intentional way. Evie describes it as *cathartic*:

> Being submissive is entrusting someone to do things to you that you wouldn't let anybody else do.... [S]o I'm dominating in the sense that I like to submit the way that I like to submit.... [I]t's like playing with societal norms and things you experience in everyday life on your terms. You don't have any control over the dudes that holler at you, grab you, hurt you, any of that stuff, but you have control over the person who you feel comfortable with doing that stuff to you. I feel like it can be somewhat cathartic.

Evie raises the question of what it is that actually feels good about submission. She describes submission as a form of control, and thus encapsulates a sentiment that many of the women I spoke with shared. For these women, controlling what might feel in a certain moment like your own destruction can be cathartic, it can be sexy. Participants' descriptions of catharsis through submission on their own terms is reminiscent of psychoanalytic theorizing that suggests that engaging in BDSM, particularly submission, can enact a "rescripting" of a trauma scenario (Brothers, 1997)—but I do not want to reduce my participants' experiences to this type of psychoanalytic theorization. What I want to focus on instead is the crucial fact that so many of the low-desiring women I interviewed shared this view of catharsis emerging from trauma, and consider how this experience might be evidence not of something constituted through Oedipal desire, but rather as imbricated with a social and sexual landscape in which femininity itself is conceived as traumatic—a point that Benjamin (1988) and Hart (1998) have alluded to. I also want to consider this landscape as productive of affective experiences, and as productive of traumatized populations, as femininity here is the product not only of dyadic interpersonal traumas but also of violent discursive configurations, mass social enactments, and pervasive shared emotional orientations (often, but not exclusively, among women and femmes)—what Cvetkovich (2003) might call traumatic "public cultures" drawn together through specific "collective sentiments" (Berlant, 2008) or "structures of feeling" (Williams, 1977).

Many of the other participants I spoke with discussed the notion of catharsis being experienced through truly consensual and safe sexual experiences. Sadie describes how an enactment of something that feels so taboo, a relinquishing of control in submission, is linked to what is most sexually stimulating for her, and frames it in terms of passion:

> What it seems like is an uninhibited safety in being with somebody, an uninhibited experience of oneself. . . . [I]t's very much about self and other for me. . . . [I]t is a sense of kind of dissolving those structures . . . that exoskeleton that is built up. . . . [W]hen I have experienced moments of passion with people, it is a dissolution of those boundaries, a safety to be vulnerable, and like an indulgence that I haven't had much of.

For Sadie, it seems like the conditions that allow for consent are so unusual that to experience them is to experience literal passion. In other words, the circumstances that structure consent also structure a form of passion—the ability to fully let go. Her description of what it feels like to relinquish control, and the vulnerability of her "exoskeleton," sounds like a page out of Freud's *Beyond the Pleasure Principle*—and also resonates deeply with Cvetkovich's (2003) discussion of the power and agency of femme receptivity alongside butch untouchability (and the intersubjective exchange of power that this framing calls up, in line with Benjamin [1988]). Sadie's desire to be vulnerable *and* cross boundaries also troubles the delineation of femme receptivity and butch untouchability, however, as it speaks to elements of both, and also to a type of passion that is borne out of or alongside trauma.

Taja expresses similar sentiments around the relinquishing of control, the crossing of boundaries, and why these things are so enticing, yet also so frightening. I ask her how these ideas have informed her feelings about BDSM, specifically:

> A lot of my fantasies revolve around ideas of ownership, [but] I would have to think somebody is really wonderful in order for that to be an okay set of circumstances, that I would give somebody that kind of agency over me. . . . [O]nce I am really comfortable with somebody, I will be very submissive. I love the idea of someone sort of using me, being selfish with me, in fantasy. I never really like it in reality, which is interesting. I love the idea of giving to somebody and being generous in that way . . . of using me for their own pleasure in some way, whatever that might be . . . or feeling like it is too good to miss, or it is too good to wait, that they can't help themselves.

Sam extends these ideas about the pleasures of vulnerability and being taken care of, explaining how the desire to relinquish control to someone she trusts has almost become a requirement for her own sexual excitement:

> I want somebody to be there to carry part of it for me, to take part of it from me, to force me to relinquish it from time to time. And that is in every facet of my life. I want someone who is like, "I will go buy groceries, I will make dinner, I will clean, I will wash your hair for you, I will pin you against the wall"—I am such a control freak that having control taken from me is important to me, I desire that, I want it.

Sadie's, Taja's, and Sam's comments all speak to the truism that all bottoms are power bottoms. Lola shares a similar sentiment about the origins of her desire to be dominated:

> Part of me thinks it's just because it's the opposite of what I'm doing in life. . . . I feel like sex is that place where like you wanna really just kick back and explore other sides of yourself that you don't normally do. . . . [I]n the real world, under no circumstances do I let anyone dominate me. It's like a thing that I cannot allow. So it's like I'm so adamantly against that, so maybe

sexually I just want the opposite, just to like balance it . . . because sometimes you just want to not always be in control.

The women I spoke with had very complex views on the place of power in sex, and nuanced thoughts on the kind of roles they like to play, with whom, and why. It is important to note that particularly women who identified as subs or who were more interested in submitting than dominating sexually were very thoughtful regarding the limits of the role-playing scene and what kinds of boundaries were being crossed. Power/play in BDSM is not something they take lightly, and most of the women I talked to were very clear on the fraught nature of their own enjoyment during submission. They were aware of the role of previous traumas, and of the violation of women's bodies as a cultural trope and as a material reality, and they actively took this into account when acting on their own desires and fantasies. Ultimately, they placed utmost importance on negotiation, intentionality, trust, and safety during any sexual encounter.

Submission without Coercion: Low-Desiring Women on Enhancing Sexual Enjoyment

Most of the women I interviewed had experienced fulfilling sex at some point in their lives, even if they identified as low-desiring and were currently not having a lot of sex—or at least not a lot of fulfilling sex. When I asked these women what gives them pleasure, what does fulfill them, and what their partners could do to help increase their desire, they had plenty of answers (and suggestions). Many of these pleasures centered on issues of time, labor, effort, and play. The women I interviewed also stated that there are many nonsexual things in their lives that give them great pleasure.

Time, Labor, Presence

Many of the women I spoke with discussed how timing or tempo affects their sexual experiences, and described wanting partners to "slow down." When I ask Sadie what gives her the most pleasure sexually, she tells me:

> I have discovered that I much prefer slower tempos, so I will have to take control, and communicate physically that I am taking control at that time, and slow it down. Because there is something about that for me that totally

changes the situation, and that will arouse me far more than just the act of "doing this thing." I feel like it shifts more from this sexual technical thing to the sensual enjoyment of what is going on. I discovered that was really exciting to me . . . with men specifically . . . when I had been so bored with guys. I think the root of that is just being able to play around with somebody.

In this statement, Sadie links "slowing it down" with both increased sensuality and a feeling of being in control—which is something that clearly turns her on a lot. This is an interesting contrast to the way mindfulness is typically deployed within the popular rhetorics of mindfulness-based sex therapy, which rarely seem to connect mindfulness in sex to *power*. What Sadie seems to enjoy, just as much as the slowing down itself, is that she gets to enact a form of control in leading the sexual exchange and changing the tempo. Taja expands on this notion, and emphasizes the importance of reciprocity in this regard, raising the specter of not only play but work: "In terms of my partner, it's about pace, patience, and willingness to put in the *time*." When I ask her if she can describe a time when she was really turned on, she tells me about a lover she had a few years back and describes an encounter in which tempo really mattered, and also suggests aspects of both labor and play. She and her partner went to the beach together, and he put in a lot of work over a long period of time to build the ambiance and set the tone:

> I remember thinking, "This is the best thing that has ever happened!" . . . [W]e could hear the waves, perfect temperature, just warm from the shower, after having this intimate experience with this person in the ocean . . . and so I was just really into it, really excited about his existence in that moment, and the fact that I was there with him. . . . [T]here had been this slow build, for a good two hours. . . . [I]t makes a difference! Like extended foreplay across different locations.

Valdivia also mentions the importance of ambiance and time, explaining that she enjoys sex with women and genderqueer, gender-nonconforming, and nonbinary individuals more than with cis men, generally, because these folks have been more willing to extend the experience, devoting a lot of time to it, whereas the cis men she has dated were more concerned with "getting to the finish line":

> And then when I started dating queer people, I definitely understood, I was like, "Oh my god! It's possible! Maybe it took this person to give me head for an hour [to make me come]"—which is the kind of time no man has

ever given me. And that can go on the record: No man has ever given me that kind of time.

Here, Valdivia reiterates the importance of allowing pleasure to build, over time, and emphasizes the importance of mutual reciprocity and shared labor in a sexual exchange. Her statement also hearkens back to the theme of sexual carework (discussed in chapter 4)—the notion that women are socialized to provide sexual, emotional, and relational care to men, as a form of release, who are generally not expected to provide the same sort of sexual care to women. This is not to say that there are not gendered sexual expectations for men; it is to say—as many of these women do—that expectations for men and women, in terms of this work, are different. According to these participants, instead of providing sexual care, men are expected to *perform* sexually, which often paradoxically indicates a rushed, (anti)climactic goal orientation toward any given sexual experience. Rose exemplifies this perspective:

> Slowing it down would take some of the pressure off that final moment, too, that like, "We have to get there!" Instead it could be like, "Well, we will get there when we get there." . . . I think men think actual penetration should take a while because that is what gets women off, even though it's not actually what gets women off.

The practitioners I spoke with also shared thoughts on altering the tempo of a sexual experience. Celeste, a tantric/yogic healer who works specifically with women, states that women *essentially* require a slower sexual pace, and she links this again (as described in chapter 4) to the notion of feminine receptivity as responsibility:

> When I talk about this [feminine receptive responsibility] in my training, I remind them of the old Pointer Sisters song "I Want a Man with a Slow Hand"—that whole thing of "slow down," that's the second chakra, the second chakra is "slow down," you can feel the wind on your skin, you can taste the cool water going inside of you, so you can feel your cells rejoicing when the water comes into your body.

In this quote, Celeste essentializes the notion of "slowing down," conceptualizing it as part of a natural female association with the second chakra and with feminine receptivity. In other passages, she also extends the issue beyond the practices of sex—she discusses the need for women to "slow down" and "enjoy life" as essential for maintaining their overall health, the health of their partners, the health of their relationships, the health of the planet, and the fitness of society and the broader populace, all as an extension of feminized social reproduction. This essentializing discourse conflicts with the narratives of most of the women I interviewed, who did not make any naturalizing claims about their desire to "slow it down" during sex. Here, there is an interesting contrast between Celeste's comments and those of the women I interviewed—there is a similarity at the level of technique, but "slowing down" signifies differently in the two framings. Importantly, participants' vision is more relational. Most of the women I interviewed spoke in terms of the socialization that men receive, which teaches them to drive toward the goal of orgasm—their own, and in some cases, their partners'. Rose exemplifies this perspective, in her comment above, and she blames men's erroneous assumptions about what "gets women off" on the fact that they watch too much (heteronormative) porn. It is illustrative to compare these women's narratives of tempo, speed, and labor (which pertain to the sexual experience itself, and which men and women have been socialized to play specific roles within) to practitioners' (both traditional clinicians' and alternative healers') views, which tend to naturalize feminine receptivity and are more likely to essentialize women's desire for "slowness" when it comes to sex. It is imperative to note that it is not only practitioners within the medical realm who reductively focus on "being in the present" (through techniques like mindfulness-based sex therapy) as the primary way to experience one's sexuality more fully and enhance sexual pleasure.[8] Celeste also frames being mindful as an apolitical tool of sensual enhancement used in tantric meditational exploration, simultaneously admonishing BDSM, fantasy, negotiations of power, and role-playing:

> To be lost in the present moment without the need for any—the deepest teachings of Tantra and Taoism, the deepest most advanced teachings, suggest *no fantasy*. It suggests staying deeply rooted in the present moment, in what's happening right here, right now. That ultimately that is the most potent form of sexual pleasure. That's when I go to the highest heights, is when I'm just lost in the present moment, and I could no more begin to have a fantasy, I couldn't even conceptualize a fantasy, I'm so in the flow of what's happening in my cells. . . . [T]hat's the real ecstasy, when you get to that.

In this very interesting passage, Celeste takes up the notion of "being in the present" in a way that resonates with the mindfulness discourse I have ana-

---

8. Mindfulness, as it taken up in Western medicine, including in MBST, is increasingly the bridge between these two previously separate groups (traditional medical practitioners and alternative or holistic healers).

lyzed in previous chapters—in which power relations, either explicitly or implicitly, tend to be disavowed in the name of staying in the moment, nonjudgmentally—a notion that sounds too much at times like either "bypassing" trauma (in the sense in which Helen Singer Kaplan originally described it) or as disregarding the reality—and potential *sexiness*—of power relations. This framing does not link up with the way these participants described slowing down and being in the moment, which can manifest as a form of control and play, and is not a disavowal of power, fantasy, or (even taboo) desire. Although some participants did describe "being in the present" in ways that are consistent with mindfulness discourse, for most, being "in the present" or "in the moment" and "slowing down" were mainly about manifesting a feeling of communion with a partner, a sense of strong compatibility, a tangible chemistry—or even a sense of control. When one is with a trusted partner and the relationship is founded upon negotiation, clear communication, and intentionality, mindfulness can clearly be a tool for sexual enhancement. But, as I have argued throughout this book, a depoliticizing of the technique, or its uncritical removal from the larger context of a woman's sexual relationships, background, and history, can pose problems for women—specifically those with histories of trauma. My participants' stories illuminate how mindfulness cannot be posited as an antidote to the larger institutionalized and relational power structures and constraints within which women's sex lives fundamentally take shape. Molly, for instance, explains how she derives the most pleasure from sex when she is acting out BDSM role-playing scenarios, and how she finds the act of submission itself meditative:

> When I am in the dom/sub relationship [subbing with her long-term dom], it's almost like I am so physically involved that my mind does not wander, it's almost like a weird meditative thing. I don't think about other stuff, I don't do a laundry list in my head, or wonder what's on TV, or watch the clock.

Molly provides a powerful example here of how incorporating BDSM, submission, and fantasy into her sex life is a mindful act, how submission is meditative for her, and how participating in sex in which she is mindfully submissive and in which power relations are clearly articulated allows her to feel more present than most other forms of sex with partners where power relations are not as clearly negotiated or intentional. In what may seem like a paradox, Molly is more likely to "check out" or dissociate during sex when the experience is uncritically assumed to be about being "in the moment" and simply feeling the sensuality of the present. Through Molly's example, we see how BDSM and mindfulness are not mutually exclusive—they need not be posed as binary when it comes to sex, with power, role-playing, and fantasy on one side of the polarity, and mindfulness, meditation, and sensually "being in the present" on the other (as they are framed in Celeste's description of the negation of fantasy in the most "ecstatic" sex). There has been some attention to the meditative state induced by BDSM in media accounts recently (LaMorgese, 2016), but mainstream sex therapy discourse rarely mentions how submission and BDSM might be meditative or mindful practices.[9] Many of my participants' traumatic sexual experiences also bring the depoliticizing and detheorizing of "meditating the (sexual) pain away" into sharp relief; their very different stories about the uses of mindfulness, meditation, BDSM, and fantasy make it clear that none of these techniques are simply apolitical tools for sexual enhancement, and instead ought to be theorized and thoughtfully considered from a perspective that takes white supremacist heteropatriarchal power relations and women's traumatic sexual histories into account (Gentile, 2017a, 2017b).

Performing Femininity, Camp, and Switching

How dominance, control, and "switchiness" could feel sexy were common themes among the women I interviewed. Often women spoke of the power of "performing femininity" on their own terms. But the freedom to play with different gendered roles, to inhabit both "masculine" and "feminine" orientations to sex, and to go back and forth between dominating and submitting, were also considered important turn-ons by many of the women I spoke with. Ava describes the pleasure she derives from inhabiting and embodying femininity: "A lot of the way that I express my sexuality is through clothing and makeup and having a really feminine appearance." Evie extends this notion, but theorizes it in terms of "camp" and actively playing with gender roles:

> It's like almost satirical. . . . [T]here is something kind of sexy about putting on an apron and like making food for your partner—it's like being aware of those gender roles and having it be something that is super normative, but

---

9. Recently, some clinical and experimental sex researchers have begun to explore the connection between mindfulness and BDSM. Brotto, for instance, has coauthored a few studies of clinical considerations regarding BDSM practitioners (see Dunkley & Brotto, 2018, 2019; Dunkley, Henshaw, Henshaw, & Brotto, 2020); I am excited and hopeful about this new line of research and hope to see Brotto and other sex researchers and therapists who have focused on mindfulness further explore the meditative components of BDSM, in addition to exploring the connections between trauma and low desire, more broadly (see O'Loughlin & Brotto, 2020).

not something super normative in *my life*. And so kind of playing into those roles is fun, it's like playing with gender in a way that's been prescribed to me my whole life but something I've never adhered to.

Taja describes a similar enjoyment with playing into prescribed gender roles, and expands on the notion of "camp" or "drag":

> I am from the South, my mother is from the South, there was a lot of cultural conditioning around feminine behavior, that included things like Girl Scouts, and majorettes, cheerleading, ballet, tap, jazz, horseback riding, you name it, the traditional schooling that you would give to a girl. . . . [A]nd I lived for all of that, I loved all of that, and wouldn't even wear pants until second grade! I was super girly about all of it. . . . [A]nd so I think there is still for me this sort of mystique to this uber-femininity, that I would love to inhabit. . . . [I]t's not necessarily what you see in an advertisement or in a movie, it's camp, it's drag. . . . I love that shit, love it! Let's inhabit something that is not even *us* at this point . . . we are playing something else. . . . [I]t's like getting closer to that [feminine] space sexually somehow, that is satisfying to me.

Taja and Evie sum up how expressing, performing, and playing with femininity can be fun and feel powerful, but they also elucidate how it is only in the context of performativity (as this concept is described in the quintessential queer theory texts of the 1990s, including in the work of Judith Butler, e.g., *Gender Trouble* [1990]) and a playful nostalgia that they tend to feel comfortable doing this—and only with partners whom they know are also "playing along." Valdivia expresses how playing with these roles might involve explicitly blurring gender boundaries within a specific sex act as well, and describes how she plays with gender and activity/receptivity by wearing a strap-on dildo and penetrating her masculine-of-center non-binary partner:

> I think that's part of the sexy thing, it's like, "Oh my God, here is this femme wearing a strap-on dick!" . . . That might be above some people's heads. I am a femme with a dick! And it's great! I am so proud! It's really empowering!

Sadie also describes how she has always felt constrained by "rules" about the femininity that was expected of her, and that it wasn't until she started experimenting with these and trying out different orientations during sexual encounters that she felt freed from these constraints:

Like an exaggerated femininity, I could put on that role, which I do like, and being totally submissive, I found out that I like that . . . [but then I can also do] that super masculine, very confident thing. I was like, "Oh, I can wear both hats, I can play with both things, and I don't have to choose one," and I think that was hanging me up for a really long time . . . because I like aspects of both, and both sides of me are totally legitimate.

Zola discusses how she enjoys playing a submissive role with women, but ultimately identifies as a "switch," as she feels more empowered dominating the men she is sexually involved with:

I prefer to be submissive to women, I don't want to be submissive to men, because of a past relationship [in which she was violated]. But I do like to dominate men. . . . I have a [cis male] friend who plays with me. And we don't have intercourse at all. He has given me oral sex once but other than that one time, we don't have any type of penetrative sex, there are no fingers, no penis, it's just like rough play, like borderline S&M, and we just kind of kiss and touch and play, and this is the first sexual relationship I have been involved with like that. But it has been bringing me more gratification and satisfaction sexually than actual intercourse sometimes will. . . . I'm in control of it. I am dominant in it. . . . [W]e kind of switch off, but it is mostly me. . . . [H]e is very attentive and intuitive to how my body feels.

Tiffany echoes a similar sentiment about the pleasures of switchiness:

I'm still figuring all this stuff out, this is all very, very new to me. I think realistically I just need someone who I can share that with [sexual exploration, including BDSM], and who will help me figure that out for myself, as well as [allowing me to help] figure that out for them. But I definitely think that I am a switch, I am both, I definitely like being dominant, I like to play that role, but I also enjoy, I'm sure I would enjoy being a submissive, serving someone and pleasing them in that way.

For some women, the ability to switch back and forth among different roles, including between "passive" and "active" roles, and between "masculine" and "feminine" roles within sexual acts, in addition to other forms of playfulness, is what makes a sexual encounter stimulating. This sense of play and the freedom to switch roles was just as important as the need to "slow down" and "be in the present"—and for many women, they seem to go hand in hand. Molly's comments in the previous section about submission as meditative again make it clear why these two orientations are not mutually exclusive.

Queerness, Enthusiastic Consent, and Rejecting Heteronormative Scripts for Sexual Pleasure

Although many of the women I spoke with identify as straight, most were very interested in exploring non-normative configurations of pleasure and intimacy, as they explicate above (this is also true for those who identify as queer). Part of this involved rejecting heteronormative scripts for sexual pleasure, a theme also identified by Cacchioni (2015), which Zola describes:

> I went to a play party late last year, and it was the first play party I'd ever been to, and I had a really good time *not* having sex; it was some of the best sex I've had without having intercourse or penetrative sex. . . . [T]here was a lot of touching, somebody gave me a massage, and I gave somebody else a really sensual massage, [and] at one point I had somebody spank me with a paddle, while her girlfriend was kissing me, and just that—it was probably fifteen minutes long—but it was some of the most amazing fifteen minutes of my whole life!

Here we have another example of how temporality affects participants' experiences of sex. Zola's comments make the limitations of the cisheteronormative cultural imperative to equate sex with penile-vaginal intercourse (Gavey, 2011; Kaye, 2011; Loe, 2004; Mamo & Fishman, 2001) explicit. When I ask her what kind of sex is most desirable to her, or what it is that turns her on about going outside of or beyond the boundaries of "normal" sexual activity, Zola states:

> When you have "alternative" sex, there is a lot of respect and negotiation that goes into that, and that adds to my ability to really appreciate it and feel satisfied by it because everyone that is involved in whatever scenario makes sure that everyone is getting what they want, that doesn't hurt anybody, doesn't offend you, doesn't make you feel used or worthless. . . . [I]t's kind of empowering to be able to have that.

Evie extends this notion:

> In order for me to want to have sex with somebody, I have to feel comfortable. . . . I have had intense sex and I'm interested in being more explorative with it, with bondage, S&M, that type of stuff, I'm not interested in haphazardly shoving a penis in my vagina. I'd like to be with someone who knows what they are doing, who is interested in *not* having heteronormative sex. . . . I'm more like, "Well, let's get to know each other, let's see if our sex lives would work together, and let's see if you're interesting, experimental . . ." I want to have it be a little bit more thoughtful and intentional.

Both Zola and Evie are clear about what turns them on, and explain that they are interested in going beyond the constraints of the hegemonic (i.e., heteronormative, linear, penetrative) sexual protocol that they have been culturally prescribed and socialized to expect over the course of their lives. Valdivia extends this explicitly to the notion of enthusiastic consent: "When somebody is like, 'Can I do this thing to you?' and you are like, 'You want to do what? Okay, cool. That's cool, I'm glad we established that!'"

Some women spoke of this in terms of advocating for oneself, of being "proactive"—specifically in the face of heteronormative constraints and rigid sexual prescriptions, including, paradoxically, for feminine flexibility and fluidity (Fischer, 2013; Rupp, Taylor, Regev-Messalem, Fogarty, & England, 2014; Valocchi, 2005; Wade, 2017). Sadie illustrates this point, returning to the notion of feeling "voiceless" during sexual encounters, and describes how she has attempted to combat this:

> I felt very inactive and submissive with a lot of guys I've been with, and really voiceless, like I was just kind of doing what the formula is, and that is the most disturbing part of the part of me that is like heterosexual, that I have to play by these hetero rules, because it is scripted, it is visible, we see it everywhere, it is the formula, it is the pattern—it is just so ridiculously formulaic! What I like about exploring things with girls is that there is so much less visibility, there's so much more new terrain, there's more spontaneity, freedom, whereas I feel more constricted with men.

Sadie's comments illustrate how she feels voiceless not only because of the formulaic nature of the heteronormative sex she has had over the course of her life but also because there has literally been very little communication between her and her partners. Many of the women I spoke with expressed similar concerns about a lack of communication, and said that some of the best sex they had happened after desires had been clearly communicated by both partners, and when they felt truly "on the same page" with and respected by a partner because of the communication that had occurred.

Kelly's and Astrid's experiences, after being involved in a treatment program for women who experience low desire and pain during intercourse, also emphasize these points about proactivity, intentionality, communication, and enthusiasm. When I ask Kelly how her sex life has been since completing treatment in the program (which she deemed unsuccessful), she describes having developed a more intentional orientation toward the process of choosing her sexual and romantic partners, which has dramatically increased her sexual desire and experience of pleasure:

> I saw a [psycho]therapist [after treatment in the program] to talk about relationships in general, and she encouraged me to be much more ruthless with who I date, to be more picky about the people who I choose to be in relationships with. . . . [B]eing more conscious of who I'm choosing to have sex with [helps]. . . . [T]here are still times when it hurts, but there are a lot of ways to get creative with sex! As long as people are open to it . . . and even just waiting, if I'm going to have intercourse, not just going ahead and doing it, but being with men who prefer to actually make you aroused and want to have sex first—which not all of them do!

Astrid's experience post-treatment is even more striking. She did not complete the treatment program and also deemed it as a failure, because she realized that the type of sex she was having with the partner she was with during that time was what was actually not working for her; she no longer identifies as having low desire because she now has a fulfilling sex life and plays the sexual roles she wants to and uses her body the way she wants to during sex. Regarding her new orientation to sex, Astrid tells me:

> I guess like in a queer understanding of sex, sex can mean a lot of different things and in the sex that I have today, this "disorder" is no disorder at all, it doesn't get in the way of my sex. . . . [L]ooking back, I thought that I was supposed to have sex in a specific way and I tried to do that and it never felt right, it always felt invasive, it always felt like I was giving in to what was expected of me, never what I really desired or wanted. . . . [A]nd the more that I acknowledged that I was not straight, the more that this "disorder" became a nonissue. The more that I started having queer sex, sex with women, the more that I realized I was completely sexually functional, that I could have all kinds of sex and that I could do all kinds of things, and that I didn't in fact have any impediments to my sexual expression, that there are

certain things that my body doesn't like, and certain kinds of touch that don't feel good and that that was fine, and that that was never a problem to communicate to queer partners.... [N]ow I only have negotiated, consensual, enthusiastic, good-feeling sex.... [I]t's just not an issue anymore.

Astrid's story makes particularly clear the importance of being able to set the terms of any given sexual encounter, to reject heteronormative scripts for sexual pleasure when they feel coercive, and to only engage in intentional, negotiated sexual experiences that she feels enthusiastic about. Although her interaction with medical discourses that pathologized her low desire (or, rather, lack of heteronormative desire) was unique among the stories of the women I interviewed, she brings home the crucial notion of sexual intentionality—something that most of the low-desiring women I interviewed felt was important, and that had been missing from their sex lives. Her comment also lays bare the myriad problems with the broad feminized responsive desire framework—including the FSIAD diagnosis, the circular sexual response cycle, plethysmographic research that emphasizes female genital/subjective discordance, and associated behavior-based treatments and therapeutic protocols (including not only MBST but also other protocols from the realms of alternative or holistic care that emphasize mindfulness/meditation as an apolitical sexual enhancement tool and that admonish fantasy). We see here how both contemporary medical and alternative approaches to treatment for low female desire fall short, precisely because they assume a cis female subject who experiences herself as reductively feminine, who desires a specific type of masculine partner, who has never been traumatized (or who has or can be healed from that trauma), and who simply needs to bridge the gap between her "subjective" and "objective" arousal—or rather who needs to deal with her naturalized feminine discordant/dissociative tendencies in order to enhance her own sexual pleasure. For most of the low-desiring women I interviewed, this model of female sexuality is, at the very least, constraining and restrictive, and in some cases, it is harmful and violent.

Reclaiming Receptivity, Subverting Submission

Through medical and scientific discourses and popular representations, women are consistently depicted as essentially receptive or responsive, and their sexuality is framed as more complex, complicated, fluid, and flexible, often in neurobiological terms. Concomitantly, their presumed desire for submission is often posited as an evolutionary predisposition, or it is not theorized at all. This is an unfortunate side effect of the dismantling and jettisoning of psychoanalytic theory from modern-day psychiatry and psychology, wherein trauma and desire—and especially the relationship between the two—are pushed out of the contemporary mainstream (including the mainstream white liberal feminist) clinical milieu. Current scientific discourses and medical treatments that address low desire in women both *rely on* and simultaneously *negate* women's trauma. Further, feminine dissociation is essentialized via its uncanny resemblance to female subjective/genital discordance, while the social and traumatizing factors that influence these phenomena are not analyzed or theorized. Through these discourses, feminine receptivity is naturalized and even romanticized, whereas the desire for submission is more often dismissed or pathologized. My findings flip this framing on its head.

My research suggests that subbing in BDSM may be experienced as more agentic than utilizing mindfulness protocols in sex therapy. Myriad feminist researchers since the "sex-positive turn" have suggested that the explicitness of power dynamics in BDSM offers a space where women can actually experience safety and agency and work through trauma, and they can do all of those things because the erotics of power are in plain sight. Conversely, the receptivity protocol of the feminized responsive desire framework functions as a new way to hide power relations in sexual life and particularly in cisheterosex. BDSM offers a much different kind of outlet, so, just like dissociation is an uncanny twin of discordance, submission is an uncanny twin of receptivity. Receptivity here might be recoded as submission, and mindfulness as a sub state. I argue that this framing is actually much more helpful, as submission here is made explicit and visible, rather than remaining hidden behind medicalized hypotheses about innate feminine receptivity.

Part of my project here has been to examine why and how sexual trauma, gendered violence, and differences in masculine and feminine socialization are consistently neglected in sexological research and associated treatment protocols; to illuminate what women themselves have to say about these discourses and about their own desire—including the desire for submission; and, finally, to excavate which populations are produced via these discourses. Foucault (1978) outlined biopolitics as concerned with the securitization of populations and with "control over relations among the human race" (p. 245), and this production and regulation of feminine receptivity arguably fits within this framework. As I have argued throughout this book, medical and scientific narratives (from the mouths and pens of clinicians who self-identify as feminists) biopolitically produce and configure feminized populations and aid in the socialization of the individuals therein into specific heterocisgendered orientations toward their own bodies, the bodies of their partners, and their relationships. This has dire consequences for women's (and others') sexual personae and for their sexual and mental health.

Unfortunately, the feminist sex wars of the 1970s and 1980s, which occurred right alongside the research that set the stage for the reworking of feminine receptivity in post-Freudian terms, have not aided the cause of women's empowerment through submission. Mainstream or popular, scholarly, political, and in some cases medical and scientific discourses framed as feminist have tended to perpetuate narratives of natural and essential feminine receptivity (which must be guarded against, in the case of the radical feminist, or which alternatively may be romanticized or celebrated, in the case of the liberal/cultural feminist—including the liberal/cultural feminist sex researcher and sex therapist), while simultaneously stripping the act of submission within BDSM of its agency. Feminism and the clinic have unfortunately worked hand in hand to take submission away from women as a legitimate avenue for self-care—an avenue that is sometimes sexual, or that sometimes might be *para*sexual (as it is situated near the sexual but cannot always be entirely encompassed by it).

My findings suggest that the naturalization and romanticization of feminine receptivity and concomitant dismissal and pathologization of submission are not adequate in accounting for women's orientations toward their own embodied experiences and praxes. Many of the low-desiring women I interviewed were interested in subbing in BDSM—sometimes as a meditational practice, sometimes as an exploration of pure sensuality, sometimes as a reclamation of trauma through submission, and sometimes for unrelated reasons. Importantly, subbing requires trust, negotiation, and communication; and so essentialized feminine receptivity or responsiveness is replaced with intentional and controlled submission, which paradoxically becomes a more empowering or agentic frame. Further, this contrasts with the way mindfulness too often appears as a means to a (cishetero)normative end by clinicians and sex therapists interested in "brief" and "efficient" treatment protocols within a cognitive behavioral tradition, and within bio-/psycho-medical and evolutionary discourses of female receptivity and responsiveness (the same could be said for alternative healers in this vein). Subbing in BDSM as intentional, negotiated, and/or as a form of meditation or a very different version of mindfulness pushes against this heteronormative framework, and thus has a queer potential (even when executed by women who do not necessarily identify as queer). Here, we can see how medical discourses of receptivity are actually disempowering and potentially retraumatizing, whereas BDSM becomes a space to rework power dynamics and reclaim agency in the face of trauma, including through submission, meditation, and other parasexual practices (which become part of a sexual-asexual-parasexual series or assemblage).

When considering the intersections of clinical medicine and white liberal or cultural feminism, and the iatrogenically retraumatizing potential of contemporary sexual medicine and sex therapy itself, women's own experiences and practices must be considered and theorized, with broader populations and technologies in mind. How do these meditations on and reclamations of receptivity—via submission—possibly exist outside of or alongside the sexual? Does this type of queer practice challenge the sexual/asexual distinction, making space for parasexuality, within a crip-asexual framework (Kim, 2014)? If so, what is the potential of being beyond sexuality in this way? And how is this potential impeded by misogynistic, racist, classist, colonialist, and ableist violence under neoliberal capitalism, and by these as facets of feminized trauma specifically? Discourses of medicine and science, of feminism and empowerment, have far-reaching effects, as do practices involving mindfulness and submission. Analyzing how these produce and configure gender in new and surprising ways in our current moment and into the future is imperative, for we are all affected (albeit to different extents and in different ways) by these population-producing regimes and technologies. The women I interviewed actively subvert, reject, queer, and sometimes take pleasure from their own experiences of feminine sexual difference socialization—even as it is a coercive experience that leaves many women with few options for pleasure. In spite of this, the conversations I had and that I have illuminated throughout this book suggest that even self-identified low-desiring women find spaces within the sexual, and sometimes somewhere alongside it, for pleasure, play, and connection. Maybe this is the kind of *feminine anarchism* we should pay more attention to.

CONCLUSION

The Freedom to Fall Apart

Feminine Fracturing and the Affective Production of Gendered Populations

In June 2015, popular Canadian news outlet *The Globe and Mail* published a piece entitled "'Arousal-First' Desire May Be More Typical for Women, and It Doesn't Need a Cure." Author Zosia Bielski interviews a number of sexual medicine celebrities in her piece (many of the same ones I have discussed in this book), presents their research that supports the new FSIAD diagnosis, and emphasizes women's desire as uniquely responsive and discordant. Bielski states:

> The current thinking builds on decades of research about the human sexual response cycle. In 2000, Rosemary Basson . . . nudged the science away from a strictly linear desire-arousal-sex-orgasm model, pioneering a cyclical model instead. The latest edition of the *DSM-5* . . . also reflects this shift, collapsing women's sexual desire and arousal disorders into a new diagnosis of "[Female] Sexual Interest/Arousal Disorder" ([F]SIAD), after clinicians reported female patients often had difficulties differentiating between desire and arousal. Today, some researchers and clinicians believe a more common experience for women might be "responsive desire": a desire that arises in response to something pleasurable, not in anticipation of it.

Later in the article, Bielski describes her own experience at Meredith Chivers's laboratory, where she was connected to a photoplethysmograph and shown a variety of different types of pornography, so that her self-reported "subjective arousal" could be compared to her "physiological arousal"—or, according to Bielski, "between what I say turns me on and what my body actually responds to." She then goes on to explain, based on her interview with Chivers, how "discordance" between self-report and objective measurement is a "mostly female phenomenon" that "researchers have been exploring since the 1970s, with women's bodies often not aligning with their words." She states that Chivers is "constantly having to correct those curious about her work who assume that what happens in a woman's body reveals what she really wants—that the vaginal plethysmograph is a lie detector test." But if the claim here is *not* that what turns women on physically explains what they truly desire, then why study the disconnect in the first place, so intensively and extensively? Why develop an "arousal-first" model of desire, and apply it disproportionately to women? Why not just listen to what women report about what turns them on? If researchers believe that physiological arousal does not equal desire, then why create a female-specific low-desire diagnosis for the *DSM-5* that collapses desire and arousal in the first place—particularly if the argument based on plethysmographic research is that physiological arousal and subjective desire operate in accordance with two entirely different logics, on two completely separate planes, for women uniquely? And most importantly, if feminist-identified sex researchers are reluctant to have plethysmographic evidence for female discordance interpreted as the "truth" of women's desire, why have they organized an entire research industry and set of treatment protocols precisely around this phenomenon?

In recent published accounts, particularly since the *DSM-5* was released in 2013, many researchers that I have cited in this book have begun to describe Rosemary Basson's circular sexual response cycle as being equally applicable to men and women, and have moved toward embracing both the gender-neutral incentive motivation model of desire and a theory of state-dependent (over trait-dependent) desire. And sometimes when these researchers describe the FSIAD diagnosis, they drop the "F," positing it as "SI/AD" instead (for an example, see Chivers & Brotto, 2017), thus giving the impression that it is gender-neutral. These researchers now also tend to only cite Basson's article in the *Journal of Sex & Marital Therapy*, "Human Sex-Response Cycles" (2001a), when discussing responsive desire and the circular sexual response cycle—but it is important to note that this is the only published research account wherein Basson described the model as gender-neutral. In all other discussions (by Basson and others)—up until very recently—it has been used to describe *women's* responsive desire, specifically. Popular analyses such as Bielski's above highlight the problematic slippage between proclaiming "women are uniquely responsive" and stating "no, men are too, we just haven't studied them enough yet," which is now often implied. Further, it doesn't really matter if researchers now argue that this model of "responsive desire" is not unique to women; the history of how the circular sexual response cycle has informed the last two decades of research on women's sexuality, the way it is linked up with the gendered use of the incentive-motivation model and with experimental research on male concordance and female *dis*cordance (which has often espoused evolutionary psychology theorizations of gender differences in desire), the use of mindfulness-based sex therapy techniques to cure women's discordance, and the sheer existence of the FSIAD diagnosis itself (as a diagnosis that, categorically, only women can receive) all tell a very different story. The feminization of receptivity and responsive desire, including in the most cutting-edge contemporary research, is undeniable, and popular analyses such as Bielski's make the lineage here, the genealogy of feminine receptivity/responsiveness/complexity, from hysteria to FSIAD, unmistakably obvious.

The feminization of this arousal-first model of responsive desire, especially as it is linked to therapy protocols that prescribe mindfulness to help women let negative thoughts "flow downstream," seems to suggest nothing less than using "the other story the plethysmograph keeps tabs on" (Bielski, 2015) to cast doubt on women's verbal accounts, and to potentially control, modify, and *change* their feelings and behaviors. Or, at the very least, it opens up these possibilities. So, even if researchers such as Chivers really don't believe that physiological arousal has anything to do with women's true subjective desires, the fact that they constantly have to correct people who think that their work in this regard represents a type of "lie detector test" is very telling indeed. And it suggests that regardless of Chivers's (or any other researcher in this domain's) intentions, the conclusions of this research are being received by the general public in a very different way.

Take, for instance, the very first comment after the Bielski article was published online (comments that have since been taken down). A commenter who goes by the name of "riksaga" states: "Ok—'responsive desire' sounds great BUT the problem seems to be how forceful do I act in activating her responsive desire? Legal and ethical considerations are dumped on me." The second commenter, "Frederick Mackenzie," responds: "A generation of epicene men, too effete to just go for it (or too quivered by possible social or legal repercussions) when he has a woman before him, and now there is a problem with a lack of arousal among women. You wonder why?" These comments alone say much about public response to this research, and the potential impact it has on women, men, and sexual relations among them. riksaga is not concerned with how women will benefit from this new "responsive desire" model; he is instead concerned with how to activate women's desire, and with how far is "too far" to go with this activation, for his own legal protection. Luckily for the women in his life, because riksaga apparently cares about not getting into trouble with the law, he suggests that he is not planning on forcing any women into sexual acts in the name of activating their desire at this time. Frederick Mackenzie is frustrated by what he believes is a cultural emasculation of men who no longer feel manly enough to just "go for it"; he believes this has caused women's desire to suffer, and thus I'd imagine he sees promise in the institution of a circular sexual response cycle for women based on the notion of responsive feminine desire. As was also suggested by commenters "George" and "David" on Bergner's 2009 *New York Times* pieces that I cited in the introduction to this book, these comments on Bielski's piece represent at least some of the broad lay interpretations of a model of female sexual desire founded upon responsiveness and receptivity. All of these comments highlight the looming threat of the normalization of sexual coercion of women, and men's responses to it. They illuminate these misogynistic trends regardless of what clinicians say their research "actually" indicates. This—the disconnect between purportedly objective, apolitical, atheoretical, and neutral science, on the one hand, and public interpretation of that research, on the other—is one type of *discordance* that really is a problem.[1]

•

In my participants' stories of their experiences of sexual difference socialization, of providing sexual carework throughout their lives, and of the circuitous ways they have come to navigate and negotiate sexual intentionality and embrace parasexual care in the face of so much harm—the omnipresence of feminized receptivity/responsiveness and the expectations and responsibilities that come along with it are the binding themes. This paradoxically and insidiously mandated receptivity can feel coercive, like a violation, and it can

---

1. In one final telling example: In January 2020, as I was working on the final revisions to this book, I came across the series *Sex, Explained* on Netflix. Episode 3 on "Attraction" features the study in which subjects watched bonobo porn in addition to other types of porn (Chivers et al., 2007) while their genital responses, as measured with plethysmographs, were compared to their subjective statements about whether or not they were turned on. The episode emphasizes that discordance is a largely female phenomenon, and that "men tend to be more rigid with the type of people they're attracted to [in terms of gender], whereas women are more flexible" (this is stated by Lisa Diamond, who is interviewed throughout the episode). The narrator reads a line about how this research, conducted by Chivers, Seto, and Blanchard in 2007, demonstrates that women are turned on by "pretty much everything" (including monkeys having sex).

result in trauma. Whether it is the experience of everyday banal incursions such as street harassment or trust being breached in intimate relationships, or the more obvious violations such as child molestation and sexual abuse, almost all of the women I spoke with were bound by a common experience of gendered and sexualized trauma. For some, their experiences as women of color, as queer, and/or as gender-nonconforming, amplified this reality. No generalizations can be made about the relationship between trauma and low desire, as this is an exploratory qualitative study, but the narratives of my low-desiring participants suggest that an important component of one's experience of femininity in a broad sense does to some extent involve the experience of violation. Thus, one central aspect of this study has been an attempt to shed light on how femininity, as an affective and biopolitical phenomenon lived at the level of the population, is traumatic, and involves the constant potential threat of violation—at least for some women and femmes, including those with whom I spoke about their experiences of low desire. This is one part of how the category and population I have sought to illuminate—*women-with-low-desire*—gets produced in everyday life.

Lynda Hart (1998) has suggested that some feminists argue that "the heteropatriarchal system as such is an ideological institution that interpellates and produces women as a traumatic category" (p. 183). This perspective on femininity is reminiscent of Kaja Silverman's (1992) notion of a "dominant fiction" regarding the ideological production of masculine and feminine subjectivity (which are produced when bodies and ways of being are equated with valuable—or not-so-valuable—symbols). I appreciate a consideration of how femininity is produced as a devalued, traumatic category, but I also think we must go further, into the realms of affect and phenomenology, to consider what the experience of that feminized trauma and violation actually feels like—and, ultimately, to reposition it in terms of agency. Thus, I want to take up a different orientation to embodiment and trauma, and push through ideology and interpellation, into the "crisis ordinariness" (Berlant, 2011) or "insidious traumas" (Cvetkovich, 2003) of everyday gendered, sexualized, and racialized violence. Although I am concerned with the way that (low-desiring) femininity is configured within the diagnostic discourse of the *DSM-5*, for instance, I am more concerned with the material-discursive relations that are played out alongside clinical and therapeutic regimes and diagnoses, and their effects on the lives of real people.

The women I interviewed who had been treated in medical programs for pain and low desire experienced specific sexual problems that they eventually identified as largely relational. This experience reveals the emptiness of diagnosis, and also of the coercive, nonconsensual nature of both treatment for low female desire and of cisheteronormative sexual and structural relations that tend to occur alongside women's low desire more broadly. Pain, discomfort, and trauma are always embodied, and thus it may be imperative to consider why we have set up such stark boundaries through these discourses between the "psychological" and the "physiological" in the first place, and concomitantly, why dissociation has been feminized in such violent ways (materially and discursively—which are always one and the same). It appears that the line between "the psychological" and "the physiological" can be drawn—and erased—at will within these protocols. But the irony here is that this violent essentializing, naturalizing, neurobiologizing, and, ultimately, *feminizing* of dissociation (or a mind/body disconnect or discordance) functions to hide the experiential realities of the actual violence women, femmes, and gender-nonconforming folks experience every day—violences that are so expected as to be banal and normal, and that are, in some cases, traumatizing, and may produce dissociative tendencies such as depersonalization and derealization during sex. Further, the biologizing and feminizing of dissociation paradoxically creates a situation in which dissociation itself is, in some cases, iatrogenically induced—for instance in the research laboratory or clinic, both of which extend into the bedroom.

Current scientific discourses and associated treatments both *depend on* and simultaneously *disavow* women's trauma. Because feminine dissociation is naturalized and essentialized *as discordance* in expert discourses about women's low desire and the feminized responsive desire framework, while social factors that influence this situation (i.e., sexual, gendered, and racialized violence and resulting traumas) are not analyzed or theorized, these therapies and treatments may actually retraumatize women. Trauma, then, is constitutive of and simultaneously denied within these regimes and by the practitioners and researchers who support them. Both the experience of women's low desire and the diagnostic category itself are melancholic and tropological (Butler, 1997)—that is, they are figurative, they are self-producing, they call up a fracturing, and in that very calling up, they fracture. This is made more starkly apparent when considering how dissociation seems to be an uncanny twin of discordance—I am not arguing that all women who are measured as discordant have experienced trauma and thus dissociate as a result of this, but the possibility that many women who are measured in this way have been traumatized (potentially by measurement apparatuses themselves) and experience dissociation as a result should not be taken lightly, nor rejected out of hand. Further, the concordance/discordance measurement protocol itself reifies a mind/body split, thus conjuring it into being—and this is part of the *work of the gap* that I have identified throughout this book.

It has been argued by some scientists and clinicians that women's sexuality is inherently fluid, flexible, and receptive or responsive; at least for the women-with-low-desire I interviewed for this project, it may be true that women's sexualities are complex. But if they are more complex than men's sexualities and desires, these interviews make it clear that this is primarily due to sociopolitical and material factors, including gendered and sexualized violence—which are completely elided in scientific research that suggests that women are "hardwired to submit" or are "evolutionarily programmed to be sexually flexible." Not only this, but trauma and low desire are held apart discursively in the *DSM-5* and in its foundational research; as it may result from "severe relational distress" (listed as a diagnostic caveat which would preclude diagnosis), being diagnosed with PTSD would likely prevent a woman from receiving the FSIAD diagnosis. What violence is done—discursively and materially—when this type of comorbidity is not explored, theorized, and politicized?

The receptivity prescribed by FSIAD and the circular sexual response cycle, within the feminized responsive desire framework more broadly, is an instantiation of the murkiness of discursive configurations of femininity, which are not only discursively nebulous but are materially, experientially, and phenomenologically confusing because of the proliferation of traumatic violence and its institutional enforcement. Being a low-desiring woman here is about facing the porous and perpetually probed boundaries of one's feminized body; it involves being forced to answer—over and over again—what one will accept inside, what one will invite within, what one will *receive*. It involves the assumption that that reception, that response, is consensual, but rarely being asked the question. And it involves knowing that others like you are also being probed in this way, that you are part of a population, but that you are discouraged, within an individualistic neoliberal milieu of blame and shame, from coming together as a community to speak to each other and to speak back against this treatment.[2]

One must only take a look at the titles of the numerous media accounts of the scientific research on women's sexuality over the last few years to see what is at stake—and under conquest—here: "Cracking The Code on Female Sexual Desire" (Madsen, 2013), "The Misunderstood Science of Female Desire" (Barmak, 2018), and "Hunting the Female Libido" (Conniff, 2010) are just a few of them. There is a consistent investment in finding the truth of female desire, the truth of sexual difference. And in all of these articles, responsiveness and receptivity are described as constitutive of feminine sexuality. The

---

2. This framing resonates with Patsavas's (2014) suggestion that the purported unnarratability of chronic pain is not due to anything unique about the condition itself, but rather to widespread cultural silencing of those who are in pain.

feminized responsive desire framework has become much bigger than any of the researchers who created it perhaps intended—and now it is increasingly hard to do away with. So regardless of anyone's intentions, this model is now deeply embedded, culturally pervasive, an indisputable truism—and the way it is being interpreted and has taken hold shouldn't be a surprise to anyone. Further, sex therapy and sexology have always been to some extent about management and control, and they have always been white, bourgeois, and hetero-/cisnormative—which is why seeking the "truth" of female desire can never be a neutral endeavor and will instead always be a project of domination, production, modification, and surveillance. And because there is no singular feminine desire, the institution of responsiveness as categorical can never be a corrective to the older linear response models of sexology. Now we have the same old tropes about feminine receptivity, simply reframed in the guise of female empowerment under neoliberalism. But, we must ask: Empowerment for whom? If we embrace a model of receptive feminine "willingness" in sexual response models and therapy, we must responsibly inquire—who gets to be willing? Much is assumed here regarding a romanticized white, cis, hetero, wealthy or middle-class lifestyle, and it is also assumed that willingness is happening in the absence of coercion. Not only is the figure of the woman who is to be helped via sex therapy always imagined as white, wealthy, normatively able-bodied, and cishet, she is also imagined to be a subject who is free of trauma. And trauma here is also conceptualized as something exceptional, extraordinary, and discrete, a rupture, break, or breach—one is either traumatized or they are not. But if we take the work of feminist madness studies and critical trauma, queer/crip of color, and disability studies scholars seriously, then it is clear that trauma is not so remarkable, and it is not something that can be recovered from so easily (Piepzna-Samarasinha, 2018). It also affects different populations differently—that is, women, femmes, and particularly trans women and gender-nonconforming folks of color are disproportionately affected by both everyday insidious traumas, on the one hand, and the more easily identifiable traumas of stranger rape and childhood sexual abuse, on the other. Not only this, but survivors are consistently expected to heal and recover from, or to *overcome* trauma—on their own.[3]

---

3. In this vein, it is also important to distinguish between *trauma* and *stress*. The sexually troubled woman is regularly framed as low in desire because she is "stressed out" (see www.debunkingdesire.com for a quintessential example of this framing)—but it is imperative to remember that *stress* (for instance, from too much "multi-tasking") and *trauma* (for instance, from experiencing everyday racialized, gendered, and sexualized violence) are not the same thing. But if we were committed to distinguishing stress from trauma in these discourses of low female desire, we would have to reckon with race, class, and other important differences among groups of women, and we would have to take seriously what types of treatments are

Through my qualitative research with low-desiring women, many of whom identify as trauma survivors, I have examined feminized experiences of violence in terms of affect and populations, but also as experiences that are felt and lived at the level of individual bodies and relations between and among them, and that are often—but not always—linked to the realm of the sexual. It is imperative to attend to the limitations of current biomedical configurations of low desire, not only because these paradigms elide gender, race, and class differences in how violence is meted out and experienced, but also because these biomedical tropes are hetero- and cisnormative, individualizing, and rooted in colonialist, neoliberal, and white formulations of the body and mind (which are held separate). These frameworks thus perpetuate antiquated ableist, cisnormative, heterosexist, and racist notions of sexual difference and gendered experience. By attending to banal, everyday, ordinary trauma, the feminization and racialization of these technologies and experiences is drawn sharply into view, and thus women, femmes, and gender-diverse folks—particularly those of color—may have their experiences validated.

•

I want to end this book by illuminating two competing—and, unfortunately, incommensurable—realities about the new science of female sexuality and the feminized responsive desire framework. On the one hand, there are lots of new technologies for enhancing desire, including neurotransmitter drugs and mindfulness-based sex therapy, and their excesses cannot be predicted or controlled. This is exciting and speaks to Chivers's notion that women can now explore their "internal playgrounds" (as cited in Martin, 2018, p. 46). To this end, we must remember that biopower (Foucault, 1978) is about control, and can be disciplinary, but that it is also always productive—of new categories, subjectivities, and ultimately, new ways of life. If we consider production within this biopolitical frame, and perhaps ironically, simultaneously turn a psychoanalytic lens to mindfulness-based sex therapy, plethysmography, and models of receptive sexual desire—in keeping with the Foucault and Freud of queer theory—we can see that there might be a queer excess, an erotic potential in these new technologies, that can never be fully accounted for,

---

appropriate for whom. I argue that "stress" has become the go-to category in this discourse precisely because it invokes a white, middle-class, cishet woman in need of sexual help, for instance through mindfulness-based sex therapy, and that treating this imagined figure (with "brief" and individualized behavior-based treatments) is inherently much easier, neater, and tidier than truly and adequately addressing feminized trauma (trauma that is sometimes incurred through these bourgeois treatments themselves).

predicted, or controlled. There is potentially something very queer and hot, for example, about meditating, along with several other low-desiring women, on the "vulva-like" contours of a raisin (Brotto, 2018, p. 77), together, in a group mindfulness session. Even technologies that are meant to train and produce heterosexual desire have a queer excess and erotic potential. Take Brotto's recounting of the story of "Gianna," a woman who is learning how to use mindfulness in her romantic relationship to enhance her own subjective/genital concordance, but who has a much harder time "being in the present" when she's at home than she does at the clinic:

> During an extended mindfulness practice one day, Gianna said, through tears, "I just don't get it, I can be so present in my body when I'm here in this isolated room with a group of strangers, and yet at home, when I try to be with my physical sensations in my comfortable and familiar environment, I feel like I get even more distracted, and I just don't feel anything in my body!" (p. 145)

It is worth noting that something sexy and unpredictable appears to happen in the clinic for Gianna, something about the mimetic, fantastic or phantasmatic, uncapturable qualities of desire, that cannot be re-created outside of this scene. Following this line of psychoanalytic thought, and the notion that mindfulness itself might be refigured as an internalized dom/sub scenario (as I alluded to at the end of chapter 2), I'd like to propose that it can also be kinky. How many women have been turned on by sitting in the meditation room with other women and the raisin? How many women have fantasized about the mindfulness-based sex therapy facilitator herself? How many women became aroused from having a plethysmographic vaginal probe inserted or other instruments attached to their bodies? How many were turned on knowing a researcher was recording their genital response, or watching them on camera from an adjacent room? How many got to play out their most unspeakable, perhaps inarticulable, fantasies when they submitted themselves to be examined in an experimental laboratory as a participant in a scientific study on sexual desire? If we apply a psychoanalytic lens to these behaviorist protocols, the possibilities are endless.

Under biopolitical regimes, while there is regulation, there is also new potential. Here, I would like to follow Jagose's analysis of the "queer trace" (2013) of orgasmic reconditioning in gay men. Just as behaviorism and queer theory have surprising resonances (as neither have a sexual subject, per se, only a grouping of behaviors used to approximate identity) and thus they make strange bedfellows, I'd like to think of these new medico-scientific technologies, on the one hand, and kink, on the other hand, in the same way—as strange bedfellows. Fantasy is constitutive of sexual desire in a way that it isn't for really any other "behavior" (including behaviors that have been treated with similar cognitive-behaviorist protocols), so whatever is intended or expected to happen as a result of the therapy (such as the cultivation of heterosexual desire) *doesn't* always happen, and thus the treatment may take surprising turns. I'd like to think of the spaces in which mindfulness-based sex therapy, photoplethysmography, and receptive sexual response cycles are enacted as uncontainable and proliferative spaces, where there will always be a kinky queer excess and erotic potential.

On the other hand, however, these new technologies *do* seek to predict and control—and often in the service of cisheteropatriarchy, white supremacy, neoliberal capitalism, colonialist medicine, and rape culture. For example, mindfulness—and it does makes sense that we want to use it, as it helps lots of us "get by" when things feel overwhelming—is now regularly used to make workers more productive. And, as an important extension, there are race and class implications regarding access to these protocols—or rather, there are racist and classist and nativist barriers to treatment. While it is a white, receptive femininity off of which these treatments are modeled, different members of forcibly feminized populations will not all benefit in the same ways from being treated—however, they will all be expected to fall in line. To this end, not all women and femmes have the *opportunity* to "explore their internal playgrounds," in Chivers's words, in the same ways or to the same extents. And what of nonbinary, gender-nonconforming, agender, and genderqueer folks who will be expected, sometimes against their will, to fall in line? I think here of the ways that some of the participants were taught about the circular sexual response cycle and how it applies to women, when they had really gone in to a clinic for treatment of vaginal pain. Why is a protocol for femininity being taught in these clinical and therapeutic spaces? And what are its potentially noxious effects for those who do not identify with these versions of femininity (or perhaps any version of femininity at all)?

In an article for the *Guardian* in 2018, Moira Donegan points to the ways that racial and class divisions in feminism have now been made clear, specifically in the context of #MeToo. This is worth articulating, as well, in relation to the field of the new science of female sexuality, the feminized responsive desire framework, and the FSIAD diagnosis. Donegan states that there is a central rift within feminism that is revealed by the #MeToo movement: "Feminism has come to contain two distinct understandings of sexism, and two wildly different, often incompatible ideas of how that problem should be solved. One approach is individualist, hard-headed, grounded in ideals of pragmatism, realism, and self-sufficiency. The other is expansive, communal, idealistic, and premised on the ideals of mutual interest and solidarity." This rift is clear in a division between, on the one hand, white liberal feminism of the type that requires one to pull oneself up by one's own bootstraps and which simultaneously erases difference; this is the typical version of "#MeToo" feminism which has now been largely constrained by discourses of liberalism, legality/consent, and individualism in the vein of neoliberal carcerality. On the other hand, however, there is a more intersectional and class-attentive version that encompasses the idea that feminism must not only be for middle-class and wealthy, able-bodied, cishet, white women in the Global North, but for the most marginalized groups, including femmes of color, genderqueer and trans folks, and other people who are brutalized under heteropatriarchal, cisnormative, white supremacist, ableist, neoliberal capitalist rape culture. This second version, this more radical ideology and praxis, also attends to the diversity of "#MeToo moments," reminding us that not all traumatic experiences are registered or *received* in the same way (Rodriguez, 2019). This second version further recognizes that many traumas do not involve a complete schism, break, or rupture, and instead may be more banal or insidious.

The version of feminism that is espoused in the new science of female sexuality and the feminized responsive desire framework is a white liberal feminism, however, insofar as it imagines a subject who can enhance her desire (or is it heal her trauma?) via individualistic treatments that she endeavors upon herself. If we chose to recognize trauma, we would also have to recognize that "consent" and "nonconsent" are not so clear and easily separable in real life, and that trauma is not so discrete—much of trauma operates as crisis ordinariness (Berlant, 2011), and is also made to be productive under neoliberalism. We live in a culture that relies on the hypostatization or othering of trauma as extraordinary and exceptional (as I argued in chapter 5)—but the reality of many of our lives is that they are characterized by mundane, banal, insidious, everyday violence. Our current conception of trauma is myopic, however, as are proposed treatments for sexual dysfunction. I argue that we need to acknowledge the diversity of relationships and trauma experiences, distinguish trauma from "stress," and ultimately recognize the myriad problems with models of sex therapy that assume a tidy, happy, consensual relationship under which "responsive desire" can easily and safely be accessed or triggered, and mindfulness techniques applied. What of those who are traumatized by the very notion of this tidiness?

Critical disability studies and madness studies scholars offer ways to crip theories of trauma, and analyze current models of dissociation as too uniform and restrictive (Johnson, 2015; Johnson & McRuer, 2014; Kafer, 2013; Spurgas, under review). We know that women and femmes are likely to be victims of sexual assault, and now we know that trans women, particularly trans women of color, are disproportionately likely to experience violence (including sexual violence) during their lives. We are now in an age of ever-present yet unspectacular violence, we are haunted by specters of violability, and so we are in a moment to rethink the importance of structures of gender, race, and class as structures of feeling (Williams, 1977). If part of living as a cis or trans woman, as a genderqueer, gender-nonconforming, or nonbinary person, as a femme-identified or AFAB individual (and particularly if one is a person of color who lives within these categories of experience) is about living with anxiety, hypervigilance, and the daily specter of a low-grade, mundane, and banal sexualized violence, then how might we understand dissociation? Maybe dissociation instead looks like anxiety, just too pervasive and partial, or it's the perpetual feeling that you're about to fall apart, to come unglued. Maybe it's having a constant lump in your throat and a racing heartbeat while also feeling completely empty and numb when you read the news, when you walk down the street.

We might take the experience of dissociation, or even more usefully of *dissociative-adjacent* experiences, of feeling threadbare, of falling apart, as a standpoint from which to theorize. Black feminist scholars such as Kimberlé Crenshaw (1991) and Patricia Hill Collins (1990) have utilized intersectional analyses to forefront the importance of standpoint, particularly for marginalized folks. How might we theorize discursive feminization via biomedical protocols, while simultaneously allowing for the real live often femme or feminized person who has experienced trauma to speak—or rather to feel—from that very real material subject position? How might we use theories of the cripistemological (Johnson & McRuer, 2014), criphystemological (Mollow, 2014), and chrononormative (Freeman, 2010) to honor this feminized experience while simultaneously taking care not to essentialize or universalize it? To think about its sociopolitical and structural, yet also embodied and relational, nature? And most importantly: What does feminine fracturing in our contemporary political terrain of slow violence and crisis ordinariness look and feel like? In order to get a better picture of what falling apart feels like—an experience akin to dissociation, derealization, and depersonalization, but not quite the same thing—I propose that we work backward (Love, 2007). If we look at the ways that traumatized people have been and continue to be *expected to recover,* we can get closer to a cripistemology of feminized fracture and falling apart, and also get beyond the white, cishet, middle-class femininity built into formulations of gendered trauma and sexual dysfunction. We must look at how feminized populations have been expected to heal themselves before we can consider more communal and radical ways of caring for each other.

Trauma has historically been conceptualized as a breach that overcomes the subject's capacity to cope, and that makes it impossible to further process distressing events. This produces long-lasting disturbances that must be recovered from. But what if there can be no recovery or rehabilitation, because there hasn't been an actual break? Anxiety, hypervigilance, fracturing, and falling-apartness may be better ways to think of how femininity is produced—and then policed, surveilled, marketed, and marketed to—under late capitalism. There is an ordinariness to both assault and assault-adjacent experiences that may not result in dissociation per se, but may result in another type of crip or dissociative-adjacent experience, with its own temporality and phenomenology. Thus: Falling-apart femininity or feminine fracturing, as a vantage point that we could learn a lot from, may be one way to think and feel this experience.

To that end, the words of the feminized and traumatized are instructive, and so I am grateful that some of these folks agreed to speak with me about their experiences for this book. We need a better feminism that isn't just about offering solutions to women-with-low-desire in the vein of "women should get treatments for sexual dysfunctions, too!" We need a feminist science, medicine, and therapy that doesn't individualize or essentialize sexual problems, and instead looks to the sociopolitical and structural ways that common experiences of violence create traumatized populations—and understand that of course these experiences affect (and produce) the desire of the members of these populations. We must think about the diversity of women and femmes and their experiences and remember that "solutions" aren't solutions for everyone, and in fact may be harmful to some. It is with an eye toward this that we might stand in solidarity as members of these populations, rather than seeking to heal ourselves—from trauma, low desire, and sexual dysfunction—as individuals, or to attempt self-rehabilitation. Caring for each other in community while also attending to difference is a radical alternative to the isolation of self-care, and a radical alternative to simply trying to survive or get by. Rather than always trying to recover, to cure ourselves, and navigating these coercive structures on our own, maybe there is a freedom in falling apart, together.

APPENDIX

TABLE 1. Participant Demographics

PARTICIPANT	AGE	SELF-IDENTIFIED RACE/ETHNICITY	NATIONALITY	SEXUALITY	SEXUAL PAIN (PHYSICAL)?	MEDICAL TREATMENT?
Annie	31	Latinx, Jewish	US	Mostly straight	No	No
Astrid	30	White	Canada	Gay/Queer	Yes	Yes
Ava	24	Palestinian	US	Queer	No	No
Bridget	54	White	US	Straight/Hetero	No	Yes
Charlie	31	White, Jewish	Canada	Asexual/Pansexual	No	No
Corinne	30	White	US	Straight/Hetero	No	No
Elaine	31	Armenian	US	Straight/Hetero	No	No
Elizabeth	30	White	US	Straight/Hetero	No	No
Evie	25	White	US	Queer	No	No
Jill	26	Russian	Russia/US	Straight/Hetero	No	No
Julia	37	White	US	Bisexual	No	No
Karen	34	White	EU	Straight/Hetero	No	No
Kelly	29	White	Canada	Mostly straight	Yes	Yes
Lisa	26	White, Jewish	US	Straight/Hetero	No	No
Lola	21	Black, African	US	Straight/Hetero	No	No
Lynn	25	Korean	US	Mostly straight	No	No
Mallory	32	White	US	Queer	No	No
Marianne	32	White	US	Straight/Hetero	No	No
Maya	30	White	US	Bisexual	Yes	No
Molly	33	White	US	Straight/Hetero	No	No
Natasha	26	White, Jewish	US	Queer	No	No
Penelope	32	White, Jewish	US	Straight/Hetero	No	No
Regina	25	White	US	Bisexual	Yes	No
Rose	33	Black, Caribbean	US	Straight/Hetero	No	No
Sadie	25	White	US	Queer/Bisexual	No	No
Sam	29	White	US	Straight/Hetero	No	No
Sarah	21	Israeli, Syrian	US	Queer	No	No
Taja	30	White	US	Queer/Bisexual	No	No
Tiffany	23	Chinese, Taiwanese, Japanese	US	Queer	No	No
Valdivia	27	Latinx	US	Queer	No	No
Zola	29	Black, Latinx, African Caribbean	US	Queer	No	No

TABLE 2. Expert Demographics

EXPERT	SPECIALTY
Amelia	Sex workshop leader at a feminist/queer sex toy store
Annette	Clinical psychologist, sex researcher, sex therapist
Betsy	Clinical director of a women's sexual health center, sex therapist
Celeste	Certified yoga teacher, Tantra/Daoism sexual energy practice specialist, workshop leader
Louise	Clinical psychologist, antimedicalization activist
Yvette	Sex workshop leader at a feminist/queer sex toy store

REFERENCES

Ahbel-Rappe, K. (2006). "I no longer believe": Did Freud abandon the seduction theory? *Journal of the American Psychoanalytic Association, 54*, 171–199.

Ahmed, S. (2006). Orientations: Toward a queer phenomenology. *GLQ: A Journal of Lesbian and Gay Studies, 12*, 543–574.

Ahmed, S. (2007). A phenomenology of whiteness. *Feminist Theory, 8*, 149–168.

Ahmed, S. (2010). *The promise of happiness*. Durham, NC: Duke University Press.

Alcoff, L. (1988). Cultural feminism vs. poststructuralism. *Signs: Journal of Women in Culture and Society, 13*, 405–436.

American Psychiatric Association. (1980). *Diagnostic and statistical manual of mental disorders* (3rd ed.). Washington, DC: Author.

American Psychiatric Association. (1987). *Diagnostic and statistical manual of mental disorders* (3rd ed., revised). Washington, DC: Author.

American Psychiatric Association. (1994). *Diagnostic and statistical manual of mental disorders* (4th ed.). Washington, DC: Author.

American Psychiatric Association. (2000). *Diagnostic and statistical manual of mental disorders* (4th ed., text revision). Washington, DC: Author.

American Psychiatric Association. (2013). *Diagnostic and statistical manual of mental disorders* (5th ed.). Arlington, VA: Author.

Angel, K. (2010). The history of "female sexual dysfunction" as a mental disorder in the 20th century. *Current Opinion in Psychiatry, 23*, 536–541.

Angel, K. (2012). Contested psychiatric ontology and feminist critique: "Female sexual dysfunction" and the Diagnostic and Statistical Manual. *History of the Human Sciences, 25*, 3–24.

Angel, K. (2013). Commentary on Spurgas's "Interest, arousal, and shifting diagnoses of female sexual dysfunction." *Studies in Gender and Sexuality*, 14, 206–216.

Ayling, K., & Ussher, J. M. (2008). "If sex hurts, am I still a woman?" The subjective experience of vulvodynia in hetero-sexual women. *Archives of Sexual Behavior*, 37, 294–304.

Bailey, J. M. (2003). *The man who would be queen*. Washington, DC: Joseph Henry Press.

Bailey, J. M. (2009). What is sexual orientation and do women have one? In D. A. Hope (Ed.), *Contemporary perspectives on lesbian, gay, and bisexual identities* (pp. 43–63). New York, NY: Springer.

Balon, R., & Clayton, A. H. (2014). Female sexual interest/arousal disorder: A diagnosis out of thin air. *Archives of Sexual Behavior*, 43, 1227–1229.

Bancroft, J., Graham, C., Janssen, E., & Sanders, S. (2009). The dual control model: current status and future directions. *Journal of Sex Research*, 46, 121–142.

Barbach, L. (1974). Group treatment of preorgasmic women. *Journal of Sex & Marital Therapy*, 1, 139–145.

Barbach, L. (1980). *Women discover orgasm*. New York, NY: Free Press.

Barker, K. (2014). Mindfulness meditation: Do-it-yourself medicalization of every moment. *Social Science & Medicine*, 106, 168–176.

Barker, M. (2013). Reflections: Towards a mindful sexual and relationship therapy. *Sexual and Relationship Therapy*, 28, 147–153.

Barmak, S. (2018, April 26). The misunderstood science of sexual desire. *The Cut*. Retrieved from https://www.thecut.com/2018/04/the-misunderstood-science-of-sexual-desire.html

Barounis, C. (2014). Compulsory sexuality and asexual/crip resistance in John Cameron Mitchell's *Shortbus*. In M. Milks & K. J. Cerankowski (Eds.), *Asexualities: Feminist and queer perspectives* (pp. 174–197). New York, NY: Routledge.

Barounis, C. (2015, November 13). *Pleasure, capacitation, and rhetorics of queer citizenship*. Paper presented at the annual conference of the National Women's Studies Association, Milwaukee, WI.

Barounis, C. (2019). *Vulnerable constitutions: Queerness, disability, and the remaking of American manhood*. Philadelphia, PA: Temple University Press.

Bartels, A., & Zeki, S. (2000). The neural basis of romantic love. *NeuroReport*, 11, 3829–3834.

Bartels, A., & Zeki, S. (2004). The neural correlates of maternal and romantic love. *NeuroImage*, 21, 1155–1166.

Basson, R. (2000). The female sexual response: A different model. *Journal of Sex & Marital Therapy*, 26, 51–65.

Basson, R. (2001a). Human sex-response cycles. *Journal of Sex & Marital Therapy*, 27, 33–43.

Basson, R. (2001b). Using a different model for female sexual response to address women's problematic low sexual desire. *Journal of Sex & Marital Therapy*, 27, 395–403.

Basson, R. (2002). Are our definitions of women's desire, arousal and sexual pain disorders too broad and our definitions of orgasmic disorder too narrow? *Journal of Sex and Marital Therapy*, 28, 289–300.

Basson, R. (2008). Comment on Janssen et al. (2008). *Archives of Sexual Behavior*, 37, 511.

Basson, R. Berman, J., Burnett, A., Derogatis, L., Ferguson, D., Fourcroy, J., . . . Whipple, B. (2001). Report of the International Consensus Development Conference on Female Sexual Dysfunction: Definitions and classifications. *Journal of Sex and Marital Therapy*, 27, 83–94.

Basson, R. Brotto, L. A., Laan, E., Redmond, G., & Utian, W. H. (2005). Assessment and management of women's sexual dysfunctions: Problematic desire and arousal. *Journal of Sexual Medicine, 2*, 291–300.

Baumeister, R. F. (2000). Gender differences in erotic plasticity: The female sex drive as socially flexible and responsive. *Psychological Bulletin, 126*, 347–374.

Baumeister, R. F. (2004). Gender and erotic plasticity: Sociocultural influences on the sex drive. *Sexual and Relationship Therapy, 19*, 133–139.

Benjamin, J. (1988). *The bonds of love: Psychoanalysis, feminism, and the problem of domination.* New York, NY: Pantheon.

Berg, B. L., & Lune, H. (2011). *Qualitative research methods for the social sciences* (8th ed.). Boston, MA: Pearson.

Bergner, D. (2009a, January 25). What do women want? *The New York Times Magazine.* Retrieved from http://www.nytimes.com/2009/01/25/magazine/25desire-t.html

Bergner, D. (2009b, November 29). Women who want to want. *The New York Times Magazine.* Retrieved from http://www.nytimes.com/2009/11/29/magazine/29sex-t.html

Bergner, D. (2013a, May 22). Unexcited? There may be a pill for that. *The New York Times Magazine.* Retrieved from http://www.nytimes.com/2013/05/26/magazine/unexcited-there-may-be-a-pill-for-that.html

Bergner, D. (2013b). *What do women want? Adventures in the science of female desire.* New York, NY: HarperCollins.

Berlant, L. (2008). *The female complaint: The unfinished business of sentimentality in American culture.* Durham, NC: Duke University Press.

Berlant, L. (2011). *Cruel optimism.* Durham, NC: Duke University Press.

Bersani, L. (1986). *The Freudian body: Psychoanalysis and art.* New York, NY: Columbia University Press.

Bersani, L. (1987). Is the rectum a grave? *October, 43*, 197–222.

Bielski, Z. (2015, June 21). "Arousal-first" desire may be more typical for women, and it doesn't need a cure. *The Globe and Mail.* Retrieved from https://www.theglobeandmail.com/life/health-and-fitness/health/arousal-first-desire-may-be-more-typical-for-women-and-it-doesnt-need-a-cure/article25039091/

Birke, L., & Hubbard, R. (1995). Learning from the new priesthood and the shrieking sisterhood: Debating the life sciences in Victorian England. In L. Birke & R. Hubbard (Eds.), *Reinventing biology: Respect for life and the creation of knowledge* (pp. 1–19). Bloomington, IN: Indiana University Press.

Blanchard, R. (1989). The concept of autogynephilia and the typology of male gender dysphoria. *Journal of Nervous and Mental Disease, 177*, 616–623.

Borck, C. R., & Moore, L. J. (2019). This is my voice on T: Synthetic testosterone, DIY surveillance, and transnormative masculinity. *Surveillance & Society, 17*, 631–640.

Bordo, S. (1993). *Unbearable weight: Feminism, Western culture, and the body.* Berkeley, CA: University of California Press.

Bossio, J., Basson, R., Driscoll, M., Correia, S., & Brotto, L. (2018). Mindfulness-based group therapy for men with situational erectile dysfunction: A mixed-methods feasibility analysis and pilot study. *Journal of Sexual Medicine, 15*, 1478–1490.

Both, S., & Everaerd, W. (2002). Comment on "The female sexual response: A different model." *Journal of Sex & Marital Therapy, 28*, 11–15.

Boyle, M. (1993). Sexual dysfunction or heterosexual dysfunction? *Feminism & Psychology, 3*, 73–88.

Braksmajer, A. (2017). "That's kind of one of our jobs": Sexual activity as a form of care work among women with sexual difficulties. *Archives of Sexual Behavior, 46*, 2085–2095.

Brody, S., & Costa, R. M. (2017). Vaginal orgasm is associated with indices of women's better psychological, intimate relationship, and psychophysiological function. *The Canadian Journal of Human Sexuality, 26*, 1–4.

Brom, M., Laan, E., Everaerd, W., Spinhoven, P., & Both, S. (2015). Extinction of aversive classically conditioned human sexual response. *Journal of Sexual Medicine, 12*, 916–935.

Brothers, D. (1997). The leather princess: Sadomasochism as the rescripting of trauma scenarios. *Progress in Self Psychology, 13*, 245–268.

Brothers, D. (2008). *Toward a psychology of uncertainty: Trauma-centered psychoanalysis*. New York, NY: The Analytic Press.

Brotto, L. A. (2010a). The *DSM* diagnostic criteria for hypoactive sexual desire disorder in women. *Archives of Sexual Behavior, 39*, 221–239.

Brotto, L. A. (2010b). The *DSM* diagnostic criteria for hypoactive sexual desire disorder in men. *The Journal of Sexual Medicine, 7*, 2015–2030.

Brotto, L. A. (2011). Non-judgmental present-moment, sex . . . as if your life depended on it. *Sexual and Relationship Therapy, 26*, 215–216.

Brotto, L. A. (2018). *Better sex through mindfulness: How women can cultivate desire*. Berkeley, CA: Greystone Books.

Brotto, L. A, Basson, R., & Luria, M. (2008). A mindfulness-based group psychoeducational intervention targeting sexual arousal disorder in women. *Journal of Sexual Medicine, 5*, 1646–1659.

Brotto, L. A., Chivers, M. L., Millman, R. D., & Albert, A. (2016). Mindfulness-based sex therapy improves genital-subjective arousal concordance in women with sexual desire/arousal difficulties. *Archives of Sexual Behavior, 45*, 1907–1921.

Brotto, L. A., Heiman, J. R., & Tolman, D. L. (2009). Narratives of desire in mid-age women with and without arousal difficulties. *Journal of Sex Research, 46*, 387–398.

Brotto, L. A, Krychman, M., & Jacobson, P. (2008). Eastern approaches for enhancing women's sexuality: Mindfulness, acupuncture, and yoga. *Journal of Sexual Medicine, 5*, 2741–2748.

Brotto, L. A., Seal, B. N., & Rellini, A. (2012). Pilot study of a brief cognitive behavioral versus mindfulness-based intervention for women with sexual distress and a history of childhood sexual abuse. *Journal of Sex & Marital Therapy, 38*, 1–27.

Buss, D. M. (1994). *The evolution of desire: Strategies of human mating*. New York, NY: Basic Books.

Butler, J. (1990). *Gender trouble: Feminism and the subversion of identity*. London, UK: Routledge.

Butler, J. (1993). *Bodies that matter: On the discursive limits of "sex."* London, UK: Routledge.

Butler, J. (1997). *The psychic life of power: Theories in subjection*. Stanford, CA: Stanford University Press.

Cacchioni, T. (2007). Heterosexuality and "the labour of love": A contribution to recent debates on female sexual dysfunction. *Sexualities, 10*, 299–320.

Cacchioni, T. (2015). *Big pharma, women, and the labor of love.* Toronto, ON: University of Toronto Press.

Cacchioni, T., & Wolkowitz, C. (2011). Treating women's sexual difficulties: The body work of sexual therapy. *Sociology of Health & Illness, 33,* 266–279.

Califia, P. (1994). *Public sex: The culture of radical sex.* San Francisco, CA: Cleis Press.

Canner, L. (2009). *Orgasm Inc.* [Motion picture]. West Groton, MA: Astrea Media.

Carey, B. (2005, July 5). Straight, gay, or lying? Bisexuality revisited. *The New York Times.* Retrieved from https://www.nytimes.com/2005/07/05/health/straight-gay-or-lying-bisexuality-revisited.html

Casper, M., & Moore, L. J. (2009). *Missing bodies: The politics of visibility.* New York, NY: New York University Press.

Charest, M., & Kleinplatz, P. J. (2018). A review of recent innovations in the treatment of low sexual desire. *Current Sexual Health Reports, 10,* 281–286.

Chivers, M. L. (2005). A brief review and discussion of sex differences in the specificity of sexual arousal. *Sexual and Relationship Therapy, 20,* 377–390.

Chivers, M. L. (2010). A brief update on the specificity of sexual arousal. *Sexual & Relationship Therapy, 25,* 407–414.

Chivers, M. L. (2017a). The specificity of women's sexual response and its relationship with sexual orientations: A review and ten hypotheses. *Archives of Sexual Behavior, 46,* 1161–1179.

Chivers, M. L. (2017b). Response to commentaries. *Archives of Sexual Behavior, 46,* 1213–1221.

Chivers, M. L., & Bailey, J. M. (2005). A sex difference in features that elicit genital response. *Biological Psychology, 70,* 115–120.

Chivers, M. L., & Brotto, L. A. (2017). Controversies of women's sexual arousal and desire. *European Psychologist, 22,* 5–26.

Chivers, M. L., Rieger, G., Latty, E., & Bailey, J. M. (2004). A sex difference in the specificity of sexual arousal. *Psychological Science, 15,* 736–744.

Chivers, M. L., Seto, M. C., & Blanchard, R. (2007). Gender and sexual orientation differences in sexual response to sexual activities versus gender of actors in sexual films. *Journal of Personality & Social Psychology, 93,* 1108–1121.

Chivers, M. L., Seto, M. C., Lalumière, M. L., Laan, E., & Grimbos, T. (2010). Agreement of self-reported and genital measures of sexual arousal in men and women: A meta-analysis. *Archives of Sexual Behavior, 39,* 5–56.

Chivers, M. L., Bouchard, K. N., & Timmers, A. D. (2015). Straight but not narrow; Within gender variation in the gender-specificity of women's sexual response. *PLoS ONE, 10,* 1–21.

Chodorow, N. (1978). *The reproduction of mothering: Psychoanalysis and the sociology of gender.* Berkeley, CA: University of California Press.

Chu, A. L. (2019). The impossibility of feminism. *differences: A Journal of Feminist Cultural Studies, 30,* 63–81.

Cixous, H., & Clément, C. (1986). *The newly born woman.* Minneapolis, MN: University of Minnesota Press. (Original work published 1975)

Clare, E. (2017). *Brilliant imperfection: Grappling with cure.* Durham, NC: Duke University Press.

Clarke, A., Shim, J., Mamo, L., Fosket, J., & Fishman, J. (2003). Biomedicalization: Technoscientific transformations of health, illness and U. S. biomedicine. *American Sociological Review, 68,* 161–194.

Clough, P. T. (2007). Introduction. In P. T. Clough and J. Halley (Eds.), *The affective turn: Theorizing the social* (pp. 1–33). Durham, NC: Duke University Press.

Clough, P. T. (2018). *The user unconscious: On affect, media, and measure*. Minneapolis, MN: University of Minnesota Press.

Collins, P. H. (1990). *Black feminist thought: Knowledge, consciousness, and the politics of empowerment*. London, UK: Routledge.

Collins, P. H. (1998). It's all in the family: Intersection of gender, race, and nation. *Hypatia*, 13, 62–82.

Collins, P. H. (2004). *Black sexual politics: African Americans, gender, and the new racism*. New York, NY: Routledge.

Comella, L. (2017). *Vibrator nation: How feminist sex-toy stores changed the business of pleasure*. Durham, NC: Duke University Press.

Conniff, R. (2010, October 5). Hunting the female libido. *Men's Health*. Retrieved from https://www.menshealth.com/sex-women/a19541894/female-libido/

Conrad, P. (1975). The discovery of hyperkinesis: Notes on the medicalization of deviant behavior. *Social Problems*, 23, 12–21.

Conrad, P. (1992). Medicalization and social control. *Annual Review of Sociology*, 18, 209–232.

Cooper, M. (2008). *Life as surplus: Biotechnology and capitalism in the neoliberal era*. Seattle, WA: Washington University Press.

Cooper, M., & Waldby, C. (2014). *Clinical labor: Tissue donors and research subjects in the global bioeconomy*. Durham, NC: Duke University Press.

Cosmides, L., & Tooby, J. (1994). Better than rational: Evolutionary psychology and the invisible hand. *The American Economic Review*, 84, 327–332.

Cossman, B. (2007). *Sexual citizens: The legal and cultural regulation of sex and belonging*. Stanford, CA: Stanford University Press.

Crawford, R. (1980). Healthism and the medicalization of everyday life. *International Journal of Health Services*, 10, 365–388.

Crenshaw, K. (1991). Mapping the margins: Intersectionality, identity politics, and violence against women of color. *Stanford Law Review*, 43, 1241–1299.

Cvetkovich, A. (1995). Recasting receptivity: Femme sexualities. In K. Jay (Ed.), *Lesbian erotics*. New York, NY: New York University Press.

Cvetkovich, A. (1998). Untouchability and vulnerability: Stone butchness as emotional style. In S. Munt (Ed.), *Butch/femme: Inside lesbian gender*. London, UK: Castell.

Cvetkovich, A. (2003). *An archive of feelings: Trauma, sexuality, and lesbian public cultures*. Durham, NC: Duke University Press.

Dalla Costa, M., & James, S. (1972). *The power of women and the subversion of the community*. London: Falling Wall Press.

Daly, M. (1990). *Gyn/ecology: The metaethics of radical feminism*. Boston, MA: Beacon Press. (Original work published 1978)

Darwin, C. (1859). *On the origin of species by means of natural selection*. Retrieved from http://en.wikisource.org/wiki/On_the_Origin_of_Species_(1859)

Dawkins, R. (1976). *The selfish gene*. New York, NY: Oxford University Press.

Dawson, S. J., & Chivers, M. L. (2014). Gender differences and similarities in sexual desire. *Current Sexual Health Reports*, 6, 211–219.

Dawson, S. J., & Chivers, M. L. (2018). The effect of static versus dynamic stimuli on visual processing of sexual cues in androphilic women and gynephilic men. *Royal Society Open Science*, 5, 172286.

Dawson, S. J., Huberman, J. S., Bouchard, K. N., McInnis, M. K., Pukall, C. F., & Chivers, M. L. (2019). Effects of individual difference variables, gender, and exclusivity of sexual attraction on volunteer bias in sexuality research. *Archives of Sexual Behavior*. https://doi.org/10.1007/s10508-019-1451-4

de Beauvoir, S. (1989). *The second sex*. New York, NY: Vintage. (Original work published 1952)

DeJesus, J. M., Callanan, M. A., Solis, G., & Gelman, S. A. (2019). Generic language in scientific communication. *PNAS*, 116, 18370–18377.

Deleuze, G. (1992). Postscript on the societies of control. *October*, 59, 3–7.

DeRogatis, L. R., Clayton, A. H., Rosen, R. C., Sand, M., & Pyke, R. E. (2011). Should sexual desire and arousal disorders in women be merged? *Archives of Sexual Behavior*, 40, 217–219.

DeVault, M. L. (1991). *Feeding the family: The social organization of caring as gendered work*. Chicago, IL: The University of Chicago Press.

Diamond, L. M. (2005). "I'm straight, but I kissed a girl": The trouble with American media representations of female-female sexuality. *Feminism & Psychology*, 15, 104–110.

Diamond, L. M. (2008). *Sexual fluidity: Understanding women's love and desire*. Cambridge, MA: Harvard University Press.

Dodson, B. (1987). *Sex for one: The joy of self-loving*. New York, NY: Crown.

Donaldson, E. J. (2002). The corpus of the madwoman: Toward a feminist disability studies theory of embodiment and mental illness. *NWSA Journal*, 14, 99–119.

Donegan, M. (2018, May 11). How #MeToo revealed the central rift within feminism today. *The Guardian*. Retrieved from https://www.theguardian.com/news/2018/may/11/how-metoo-revealed-the-central-rift-within-feminism-social-individualist

Downing, L. (2007). Beyond safety: Erotic asphyxiation and the limits of SM discourse. In D. Langdridge & M. Barker (Eds.), *Safe sane and consensual: Contemporary perspectives on sadomasochism* (pp. 119–132). Basingstoke, UK: Palgrave MacMillan.

Downing, L. (2013). Safewording! Kinkphobia and gender normativity in *Fifty shades of grey*. *Psychology and Sexuality*, 4, 92–102.

Duncombe, J., & Marsden, D. (1996). "Whose orgasm is this anyway"? Sex work in long-term couple relationships. In J. Weeks & J. Holland (Eds.), *Sexual cultures: Communities, values, and intimacy* (pp. 220–238). New York, NY: St. Martin's Press.

Dunkley, C. R., & Brotto, L. A. (2018). Clinical considerations in treating BDSM practitioners: A review. *Journal of Sex & Marital Therapy*, 44, 701–712.

Dunkley, C. R., & Brotto, L. A. (2019). The role of consent in the context of BDSM. *Sexual Abuse*, 1–22.

Dunkley, C. R., Henshaw, C. D., Henshaw, S. K. & Brotto, L. A. (2020). Physical pain as pleasure: A theoretical perspective. *The Journal of Sex Research*, 57, 421–437.

Dworkin, A. (1987). *Intercourse*. New York, NY: Basic Books.

Dymock, A. (2012). But femsub is broken too! On the normalisation of BDSM and the problem of pleasure. *Psychology & Sexuality*, 3, 54–68.

Dymock, A. (2013). Flogging sexual transgression: Interrogating the costs of the "Fifty Shades effect." *Sexualities*, 16, 880–895.

Dymock, A. (2018). Anti-communal, anti-egalitarian, anti-nurturing, anti-loving: Sex and the "irredeemable" in Andrea Dworkin and Catharine MacKinnon. *Paragraph*, 41, 349–363.

Ehrenreich, B., & English. D. (1978). *For her own good: Two centuries of the experts' advice to women*. New York, NY: Anchor Books.

Elton, C. (2010, May/June). Learning to lust. *Psychology Today*, 70–77.

Fahs, B. (2011). *Performing sex: The making and unmaking of women's erotic lives*. Albany, NY: SUNY Press.

Fahs, B. (2016). Naming sexual trauma: On the political necessity of nuance in rape and sex offender discourses. In E. Wertheimer & M. J. Casper (Eds.), *Critical trauma studies: Understanding violence, conflict, and memory in everyday life* (pp. 61–77). New York, NY: New York University Press.

Faludi, S. (1991). *Backlash: The undeclared war against American women*. New York, NY: Vintage Books.

Fausto-Sterling, A. (1992). *Myths of gender: Biological theories about women and men*. New York, NY: Basic Books.

Fausto-Sterling, A. (1994). Gender, race, and nation: The comparative anatomy of "Hottentot" women in Europe, 1815–1817. In J. Terry & J. Urla (Eds.), *Deviant bodies: Critical perspectives on difference in science and popular culture* (pp. 19–48). Bloomington, IN: Indiana University Press.

Fausto-Sterling, A. (1997). Beyond difference: A biologist's perspective. *Journal of Social Issues*, 53, 233–258.

Fausto-Sterling, A. (2000). *Sexing the body: Gender politics and the construction of sexuality*. New York, NY: Basic Books.

Federici, S. (2004). *Caliban and the witch: Women, the body, and primitive accumulation*. Brooklyn, NY: Autonomedia.

Federici, S. (2012). *Revolution at point zero: Housework, reproduction, and feminist struggle*. Oakland, CA: PM Press.

Feher, M. (2009). Self-appreciation; or, the aspirations of human capital. *Public Culture*, 21, 21–41.

Feher, M. (2018). *Rated agency: Investee politics in a speculative age*. New York, NY: Zone Books.

Ferenidou, F., Kirana, P., Fokas, K., Hatzichristou, D., & Athanasiadis, L. (2016). Sexual response models: Toward a more flexible pattern of women's sexuality. *Journal of Sexual Medicine*, 13, 1369–1376.

Ferguson, R. A. (2004). *Aberrations in black: Toward a queer of color critique*. Minneapolis, MN: University of Minnesota Press.

Fine, C. (2010). *Delusions of gender: How our minds, society, and neurosexism create difference*. New York, NY: W. W. Norton.

Fine, C. (2013, December 4). New insights into gendered brain wiring, or a perfect case study in neurosexism? *The Conversation*. Retrieved from http://theconversation.com/newinsights-into-gendered-brain-wiring-or-a-perfect-case-study-in-neurosexism-21083

Fine, M. (1988). Sexuality, schooling, and adolescent females: The missing discourse of desire. *Harvard Educational Review*, 58, 29–53.

Fischer, N. L. (2013). Seeing "straight," contemporary critical heterosexuality studies and sociology: An introduction. *The Sociological Quarterly*, 54, 501–510.

Flore, J. (2014). Mismeasures of asexual desires. In M. Milks & K. J. Cerankowski (Eds.), *Asexualities: Feminist and queer perspectives* (pp. 17–34). New York, NY: Routledge.

Flore, J. (2016). The problem of sexual imbalance and techniques of the self in the *Diagnostic and statistical manual of mental disorders*. *History of Psychiatry, 27*, 320–335.

Flore, J. (2018). Pharmaceutical intimacy: Managing female sexuality through Addyi. *Sexualities, 2*, 569–586.

Floyd, K. (2009). *The reification of desire: Toward a queer Marxism*. Minneapolis, MN: University of Minnesota Press.

Fortunati, L. (1995). *The arcane of reproduction: Housework, prostitution, labor, and capital*. Brooklyn, NY: Autonomedia.

Foucault, M. (1965). *Madness and civilization: A history of insanity in the age of reason*. London: Tavistock.

Foucault, M. (1972). *The archaeology of knowledge and the discourse on language*. New York, NY: Pantheon.

Foucault, M. (1973). *The birth of the clinic: An archaeology of medical perception*. New York, NY: Random House.

Foucault, M. (1977). *Discipline and punish: The birth of the prison*. New York, NY: Pantheon.

Foucault, M. (1978). *The history of sexuality, volume 1: An introduction*. New York, NY: Random House.

Foucault, M. (2000). Governmentality. In J. Faubion (Ed.), *Power: Essential works of Foucault 1954–1984* (pp. 201–222). New York, NY: New Press.

Foucault, M. (2003). *"Society must be defended": Lectures at the Collège de France, 1975–1976*. New York, NY: Picador.

Francisco-Menchavez, V. (2018). *The labor of care: Filipina migrants and transnational families in the digital age*. Chicago, IL: University of Illinois Press.

Frank, A., & Jones, T. (2003). Bioethics and the later Foucault. *Journal of Medical Humanities, 24*, 179–86.

Freeman, E. (2010). *Time binds: Queer temporalities, queer histories*. Durham, NC: Duke University Press.

Freud, S. (1952). Female sexuality. In J. Strachey (Ed.), *Sigmund Freud: Collected papers: Miscellaneous papers, 1888–1938* (Vol. 5, pp. 252–272). London, UK: Hogarth and Institute of Psycho-Analysis. (Original work published 1931)

Freud, S. (1961). *Beyond the pleasure principle*. New York, NY: W. W. Norton.

Friedan, B. (1963). *The feminine mystique*. New York, NY: W. W. Norton.

Gannon, L. (2002). A critique of evolutionary psychology. *Psychology, Evolution & Gender, 4*, 173–218.

Garland-Thomson, R. (2002). Integrating disability, transforming feminist theory. *NWSA Journal, 14*, 1–32.

Gavey, N. (2005). *Just sex? The cultural scaffolding of rape*. London, UK: Routledge.

Gavey, N. (2011). Viagra and the coital imperative. In S. Seidman, N. Fischer, & C. Meeks (Eds.), *Introducing the New Sexuality Studies* (2nd ed., pp. 119–124). New York, NY: Routledge.

Geer, J. H., Morokoff, P., & Greenwood, P. (1974). Sexual arousal in women: The development of a measurement device for vaginal blood volume. *Archives of Sexual Behavior, 3*, 559–564.

Gentile, K. (2017a). Collectively creating conditions for emergence. In S. Grand & J. Salzberg (Eds.), *Wounds of history: Repair and resilience in the trans-generational transmission of trauma* (pp. 169–188). New York, NY: Routledge.

Gentile, K. (2017b, September 18). *Commentary on Spurgas' (2017) "Queering receptivity: Parasexual pleasure in the face of compulsory and feminized trauma."* Presented at Women and Society Seminar, University Seminars, Columbia University, New York, NY.

Gilligan, C. (1982). *In a different voice: Psychological theory and women's development.* Cambridge, MA: Harvard University Press.

Giraldi, A., Kristensen, E., & Sand, M. (2015). Endorsement of models describing sexual response of men and women with a sexual partner: An online survey in a population sample of Danish adults ages 20–65 years. *Journal of Sexual Medicine, 12,* 116–128.

Goffman, E. (1961). *Asylums: Essays on the social situation of mental patients and other inmates.* Garden City, NY: Anchor Books/Doubleday.

Goffman, E. (1978). *Stigma: Notes on the management of spoiled identity.* New York, NY: Jason Aronso Press.

Goldey, K. L., & van Anders, S. M. (2012). Sexual arousal and desire: Interrelations and responses to three modalities of sexual stimuli. *Journal of Sexual Medicine, 9,* 2315–2329.

Gottlieb, L. (2014, February 6). Does a more equal marriage mean less sex? *The New York Times.* Retrieved from http://www.nytimes.com/2014/02/09/magazine/does-a-more-equal-marriage-mean-less-sex.html

Gould, S. J. (2002). *The structure of evolutionary theory.* Cambridge, MA: Harvard University Press.

Gowaty, P. A. (2000). Sexual natures: How feminism changed evolutionary biology. *Signs: Journal of Women in Culture and Society, 28,* 901–921.

Graham, C. A. (2010). The *DSM* diagnostic criteria for female sexual arousal disorder. *Archives of Sexual Behavior, 39,* 240–255.

Graham, C. A. (2016). Reconceptualising women's sexual desire and arousal in *DSM-5. Psychology & Sexuality, 7,* 34–47.

Graham, C. A., Sanders, S. A., Milhausen, R. R., & McBride, K. R. (2004). Turning on and turning off: A focus group study of the factors that affect women's sexual arousal. *Archives of Sexual Behavior, 33,* 527–538.

Grant, M. G. (2014). *Playing the whore: The work of sex work.* New York, NY: Verso Books.

Gray, J. (1992). *Men are from Mars, women are from Venus: A practical guide for improving communication and getting what you want in your relationships.* New York, NY: Harper Collins.

Green, S. (2017, July 13). Violence against black women—many types, far-reaching effects. Retrieved from Institute for Women's Policy Research website: https://iwpr.org/violence-black-women-many-types-far-reaching-effects/

Gregg, M. (2018). *Counterproductive: Time management in the knowledge economy.* Durham, NC: Duke University Press.

Grosz, E. (1990). *Jacques Laçan: A feminist introduction.* London, UK: Routledge.

Grosz, E. (1994). *Volatile bodies: Toward a corporeal feminism.* Bloomington, IN: Indiana University Press.

Gupta, K. (2011). "Screw health": Representations of sex as a health-promoting activity in medical and popular literature. *Journal of Medical Humanities, 32,* 127–140.

Gupta, K. (2015). Compulsory sexuality: Evaluating an emerging concept. *Signs: Journal of Women in Culture and Society, 41,* 131–154.

Gupta, K. (2017). What does asexuality teach us about sexual disinterest? Recommendations for health professionals based on a qualitative study with asexually identified people. *Journal of Sex & Marital Therapy, 43,* 1–14.

Gupta, K., & Cacchioni, T. (2013). Sexual improvement as if your health depends on it: An analysis of contemporary sex manuals. *Feminism & Psychology, 23,* 442–458.

Halberstam, J. (2011). *The queer art of failure.* Durham, NC: Duke University Press.

Hamilton, W. D. (1964). The genetical evolution of social behaviour. *Journal of Theoretical Biology, 7,* 1–16.

Hammonds, E. (1994). Black (w)holes and the geometry of Black black female sexuality. *differences: A Journal of Feminist Cultural Studies, 6,* 126–145.

Hammonds, E. (1999). Toward a genealogy of black female sexuality: The problematic of Silence. In J. Price & M. Shildrick (Eds.), *Feminist theory and the body: A reader* (pp. 93–104. New York, NY: Routledge.

Harding, S. (1986). *The science question in feminism.* Ithaca, NY: Cornell University Press.

Hardt, M., & Negri, A. (2000). *Empire.* Cambridge, MA: Harvard University Press.

Hardt, M., & Negri, A. (2004). *Multitude: War and democracy in the age of empire.* New York, NY: Penguin Books.

Hart, L. (1998). *Between the body and the flesh: Performing sadomasochism.* New York, NY: Columbia University Press.

Hartman, S. (1997). *Scenes of subjection: Terror, slavery, and self-making in nineteenth-century America.* New York, NY: Oxford.

Heiman, J. (1977). A psychophysiological exploration of sexual arousal patterns in females and males. *Psychophysiology, 14,* 266–274.

Heiman, J. (1980). Female sexual response patterns: Interactions of physiological, affective, and contextual cues. *Archives of General Psychiatry, 37,* 1311–1316.

Heiman, J. (2002). Sexual dysfunction: Overview of prevalence, etiological factors, and treatments. *Journal of Sex Research, 39,* 73–78.

Heiman, J., Lo Piccolo, L., & Lo Piccolo J. (1976). *Becoming orgasmic: A sexual growth program for women.* New York, NY: Prentice Hall.

Henrich, J., Heine, S. J., & Norenzayan, A. (2010). The weirdest people in the world?. *Behavioral and brain sciences, 33,* 61–83.

Hite, S. (1976). *The Hite report.* New York, NY: Dell.

Hochschild, A. R. (1985). *The managed heart: Commercialization of human feeling.* Berkeley, CA: University of California Press.

Hochschild, A. R. (1997). *The time bind: When work becomes home and home becomes work.* New York, NY: Henry Holt Books.

Hochschild, A. R., & Machung, A. (1989). *The second shift: Working parents and the revolution at home.* New York, NY: Viking Books.

Hollibaugh, A. (2000). *My dangerous desires: A queer girl dreaming her way home.* Durham, NC: Duke University Press.

Hondagneu-Sotelo, P. (2002). Blowups and other unhappy endings. In B. Ehrenreich & A. R. Hochschild (Eds.), *Global woman: Nannies, maids, and sex workers in the new economy* (pp. 55–69). New York, NY: Owl Books.

Hoon, P. W., Wincze, J. P., & Hoon, E. F. (1976). Physiological assessment of sexual arousal in women. *Psychophysiology*, 13, 196–204.

Hoskin, R. A., & Taylor, A. (2019). Femme resistance: The fem(me)inine art of failure. *Psychology & Sexuality*, 10, 281–300.

Hubbard, R. (1990). *The politics of women's biology*. New Brunswick, NJ: Rutgers University Press.

Huberman, J. S., & Chivers, M. L. (2015). Examining gender specificity of sexual response with concurrent thermography and plethysmography. *Psychophysiology*, 52, 1382–1395.

Huffer, L. (2013). *Are the lips a grave?: A queer feminist on the ethics of sex*. New York, NY: Columbia University Press.

Human Rights Campaign. (2019). A national epidemic: Fatal anti-transgender violence in the United States in 2019. Retrieved from https://www.hrc.org/resources/a-national-epidemic-fatal-anti-trans-violence-in-the-united-states-in-2019

Hyde, J. S., & Durik, A. (2000). Gender differences in erotic plasticity: Evolutionary or sociocultural forces? Comment on Baumeister (2000). *Psychological Bulletin*, 126, 375–379.

Ingraham, C. (2008). *White weddings: Romancing heterosexuality in popular culture*. New York, NY: Routledge.

Irigaray, L. (1985). *This sex which is not one*. Ithaca, NY: Cornell University Press.

Irvine, J. M. (2002). *Talk about sex: The battles over sex education in the United States*. Berkeley, CA: University of California Press.

Irvine, J. M. (2005). *Disorders of desire: Sexuality and gender in modern American sexology*. Philadelphia, PA: Temple University Press.

Jagose, A. (2013). *Orgasmology*. Durham, NC: Duke University Press.

James, E. L. (2011). *Fifty shades of grey*. New York, NY: Vintage Books.

James, S. (2012). *Sex, race, and class: The perspective of winning. A selection of writings 1952—2011*. Oakland, CA: PM Press.

Janssen, E., Everaerd, W., Spiering, M., & Janssen, J. (2000). Automatic processes and the appraisal of sexual stimuli: Toward an information processing model of sexual arousal. *Journal of Sex Research*, 37, 8–23.

Janssen, E., McBride, K. R., Yarber, W., Hill, B. J., & Butler, S. M. (2008). Factors that influence sexual arousal in men: A focus group study. *Archives of Sexual Behavior*, 37, 252–265.

Johnson, M. L. (2010). *Girl in need of a tourniquet: Memoir of a borderline personality*. Berkeley, CA: Seal Press.

Johnson, M. L. (2013, October 24). Label C/Rip. *Social Text: Periscope*. Retrieved from http://socialtextjournal.org/periscope_article/label-crip/

Johnson, M. L. (2015). Bad romance: A crip feminist critique of queer failure, *Hypatia*, 30, 251–267.

Johnson, M. L., & R. McRuer. (2014). Cripistemologies: Introduction. *Journal of Literary & Cultural Disability Studies*, 8, 127–147.

Jones, L. (2011, March 24). Why bad sex is shortening your life. *Cosmopolitan*. Retrieved from http://www.cosmopolitan.com/sex-love/tips-moves/orgasm-news

Jordan-Young, R. M. (2011). *Brain storm: The flaws in the science of sex differences*. Cambridge, MA: Harvard University Press.

Jordan-Young, R. M., & Karkazis, K. (2019). *Testosterone: An unauthorized biography*. Cambridge, MA: Harvard University Press.

Jutel, A. (2010). Framing disease: The example of female hypoactive sexual desire disorder. *Social Science & Medicine*, 70, 1084–1090.

Kabat-Zinn, J. (1990). *Full catastrophe living: How to cope with stress, pain and illness using mindfulness meditation*. New York, NY: Piatkus.

Kafer, A. (2013). *Feminist, queer, crip*. Bloomington, IN: Indiana University Press.

Kaler, A. (2006). Unreal women: Sex, gender, identity, and the lived experience of vulvar pain. *Feminist Review*, 82, 50–75.

Kang, M. (2010). *The managed hand: Race, gender, and the body in beauty service work*. Berkeley, CA: University of California Press.

Kaplan, H. S. (1974). *The new sex therapy: Active treatment of sexual dysfunctions*. New York, NY: Brunner/Mazel.

Kaplan, H. S. (1977). Hypoactive sexual desire. *Journal of Sex & Marital Therapy*, 3, 3–9.

Kaplan, H. S. (1979). *Disorders of sexual desire: And other new concepts and techniques in sex therapy*. New York, NY: Simon & Schuster.

Karama, S., Lecours, A. R., Leroux, J., Bourgouin, P., Beaudoin, G., Joubert, S., & Beauregard, M. (2002). Areas of brain activation in males and females during viewing of erotic film excerpts. *Human Brain Mapping*, 16, 1–13.

Karkazis, K. (2008). *Fixing sex: Intersex, medical authority, and lived experience*. Durham, NC: Duke University Press.

Kaye, K. (2011). Sexual intercourse. In S. Seidman, N. Fischer, & C. Meeks (Eds.), *Introducing the New Sexuality Studies* (2nd ed., pp. 113–118). New York, NY: Routledge.

Kim, E. (2014). Asexualities and disabilities in constructing sexual normalcy In M. Milks & K. J. Cerankowski (Eds.), *Asexualities: Feminist and queer perspectives* (pp. 249–282). New York, NY: Routledge.

Kim, J. (2017). Toward a crip-of-color critique: Thinking with Minich's "Enabling Whom?" *Lateral* 6.1, online, https://doi.org/10.25158/L6.1.14

Klein, M. (2002). *Love, guilt, and reparation: And other works, 1921-1945 (The writings of Melanie Klein, volume 1)*. New York, NY: Free Press. (Original work published 1975)

Kleinplatz, P. J. (2006). Learning from extraordinary lovers: Lessons from the edge. In P. J. Kleinplatz & C. Moser (Eds.), *Sadomasochism: Powerful pleasures* (pp. 325–348). New York, NY: Routledge.

Kleinplatz, P. J. (2011). Arousal and desire problems: Conceptual, research and clinical considerations or the more things change the more they stay the same. *Sexual and Relationship Therapy*, 26, 3–15.

Kleinplatz, P. J. (2018). History of the treatment of female sexual dysfunction(s). *Annual Review of Clinical Psychology*, 14, 1–25.

Kleinplatz, P. J., Ménard, A. D., Paquet, M.-P., Paradis, N., Campbell, M., Zuccarini, D., & Mehak, L. (2009). The components of optimal sexuality: A portrait of "great sex." *Canadian Journal of Human Sexuality*, 18, 1–13.

Kleinplatz, P. J., Paradis, N., Charest, M., Lawless, S., Neufeld, M., Neufeld, R., . . . Rosen, L. (2018). From sexual desire discrepancies to desirable sex: Creating the optimal connection. *Journal of Sex & Marital Therapy*, 44, 438–449.

Kleinplatz, P. J., Rosen, L., Charest, M., & Spurgas, A. K. (2020). Sexuality and sexual dysfunctions: Critical analyses. In J. Ussher, J. Chrisler, & J. Perz (Eds.), *The Routledge interna-

tional handbook of women's sexual and reproductive health (pp. 443–454). New York, NY: Routledge.

Kornrich, S., Brines, J., & Leupp, K. (2012). Egalitarianism, housework, and sexual frequency in marriage. *American Sociological Review,* 78, 26–50.

Koscis, A., & Newbury-Helps, J. (2016). Mindfulness in sex therapy and intimate relationships (MSIR): Clinical protocol and theory development. *Mindfulness,* 7, 690–699.

Kristeva, J. (1982). *Powers of horror: An essay on abjection.* New York, NY: Columbia University Press.

Laan, E. (2007, August). *A functional MRI study on gender differences in conscious self regulation of sexual arousal.* Presented at the meeting of the International Academy of Sex Research, Vancouver, Canada.

Laan, E., & Both, S. (2008). What makes women experience desire? *Feminism & Psychology,* 18, 505–514.

Laan, E., & Everaerd, W. (1995). Determinants of female sexual arousal: Psychophysiological theory and data. *Annual Review of Sex Research,* 6, 32–76.

Laan, E., & Everaerd, W. (1998). Physiological measures of vaginal vasocongestion. *International Journal of Impotence Research,* 10, S107–S110.

Laan, E., Scholte, H. S., & van Stegeren, A. (2006, September). *Brain imaging of gender differences in sexual excitation and inhibition.* Invited presentation for the 12th annual World Congress of the International Society for Sexual Medicine, Cairo, Egypt.

Labuski, C. M. (2014). Deferred desire: The asexuality of chronic genital pain. In M. Milks & K. J. Cerankowski (Eds.), *Asexualities: Feminist and queer perspectives* (pp. 301–327). New York, NY: Routledge.

Labuski, C. M. (2015). *It hurts down there: The bodily imaginaries of female genital pain.* Albany, NY: SUNY Press.

Labuski, C. M. (2017). A black and white issue? Learning to see the intersectional and racialized dimensions of gynecological pain. *Social Theory & Health,* 15, 160–181.

Lalumière, M. L. (2017). On the concept of category-specificity. *Archives of Sexual Behavior,* 46, 1187–1190.

Lalumière, M. L., Sawatsky, M. L., Dawson, S. J., & Suschinsky, K. D. (2020). The empirical status of The Preparation Hypothesis: Explicating women's genital responses to sexual stimuli in the laboratory. *Archives of Sexual Behavior,* online, https://doi.org/10.1007/s10508-019-01599-5

LaMorgese, S. (2016, July 1). Dominatrix explains how "BDSM can be a form of meditation." *Huffington Post.* Retrieved from https://www.huffpost.com/entry/bdsm-meditation_b_10673686

Langdridge, D. (2011). The time of the sadomasochist: Hunting with(in) the "tribus." In S. Seidman, N. Fischer, & C. Meeks (Eds.), *Introducing the New Sexuality Studies* (2nd ed., pp. 372–379). New York, NY: Routledge.

Laplanche, J. (1976). *Life & death in psychoanalysis.* Baltimore, MD: The Johns Hopkins University Press.

Laqueur, T. (1992). *Making sex: Body and gender from the Greeks to Freud.* Cambridge, MA: Harvard University Press.

Laumann, E. O., Paik, A., & Rosen, R. (1999). Sexual dysfunctions in the United States: Prevalence and predictors. *Journal of the American Medical Association,* 281, 537–544.

Lawrence, A. A., Latty, E. M., Chivers, M. L., & Bailey, J. M. (2005.) Measurement of sexual arousal in postoperative male-to-female transsexuals using vaginal photoplethysmography. *Archives of Sexual Behavior, 34*, 135–145.

Leiblum, S. R., & Rosen, R. C. (1988). Introduction: Changing perspectives on sexual desire. In S. Leiblum, & R. Rosen (Eds.), *Sexual desire disorders* (pp. 1–17). New York, NY: Guilford Press.

Lewontin, R. C. (1991). *Biology as ideology: The doctrine of DNA*. New York, NY: HarperCollins.

Lief, H. I. (1977). Inhibited sexual desire. *Medical Aspects of Human Sexuality, 7*, 94–95.

Liesen, L. T. (2007). Women, behavior, and evolution: Understanding the debate between feminist evolutionists and evolutionary psychologists. *Politics and the Life Sciences, 26*, 51–70.

Lindemann, D. (2011). BDSM as therapy? *Sexualities, 14*, 151–172.

Linden, R. R. (1983). *Against sadomasochism: A radical feminist analysis*. East Palo Alto, CA: Frog in the Well.

Loe, M. (2004). *The rise of Viagra: How the little blue pill changed sex in America*. New York, NY: New York University Press.

Lorde, A. (2007). *Sister outsider*. New York, NY: Random House. (Original work published 1984)

Lorde, A. (2015). An open letter to Mary Daly. In C. Moraga & G. Anzaldúa (Eds.), *This bridge called my back: Writings by radical women of color* (4th ed., pp. 90–93). Albany, NY: SUNY Press. (Original work published 1979)

Love, H. (2007). *Feeling backward: Loss and the politics of queer history*. Cambridge, MA: Harvard University Press.

Mac, J., & Smith, M. (2018). *Revolting prostitutes: The fight for sex workers' rights*. New York, NY: Verso Books.

MacDonald, C. L. (2015). Nannies on the market. In A. S. Wharton (Ed.), *Working in America: Continuity, conflict, and change in a new economic era* (pp. 103–120). London, UK: Routledge.

MacKinnon, C. A. (1982). Feminism, Marxism, method, and the state: An agenda for theory. *Signs: A Journal of Women in Culture and Society, 7*, 515–544.

Madsen, P. (2013, January 18). Cracking the code on female sexual desire. *Psychology Today*. Retrieved from https://www.psychologytoday.com/us/blog/shameless-woman/201301/cracking-the-code-female-sexual-desire

Malabou, C. (2012). *The new wounded: From neurosis to brain damage*. New York, NY: Fordham University Press.

Maltz, W., & Holman, B. (1987). *Incest and sexuality: A guide to understanding and healing*. Lexington, MA: Lexington Books.

Mamo, L., & Fishman, J. R. (2001). Potency in all the right places: Viagra as a technology of the gendered body. *Body & Society, 7*, 13–35.

Maravilla, K., & Yang, C. (2008). Magnetic resonance imaging and the female sexual response: Overview of techniques, results, and future directions. *Journal of Sexual Medicine, 5*, 1559–1571.

Markowitz, S. (2001). Pelvic politics: Sexual dimorphism and racial difference. *Signs, 26*, 389–414.

Martin, W. (2018). *Untrue: Why nearly everything we believe about women, lust, and infidelity is wrong and how the new science can set us free*. New York, NY: Little Brown Sparks.

Martínez-Guzmán, A., & Lara, A. (2019). Affective modulation in positive psychology's regime of happiness. *Theory & Psychology, 29*, 336–357.

Marx, K. (1990). *Capital: Volume 1: A critique of political economy* (Reprint ed.). New York, NY: Penguin Classics.

Masters, W. H., & Johnson, V. E. (1966). *Human sexual response.* New York, NY: Bantam Books.

Masters, W. H., & Johnson, V. E. (1970). *Human sexual inadequacy.* New York, NY: Bantam Books.

Mbembe, A. (2003). Necropolitics. Public Culture, 15, 11–40.

Mbembe, A. (2019). *Necropolitics.* Durham, NC: Duke University Press.

McClelland, S. I. (2010). Intimate justice: A critical analysis of sexual satisfaction. *Social and Personality Psychology Compass.* https://doi.org/10.1111/j.1751-9004.2010.00293.x

McClintock, A. (1995). *Imperial leather: Race, gender, and sexuality in the colonial contest.* New York, NY: Routledge.

McKinnon, S. (2006). *Neo-liberal genetics: The myths and moral tales of evolutionary psychology.* Chicago, IL: University of Chicago Press.

McRuer, R. (2006). *Crip theory: Cultural signs of queerness and disability.* New York, NY: New York University Press.

McWhorter, L. (2004). Sex, race, and biopower: A Foucauldian genealogy. *Hypatia, 19*, 38–62.

McWhorter, L. (2009). *Racism and sexual oppression in Anglo-America: A genealogy.* Bloomington, IN: Indiana University Press.

Meana, M. (2010). Elucidating women's (hetero)sexual desire: Definitional challenges and content expansion. *Journal of Sex Research, 47*, 104–122.

Merleau-Ponty, M. (1995). *Phenomenology of perception.* New York, NY: Routledge. (Original work published 1962)

Meston, C. M., & Buss, D. M. (2007). Why humans have sex. *Archives of Sexual Behavior, 36*, 477–507.

Meston, C. M., & Buss, D. M. (2009). *Why women have sex: Understanding sexual motivations from adventure to revenge (and everything in between).* New York, NY: Times Books.

Mies, M. (2010, December 29). Colonization and housewifization. *Caring labor: An archive.* Retrieved from http://caringlabor.wordpress.com/2010/12/29/maria-mies-colonization-and-housewifization/

Miles, M. B., Huberman, A. M., & Saldaña, J. (2013). *Qualitative data analysis: A methods sourcebook* (3rd ed.). Thousand Oaks, CA: Sage.

Milks, M., & Cerankowski, K. J. (2014). Introduction: Why asexuality? Why now? In M. Milks & K. J. Cerankowski (Eds.), *Asexualities: Feminist and queer perspectives* (pp. 1–16). New York, NY: Routledge.

Miller, J. B. (1976). *Toward a new psychology of women.* Boston, MA: Beacon Press.

Mitchell, J., & Rose, J. (Eds.). (1985). *Feminine sexuality: Jacques Lacan and the école freudienne.* New York, NY: W. W. Norton.

Mitchell, K. R., Mercer, C. H., Ploubidis, G. B., Jones, K. G., Datta, J., Field, N., &Wellings, K. (2013). Sexual function in Britain: Findings from the Third National Survey of Sexual Attitudes and Lifestyles (Natsal-3). *Lancet, 382*, 1817–1829.

Moir, J. (2012, June 21). Sorry, sisters, there's nothing liberating about mummy porn. *The Daily Mail.* Retrieved from https://www.dailymail.co.uk/debate/article-2162998/Fifty-Shades-Grey-Sorry-sisters-theres-liberating-mummy-porn.html

Mollow, A. (2014). Criphystemologies: What disability theory needs to know about hysteria. *Journal of Literary & Cultural Disability Studies*, 8, 185–201.

Moore, L. J., & Clarke, A. E. (1995). Clitoral conventions and transgressions: Graphic representations of female genital anatomy, c1900–1991. *Feminist Studies*, 21, 255–301.

Moraga, M., & Anzaldúa, G. (2015). *This bridge called my back: Writings by radical women of color*. Albany, NY: SUNY Press.

Moser, C., & Kleinplatz, P. J. (2006). Introduction: The state of our knowledge on SM. In P. J. Kleinplatz & C. Moser (Eds.), *Sadomasochism: Powerful pleasures* (pp. 1–16). New York, NY: Routledge.

Moynihan, R. (2005). The marketing of a disease: Female sexual dysfunction. *BMJ*, 330, 192–194.

Moynihan, R., & Mintzes, B. (2010). *Sex, lies, and pharmaceuticals: How drug companies plan to profit from female sexual dysfunction*. Berkeley, CA: Greystone Books.

Murphy, M. (2012). *Seizing the means of reproduction: Entanglements of feminism, health, and technoscience*. Durham, NC: Duke University Press.

Murphy, M. (2017.) *The economization of life*. Durham, NC: Duke University Press.

Murray, S. H. (2019). *Not always in the mood: The new science of men, sex, and relationships*. New York, NY: Rowman & Littlfield.

Musser, A. J. (2014). *Sensational flesh: Race, power, and masochism*. New York, NY: New York University Press.

Nagoski, E. (2015). *Come as you are: The surprising new science that will transform your sex life*. New York, NY: Simon & Schuster.

Nash, J. C. (2014). *The black body in ecstasy*. Durham, NC: Duke University Press.

Nash, J. C. (2019). *Black feminism reimagined: After intersectionality*. Durham, NC: Duke University Press.

Nelson, T., Cardemil, E. V., & Adeoye, C. T. (2016). Rethinking strength: Black women's perceptions of the "strong black woman" role. *Psychology of Women Quarterly*, 40, 551–563.

New View Campaign. (2018). Welcome. Retrieved from http://www.newviewcampaign.org/

Newman, Andy. (2008, June 12). What women want (maybe). *The New York Times*. Retrieved from https://www.nytimes.com/2008/06/12/fashion/12bisex.html

Ngai, S. (2005). *Ugly feelings*. Cambridge, MA: Harvard University Press.

O'Loughlin, J. I., & Brotto, L. A. (2020). Women's sexual desire, trauma exposure, and posttraumatic stress disorder. *Journal of Traumatic Stress*, online, https://doi.org/10.1002/jts.22485

Ogas, O., & Gaddam, S. (2011). *A billion wicked thoughts: What the internet tells us about sexual relationships*. New York, NY: Plume Books.

Ogden, G. (2001). Integrating sexuality and spirituality: A group approach to women's sexual dilemmas. In P. J. Kleinplatz (Ed.), *New directions in sex therapy: Innovations and alternatives* (pp. 322–346). Philadelphia, PA: Brunner-Routledge.

Oliver, K. (2001). *Witnessing: Beyond recognition*. Minneapolis, MN: University of Minnesota Press.

Oudshoorn, N. (1994). *Beyond the natural body: An archaeology of sex hormones*. New York, NY: Routledge.

Owens, D. C. (2017). *Medical bondage: Race, gender, and the origins of American gynecology*. Athens, GA: University of Georgia Press.

Owens, E. A. (2019). Keyword 7: Consent. *differences: A Journal of Feminist Cultural Studies*, 30, 148–156.

Parreñas, R. S. (2002). The care crisis in the Philippines: Children and transnational families in the new global economy. In B. Ehrenreich & A. R. Hochschild (Eds.), *Global woman: Nannies, maids, and sex workers in the new economy* (pp. 39–54). New York, NY: Owl Books.

Pascoe, C. J. (2011). *Dude, you're a fag: Masculinity and sexuality in high school*. Berkeley, CA: University of California Press.

Patsavas, A. (2014). Recovering a cripistemology of pain: Leaky bodies, connective tissue, and feeling discourse. *Journal of Literary & Cultural Disability Studies*, 8, 203–218.

Perel, E. (2006). *Mating in captivity: Reconciling the erotic & the domestic*. New York, NY: HarperCollins.

Perel, E. (2017). *The state of affairs: Rethinking infidelity*. New York, NY: HarperCollins.

Peterson, Z. D., & Muehlenhard, C. L. (2007). Conceptualizing the "wantedness" of women's consensual and nonconsensual sexual experiences: Implications for how women label their experiences with rape. *Journal of Sex Research*, 44, 72–88.

Piepzna-Samarasinha, L. L. (2018). *Care work: Dreaming disability justice*. Vancouver, BC: Arsenal Pulp Press.

Pitts-Taylor, V. (2003). *In the flesh: The cultural politics of body modification*. New York, NY: Palgrave Macmillan.

Pitts-Taylor, V. (2007). *Surgery junkies: Wellness and pathology in cosmetic culture*. New Brunswick, NJ: Rutgers University Press.

Pitts-Taylor, V. (2016). *The brain's body: Neuroscience and corporeal politics*. Durham, NC: Duke University Press.

Preciado, P. B. (2013). *Testo junkie: Sex, drugs, and biopolitics in the pharmacopornographic era*. New York, NY: Feminist Press.

Przybylo, E. (2013). Producing facts: Empirical asexuality and the scientific study of sex. *Feminism & Psychology*, 23, 224–242.

Przybylo, E. (2014). Masculine doubt and sexual wonder: Asexually-identified men talk about their (a)sexualities. In M. Milks & K. J. Cerankowski (Eds.), *Asexualities: Feminist and queer perspectives* (pp. 225–247). New York, NY: Routledge.

Puar, J. (2007). *Terrorist assemblages: Homonationalism in queer times*. Durham, NC: Duke University Press.

Puar, J. (2011). The cost of getting better: Suicide, sensation, switchpoints. *GLQ*, 18, 149–158.

Puar, J. (2017). *The right to maim: Debility, capacity, disability*. Durham, NC: Duke University Press.

Purser, R. E. (2019). *McMindfulness: How mindfulness became the new capitalist spirituality*. London, UK: Repeater.

Rabinow, P. (1996.) Artificiality and enlightenment: From sociobiology to biosociality. In J. Crary and S. Kwinter (Eds.), Incorporations (pp. 234–252). New York, NY: Zone.

Race, K. (2009). *Pleasure consuming medicine: The queer politics of drugs*. Durham, NC: Duke University Press.

Repo, J. (2016). *The biopolitics of gender*. New York, NY: Oxford University Press.

Rich, A. (1980). Compulsory heterosexuality and lesbian existence. *Signs: Journal of Women in Culture and Society*, 5, 631–660.

Richardson, S. (2012). Sexing the X: How the X became the 'female chromosome'. *Signs: Journal of Women in Culture and Society*, 37, 909–933.

Ridley, M. (2003). *The red queen: Sex and the evolution of human nature* (Reprint ed.). New York, NY: Harper Perennial.

Rieger, G., Chivers, M. L., & Bailey, J. M. (2005). Sexual arousal patterns of bisexual men. *Psychological Bulletin*, 16, 579–584.

Roberts, D. (1997). *Killing the black body: Race, reproduction, and the meaning of liberty*. New York, NY: Vintage Books.

Rodriguez, J. M. (2019). Keyword 6: Testimony. *differences: A Journal of Feminist Cultural Studies*, 30, 119–125.

Rogak, H. M. E., & Connor, J. J. (2018). Practice of consensual BDSM and relationship satisfaction. *Sexual and Relationship Therapy*, 33, 454–469.

Roiphe, K. (2012, April 16). Working women's fantasies. *Newsweek*. Retrieved from http://www.newsweek.com/working-womens-fantasies-63915

Rose, N. (2001). The politics of life itself. *Theory, Culture & Society*, 18, 1–30.

Rose, N. (2007). *The politics of life itself: Biomedicine, power, and subjectivity in the twenty first century*. Princeton, NJ: Princeton University Press.

Rose, S., Kamin, L. J., & Lewontin, R. C. (1984). *Not in our genes: Biology, ideology and human nature*. Harmondsworth, UK: Penguin Books.

Rosenthal, A. M., Sylva, D., Safron, A., & Bailey, J. M. (2011). Sexual arousal patterns of bisexual men revisited. *Biological Psychology*, 88, 112–115.

Rubin, G. (1975). The traffic in women: Notes on the "political economy" of sex. In L. Nicholson (Ed.), *The second wave: A reader in feminist theory* (pp. 27–62). New York, NY: Routledge.

Rubin, G. (1984). Thinking sex: Notes for a radical theory of the politics of sexuality. In C. Vance (Ed.), *Pleasure and danger: Exploring female sexuality* (pp. 267–319). London: Routledge.

Ruído, M. (2011, February 8). Just do it! Bodies and images of women in the new division of labor. *Caring labor: An archive*. Retrieved from http://caringlabor.wordpress.com/2011/02/08/maria-ruido-just-do-it-bodies-and-images-of-women-in-the-new-division-of-labor/

Rupp, L., Taylor, V., Regev-Messalem, S., Fogarty, A. C. K., & England, P. (2014). Queer women in the hookup scene: Beyond the closet? *Gender & Society*, 28, 212–235.

Safron, A., Sylva, D., Klimaj, V., Rosenthal, A. M., & Bailey, J. M. (2019). Neural responses to sexual stimuli in heterosexual and homosexual men and women: Men's responses are more specific. *Archives of Sexual Behavior*. https://doi.org/10.1007/s10508-019-01521-z

Schreiber, K. (2012, July/August). Flex appeal. *Psychology Today*, 36–37.

Schuller, K. (2018). *The biopolitics of feeling: Race, sex, and science in the nineteenth century*. Durham, NC: Duke University Press.

Segal, Z., Williams, J., & Teasdale, J. (2001). *Mindfulness-based cognitive therapy for depression: A new approach to preventing relapse*. New York, NY: Guilford Press.

Seltzer, L. (2012a, May 11). The triggers of sexual desire: Men vs. women [Blog post]. Retrieved from https://www.psychologytoday.com/us/blog/evolution-the-self/201205/the-triggers-sexual-desire-men-vs-women

Seltzer, L. (2012b, May 14). The triggers of sexual desire Pt 2: What's erotic for women? [Blog post]. Retrieved from https://www.psychologytoday.com/us/blog/evolution-the-self/201205/the-triggers-sexual-desire-pt-2-what-s-erotic-women

Seltzer, L. (2012c, May 17). Paradox and pragmatism in women's sexual desire [Blog post]. Retrieved from http://www.psychologytoday.com/blog/evolution-the-self/201205/paradox-and-pragmatism-in-women-s-sexual-desire

Shedler, J. (2010). The efficacy of psychodynamic psychotherapy. *American Psychologist, 65*, 98–109.

Shifren, J. L., Monz, B. U., Russo, P. A., Segreti, A., & Johannes, C. B. (2008). Sexual problems and distress in United States women: Prevalence and correlates. *Obstetrics and Gynecology, 112*, 970–978.

Silverman, K. (1992). *Male subjectivity at the margins.* New York, NY: Routledge.

Sims, K., & Meana, M. (2010). Why did passion wane? A qualitative study of married women's attributions for declines in sexual desire. *Journal of Sex & Marital Therapy, 36*, 360–380.

Skinner, B. F. (1938). *The behavior of organisms: An experimental analysis.* Minneapolis, MN: University of Minnesota.

Snorton, C. R. (2017). *Black on both sides: A racial history of trans identity.* Minneapolis, MN: University of Minnesota.

Somerville, S. (1994). Scientific racism and the emergence of the homosexual body. *Journal of the History of Sexuality, 5*, 243–266.

Somerville, S. (2000). *Queering the color line: Race and the invention of homosexuality in American culture.* Durham, NC: Duke University Press.

Spillers, H. (1987). Mama's baby, Papa's maybe: An American grammar book. *Diacritics, 17*, 64–81.

Spurgas, A. K. (2013a). Interest, arousal, and shifting diagnoses of female sexual dysfunction, or: How women learn about desire. *Studies in Gender and Sexuality, 14*, 187–205.

Spurgas, A. K. (2013b). Gendered populations and trauma beyond Oedipus: Reply to Angel's commentary. *Studies in Gender and Sexuality, 14*, 217–223.

Spurgas, A. K. (2016a). Low desire, trauma, and femininity in the *DSM-5*: A case for sequelae. *Psychology & Sexuality, 7*, 48–67.

Spurgas, A. K. (2016b, March 9). Solving desire. *The New Inquiry.* Retrieved from http://thenewinquiry.com/essays/solving-desire/

Spurgas, A. K. (under review). The Freedom to Fall Apart: A Crip Theory of Feminine Fracture.

Stahl, S., Sommer, B., & Allers, K. (2011). Multifunctional pharmacology of flibanserin: Possible mechanism of therapeutic action in hypoactive sexual desire disorder. *Journal of Sexual Medicine, 8*, 15–27.

Stekel, W. (1926). *Frigidity in woman in relation to her love life.* New York, NY: Liveright.

Stockton, K. B. (2006). *Beautiful bottom, beautiful shame: Where "black" meets "queer."* Durham, NC: Duke University Press.

Stoler, A. L. (1995). *Race and the education of desire: Foucault's history of sexuality and the colonial order of things.* Durham, NC: Duke University Press.

Subramaniam, B., & Willey, A. (2016). Fighting the *derpy* science of sexuality. *Archives of Sexual Behavior, 45*, 513–515.

Suschinksy, K. D., Dawson, S. J., & Chivers, M. L. (2020). Assessing gender-specificity of clitoral responses. *The Canadian Journal of Human Sexuality, 29*, 57–64.

Suschinsky, K. D., Fisher, T. D., Maunder, L., Hollenstein, T., & Chivers, M. L. (2020). Use of the bogus pipeline increases sexual concordance in women but not men. *Archives of Sexual Behavior, 49*, 1517–1532.

Suschinsky, K. D., Huberman, J. S., Maunder, L., Brotto, L. A., Hollenstein, T., & Chivers, M. L. (2019). The relationship between sexual functioning and sexual concordance in women. *Journal of Sex & Marital Therapy, 45*, 230–246.

Suschinsky, K. D., & Lalumière, M. L. (2011). Prepared for anything? An investigation of female genital arousal in response to rape cues. *Psychological Science, 22*, 159–165.

Suschinsky, K. D., Lalumière, M. L., & Chivers, M. L. (2009). Sex differences in patterns of genital arousal: Measurement artifact or true phenomenon? *Archives of Sexual Behavior, 38*, 559–573.

Symons, D. (1979). *The evolution of human sexuality.* New York, NY: Oxford University Press.

Szasz, T. (1960). The myth of mental illness. *The American Psychologist, 15*, 113–118.

Terranova, T. (2004). *Network culture: Politics for the information age.* London, UK: Pluto.

Thornhill, R., & Palmer, C. T. (2000). *A natural history of rape: Biological bases of sexual coercion.* Cambridge, MA: MIT Press.

Tiefer, L. (1991). Historical, scientific, clinical and feminist criticisms of "the human sexual response cycle" model. *Annual Review of Sex Research, 2*, 1–23.

Tiefer, L. (1995). *Sex is not a natural act and other essays.* Boulder, CO: Westview Press.

Tiefer, L. (1996). The medicalization of sexuality: Conceptual, normative, and professional issues. *Annual Review of Sex Research, 7*, 252–282.

Tiefer, L. (2001). A new view of women's sexual problems: Why new? Why now? *Journal of Sex Research, 38*, 89–96.

Tiefer, L. (2006). Female sexual dysfunction: A case study of disease mongering and activist resistance. *PLoS Medicine, 3*, e178.

Tiefer, L. (2012). Medicalizations and demedicalizations of sexuality therapies. *Journal of Sex Research, 49*, 311–318.

Toates, F. (2014). *How sexual desire works: The enigmatic urge.* Cambridge, MA: Cambridge University Press.

Tolman, D. L. (1994). Doing desire: Adolescent girls' struggles for/with sexuality. *Gender & Society, 8*, 324–342.

Tolman, D. L. (2005). *Dilemmas of desire: Teenage girls talk about sexuality.* Cambridge, MA: Harvard University Press.

Tolman, D. L. (2006). In a different position: Conceptualizing female adolescent sexuality development within compulsory heterosexuality. *New Directions for Child and Adolescent Development, 112*, 71–89.

Tolman, D. L., & McClelland, S. I. (2011). Normative sexuality development in adolescence: A decade in review, 2000-2009. *Journal of Research on Adolescence, 21*, 242–255.

Travis, C. B. (2003). *Evolution, gender, and rape.* Cambridge, MA: MIT Press.

Trivers, R. L. (1972). Parental investment and sexual selection. In B. Campbell (Ed.), *Sexual selection and the descent of man* (pp. 136–179). New York, NY: Aldine DeGruyter.

Tyler, M. (2009). No means yes? Perpetuating myths in the sexological construction of women's desire. *Women & Therapy, 32*, 40–50.

Ussher, J. M. (2011). *The madness of women: Myth and experience.* London, UK: Routledge.

Ussher, J. M. (2017). Unraveling the mystery of "The specificity of women's sexual response and its relationship with sexual orientations": The social construction of sex and sexual identities. *Archives of Sexual Behavior, 46*, 1207–1211.

Valocchi, S. (2005). Not yet queer enough: The lessons of queer theory for the sociology of gender and sexuality. *Gender & Society*, 19, 750–770.

Van Anders, S. M. (2015). Beyond sexual orientation: Integrating gender/sex and diverse sexualities via sexual configurations theory. *Archives of Sexual Behavior*, 44, 1177–1213.

Vance, C. S. (Ed.). (1992). *Pleasure and danger: Exploring female sexuality.* New York, NY: New York University Press.

Velten, J. Scholten, S., Graham, C. A., Adolph, D., & Margraf, J. (2016). Investigating female sexual concordance: Do sexual excitation and sexual inhibition moderate the agreement of genital and subjective sexual arousal in women? *Archives of Sexual Behavior*, 45, 1957–1971.

Vidal, F., & Ortega, F. (2017). *Being brains: Making the cerebral subject.* New York, NY: Fordham University Press.

von Werlhof, C. (1988). On the concept of nature and society in capitalism. In M. Mies, V. Bennholdt-Thomsen, & C. von Werlhof (Eds.), *Women: The last colony,* 96–112. London, UK: Zed Books.

Wade, L. (2017). *American hookup: The new culture of sex on campus.* New York: W. W. Norton.

Waidzunas, T., & Epstein, S. (2015). "For men, arousal is orientation": Bodily truthing, technosexual scripts, and the materialization of sexualities through the phallometric test. *Social Studies of Science*, 45, 187–213.

Ward, J. (2015). *Not gay: Sex between straight white men.* New York, NY: New York University Press.

Warner, M. (1991). Introduction: Fear of a queer planet. *Social Text*, 9, 3–17.

Washington, H. A. (2006). *Medical apartheid: The dark history of medical experimentation on black Americans from colonial times to the present.* New York, NY: Broadway Books.

Weeks, K. (2011). *The problem with work: Feminism, Marxism, antiwork politics, and postwork Imaginaries.* Durham, NC: Duke University Press.

Weheliye, A. G. (2014). *Habeas viscus: Racializing assemblages, biopolitics, and black feminist theories of the human.* Durham, NC: Duke University Press.

Weiner, L., & Avery-Clark, C. (2014). Sensate focus: Clarifying the Masters and Johnson's model. *Sexual and Relationship Therapy*, 1–13.

Weiner-Davis, M. (2003). *The sex-starved marriage: Boosting your marriage libido, a couple's guide.* New York, NY: Simon & Schuster.

Weiss, M. (2011). *Techniques of pleasure: BDSM and the circuits of sexuality.* Durham, NC: Duke University Press.

Wertheimer, E., & Casper, M. (2016). Within trauma: An introduction. In E. Wertheimer & M. J. Casper (Eds.), *Critical trauma studies: Understanding violence, conflict, and memory in everyday life* (pp. 1–18). New York, NY: New York University Press.

West, S. L., D'Aloisio, A., Agans, R., Kalsbeek, W., Borisov, N., & Thorp, J. (2008). Prevalence of low sexual desire and hypoactive sexual desire disorder in a nationally representative sample of U. S. women. *Archives of Internal Medicine*, 168, 1441–1449.

Williams, R. (1977). *Marxism and literature.* New York, NY: Oxford University Press.

Wilson, D. (2010, June 18). Drug for sexual desire disorder opposed by panel. *The New York Times.* Retrieved from http://www.nytimes.com/2010/06/19/business/19sexpill.html

Wilson, E. A. (2004). *Psychosomatic: Feminism and the neurological body.* Durham, NC: Duke University Press.

Wilson, E. A. (2015). *Gut feminism*. Durham, NC: Duke University Press.

Wilson, E. O. (2000). *Sociobiology: The new synthesis* (25th anniversary ed.). Cambridge, MA: Belknap Press.

Wingfield, A. H. (2015). Are some emotions marked "whites only"? Racialized feeling rules in professional workplaces. In A. S. Wharton (Ed.), *Working in America: Continuity, conflict, and change in a new economic era* (pp. 201–214). London, UK: Routledge.

Working Group for the New View of Women's Sexual Problems. (2002). A new view of women's sexual problems. *Women & Therapy*, 24, 1–8.

Yehuda, R., Lehrner, A, & Rosenbaum, T. Y. (2015). PTSD and sexual dysfunction in men and Women. *Journal of Sexual Medicine*. https://doi.org/10.1111/jsm.12856

Young, I. M. (2005). *On female body experience: "Throwing like a girl" and other essays*. New York, NY: Oxford University Press.

Zola, I. K. (1972). Medicine as an institution of social control. *The Sociological Review*, 20, 487–504.

INDEX

abuse, sexual. *See* trauma and gendered violence
active passivity, 125–26
Addyi (flibanserin), 66, 92–95, 98
affective labor. *See* carework and embodied labor
Against Sadomasochism (Linden), 193
agency, sexual, 24, 126, 172n3, 194–95, 204–5, 218–20, 225
agender people, 9, 88, 231–33
Allison, Dorothy, 194
"ambiphilic" women, 76–78
anarchism, feminine, 220
anatomopolitics, 151, 157
"androphilic" women, 76–78
arousal: category-specific, 73–78; FSAD (female sexual arousal disorder), 84–85; incentive motivation model, 65n2, 69–72, 83, 91, 222–23; information processing model (IPM) of, 69n4; interest and desire linked to, 118–24; interest vs., 85; preceding or co-occurring with desire, 70, 118–21; subjective arousal merged with desire in FSAD, 85. *See also* concordance and discordance; FSIAD diagnosis; plethysmography and mind/body disjuncture; receptivity; responsiveness
"'Arousal-First' Desire May Be More Typical for Women, and It Doesn't Need a Cure" (Bielski), 221–24
arousal-first sexual response model. *See* circular sexual response cycle
arousometer, 4, 73
asexuality, 89, 188, 195
Avery-Clark, Constance, 43

Bailey, J. Michael, 74
Barbach, Lonnie, 51n8, 114–15
barter logic, 161–63, 176
Basson, Rosemary, 6, 67–69, 96, 164–65. *See also* circular sexual response cycle
Bataille, Georges, 194
Baumeister, Roy, 31, 57–61, 83
BDSM (bondage and discipline/dominance and submission/sadism and masochism). *See* parasexuality, submission, and BDSM
Becoming Orgasmic (Heiman, Lo Piccolo, and Lo Piccolo), 114–15
behaviorist perspective: cognitive behavioral therapy (CBT), 95, 97, 100; cognitive

263

behaviorism, 43, 48, 53; conversion therapy, 75; cost-benefit analysis and conditioning models, 2–3; desensitization approach, 42–43; desire in, 52; Masters and Johnson Institute, 43; receptivity management and, 98–100; sensate focus technique, 43–44, 96–97; sexual self-management and, 100–106

Benjamin, Jessica, 104, 204

Bergner, Daniel, 1–2, 4–7, 74, 224

Berlant, Lauren, 122, 225

Bersani, Leo, 187, 193n4

Bielski, Zosia, 221–24

Billion Wicked Thoughts, A (Ogas and Gaddam), 78

biopolitical regimes: cultural feminism and, 115; Foucault on, 6, 20–21, 218; neoliberal form of labor, 150–51, 178, 182–83; population production, 151, 157; regulation and new potential, 230–31; regulatory control and sexual self-management, 101–6; self-optimization, 101–2, 150, 151, 182; sexual carework and, 176–81. *See also* mindfulness-based sex therapy

biopsychosocial model, 42, 71

bisexuality, 29, 36, 74

Black femininity and sexual difference, 11–14. *See also* race and racialization

Blanchard, Ray, 74

body and bodily processes, gendered experience of, 135–37

bodyminds, 109

body modification, 194–95

body shutting down as resistance, 143–47

Both, Stephanie, 69, 70n5

Braksmajer, Amy, 150, 152, 164

bremelanotide (Vyleesi), 93

Brody, Stuart, 58

Brothers, Doris, 194

Brotto, Lori: on BDSM, 211n9; Bergner on, 1–2, 6; on discordance, 142–43; *DSM-5*, FSIAD, and, 82–86; mindfulness-based sex therapy (MBST) and, 96–100, 103n19; on responsiveness in men, 87n14; story of "Gianna," 230; on trauma, 122

Buss, David, 54–57, 83

Butler, Judith, 212

bypassing, 48–49, 105, 210

Cacchioni, Thea, 131, 150–52, 164, 169, 214

camp, 211–12

capacitation, regimes of, 181–83

carework and embodied labor: barter and "men only want one thing" logic, 161–64; beyond the bedroom, 174–75; biopolitics of, 176–81; carework, defined, 153; in childhood and youth, 158–61; as coercion, 175–76; Cossman's sexual citizenship and Cacchioni's "sex work," 151; "doing it anyway" and "going through the motions," 164–69; egalitarianism and, 148, 155–56; faking it and affective performances of pleasure, 169–74; liberal capitalist and neoliberal biopolitical forms of work, 149–53, 178, 182–83; regimes of capacitation, 181–83; social reproduction, receptivity, and feminized labor under capitalism, 153–57, 182

castration complex, 34–35

category-specificity, 73–78

Charest, Maxime, 16

Chivers, Meredith, 4–5, 74–82, 97–98, 190–91, 221–23, 231

Chodorow, Nancy, 112

Chu, Andrea Long, 112n4, 193n4

circular sexual response cycle: about, 68–69; Brotto and, 83; critiques of, 89–91; defined, 6; feminism and, 115; gender neutrality and, 222–23; incentive motivation model and, 71n6; MBST and, 97; mindfulness and, 117; Weiner-Davis and, 177

cisnormativity: biomedical frameworks and, 229; evolutionary narratives and, 109; feminized receptivity models and, 72; feminized responsive desire framework and, 8, 25; Masters & Johnson and, 41; sex therapy, sexology, and, 228; sexual difference and, 54, 135; volumetric studies and, 4n1

citizenship, sexual, 151, 179, 182

Clare, Eli, 109n2

clitoral photoplethysmography, 73

clitoris: Freud on shift to vagina, 35–36; Masters & Johnson on, 40, 41, 46; orgasm and, 40, 41, 46, 58, 132; plethysmography and, 4, 73

cognitive behavioral therapy (CBT), 95, 97, 100

cognitive behaviorism, 43, 48, 53. *See also* behaviorist perspective
cognitive conditioning, 3
Collins, Patricia Hill, 159, 197, 233
Comella, Lynn, 179n4
complexity of female sexuality: Baumeister's erotic plasticity hypothesis, 59–61, 83; in evolutionary psychology, 58–61; Freud on, 36–37; FSIAD and, 87; Kaplan and, 47, 49; pathologizing-healing dialectic and, 137–39; political and material factors, 227; socialization and, 133–34
compulsory (hetero)sexuality: asexuality studies and, 19, 195; carework and, 25, 150; evolutionary psychology and, 52–53; feminism and, 110, 115; naturalness and, 40n5; parasexuality and, 26; self-optimization and, 102; sexual difference and, 38–39; Viagra and, 93
concordance and discordance: Baumeister and, 60; Bielski on, 222; biological-psychological-social feedback loops, 141–47; category-specificity, 73–78; Chivers on, 76; consent and, 142; discordance vs. concordance, 4–5, 23, 63; evolutionary psychology and, 58; excessive concordance, 81; MBST and, 97; plethysmography and, 7, 75, 80–81; reverse discordance, 143; submission linked to, 190–91; trauma and, 99. *See also* plethysmography and mind/body disjuncture
Conniff, Richard, 63
Conrad, Peter, 18
consent: Brotto on arousal and, 142; carework and, 176; Chivers on, 78; desire-interest-arousal linkage and, 120–24; enthusiastic, 215; fantasy about, 201; feminized responsive desire framework and, 169; foreclosure of, 196; MBST and, 99; murkiness of nonconsent vs., 232; parasexuality and, 199, 219; passion and, 204; trust and, 186, 201, 201n7
conversion therapy and orgasmic reconditioning, 3, 75, 102, 230
Cosmides, Leda, 55
Cossman, Brenda, 151
cost-benefit analysis, 2
couples, research focus on, 41–42, 46
Crenshaw, Kimberlé, 233
crip theory and cripistemology, 19, 109, 144, 232–33

cue-specificity, 73n7
cultural feminism, 110–18, 142, 193n4
Cvetkovich, Ann, 122, 126, 187, 193n4, 194, 200, 204–5, 225

Daly, Mary, 111
Darwin, Charles, 53
Dawkins, Richard, 55
Deleuze, Gilles, 101, 194
depersonalization, 120
desensitization technique, 42–43
desire: all human desire as responsive, 69; arousal preceding or co-occurring with, 70, 118–21; biopolitical control and, 102; egalitarianism and, 148; in evolutionary sexology, 52–61; husbandry and, 105–6; interest and arousal linked to, 118–24; Kaplan and, 45; Kaplan's, *Disorders of Sexual Desire*, 46; nonsexual, 186–87; in post-psychoanalytic milieu, 52; psychoanalytic accounts after Freud, dismissal of, 104; seeking the "truth" of female desire, 227–28; spontaneous vs. responsive, 14–15, 65, 127–29; subjective arousal merged with, in FSIAD, 85. *See also* arousal; FSIAD diagnosis; low female sexual desire; plethysmography and mind/body disjuncture; receptivity; responsiveness
determinism, biological, 51–52
DeVault, Marjorie L., 167
Diagnostic and Statistical Manual of Mental Disorders (*DSM*): biopolitical control and, 102–3; desire disorders and compulsory sexuality, 52–53; FSIAD in *DSM-IV* and *DSM-5*, 7, 84; New View Campaign protest against, 116–17; sexual disorders in history of, 15. *See also* FSIAD diagnosis
difference, gender. *See* sexual difference
dilators, 42–43
disability studies, 19, 144, 232–33
discordance. *See* concordance and discordance
Disorders of Sexual Desire (Kaplan), 46
dissociation: essentialization of, 190, 218; feminizing of, 226; low desire and, 165–67; rethinking, 232–34; trauma and, 99, 120–23, 160; voicelessness and, 200. *See also* concordance and discor-

dance; plethysmography and mind/body disjuncture
distributive ontologies, 33
Dodson, Betty, 51n8, 114
Donegan, Moira, 231–32
drugs. *See* pharmaceuticals
dual control model, 70n4
Duncombe, Jean, 151n1, 169
Dworkin, Andrea, 110–11, 193n4
dyspareunia, 146, 150

egalitarianism, 148, 155–56, 191
Ellis, Havelock, 12
embodied labor, invisible. *See* carework and embodied labor
erectile disorder (ED), 66, 132
erection, 132, 135
erotic plasticity hypothesis, 59–61, 83
estrogen, 37
Everaerd, Walter, 69, 70n5
evolutionary psychology (EP): Baumeister's erotic plasticity hypothesis, 59–61, 83; *DSM-5* and, 83; Freud, affinity with, 37, 38; history of, 53–54; impact of, 57–58; in popular sphere, 56, 58; preparation hypothesis, 31, 77, 143, 143n10, 189, 190n2; "quality over quantity" and, 30; racialized sexual difference and, 11–12; rape and, 30; sexually dimorphic desire in, 52–61; as uncritiqueable, 55; as universal and ubiquitous, 56–57

Fahs, Breanne, 169, 196–97
fantasy, 127–29, 201–2, 231
Fausto-Sterling, Anne, 12
Federici, Silvia, 154–55
feedback loops, 50–51, 105, 141–47
female-friendly sexual response models, 66–72
female sexual arousal disorder (FSAD), 84–85
"Female Sexuality" (Freud), 29–30
Feminine Mystique, The (Friedan), 153
feminism: Baumeister and, 60–61; BDSM and, 192–95, 219; cultural, 110–18, 142, 193n4; *DSM* desire diagnoses and, 52–53; feminized responsive desire framework and, 8; heteronormativity and, 110–11; medicalization and, 18–19; #MeToo movement and, 231–32; protocol feminism, 115–16; psychoanalysis and, 32; sex-positive, 61, 111, 179, 194, 218
feminized responsive desire framework: behaviorist perspective and conditioning models, 2–3; cultural embeddedness of, 227–28; feminism and, 8; FSIAD diagnosis and, 6–7; heteronormativity in, 91; prediction, control, and, 229–32; techniques and circular sexual response cycle (overview), 5–6; ugly side of, 165–66; volumetric studies and plethysmography (overview), 3–4; whiteness as foundation of, 13–14. *See also* circular sexual response cycle; concordance and discordance; FSIAD diagnosis; plethysmography and mind/body disjuncture; receptivity; responsiveness
femmes: andro-femme, 185n1; Cvetkovich on, 126, 187, 204–5; interview participants, 125–26, 204–5; pathologizing of, 8; queer femme receptivity, 126; strap-on dildos and, 212; tempo and, 207; trauma and, 185, 188, 197, 225–26, 228–29, 232–33
fertility-dependent change hypothesis, 77
Fifty Shades of Grey (James), 190–92
Fine, Cordelia, 61–62
Fishman, Jennifer R., 93, 132
flashbacks, 49–50
flibanserin (Addyi), 66, 92–95, 98
Flore, Jacinthe, 89
Foucault, Michel, 6, 18n5, 20–21, 101, 218
four-dimensional model of sexuality, 115
frequency of sex, 168
Freud, Sigmund, 29–30, 34–39, 48, 194, 204. *See also* psychoanalysis
Freund, Kurt, 75
Friedan, Betty, 153
FSIAD diagnosis (female sexual interest/arousal disorder): criteria and diagnostic terminology, 84–89; critiques of, 89–92; in *DSM*, 7; as gender-neutral SI/AD, 222–23; MHSDD compared to, 84, 87–89; rationale for changes in *DSM-5*, 82–83; as relational diagnosis, 129; trauma and, 99; undertheorization and implications of, 102–5

Gaddam, Sai, 78, 190–91
gap, mind/body. *See* concordance and discordance; plethysmography and mind/body disjuncture
gatekeeper role, 59

Gavey, Nicola, 131
gender differences. *See* sexual difference
gender neutrality of sexual response models, 222–23
gender-nonconforming people, 8–9, 49, 196n5, 207, 225, 231–33
genderqueer people, 4, 9, 22, 134, 179, 181, 183, 196n5, 207–8, 231–33
genito-pelvic pain/penetration disorder (GPPPD), 43
Gilligan, Carol, 113, 115
Goffman, Erving, 18n5
Gottlieb, Lori, 148
Gould, Stephen Jay, 53n10
Graham, Cynthia, 83
Grant, Melissa Gira, 152
Gray, John, 62n12
"gynephilic" women, 76–78

Hart, Lynda, 193, 194, 204, 225
Hartman, Saidiya, 12
Heiman, Julia, 114
heteronormativity: biomedical frameworks and, 229; carework and, 150, 178–79; evolutionary narratives and, 109; feminism and, 110–11; feminized receptivity models and, 72; feminized responsive desire framework and, 8, 25, 91; male aggression and, 199; Masters & Johnson and, 40, 41; parasexuality and rejection of heteronormative scripts, 214–17; penile-vaginal intercourse as norm, 131–33; sex therapy, sexology, and, 228; sexual difference and, 54, 135; volumetric studies and, 4n1
history of therapeutic models. *See* sex therapy models, history of
Hite Report, 114
Hochschild, Arlie Russell, 149
hormonal cycles, 136–37
Human Sexual Response (Masters and Johnson), 39
human sexual response cycle (HSRC), 39–40, 46, 65, 67, 116
husbandry, 105–6, 183
hypoactive sexual desire disorder (HSDD), 15, 52–53, 67, 84–85
hysteria, 29, 32–33, 143–44

In a Different Voice (Gilligan), 113

incentive motivation model (IMM), 65n2, 69–72, 83, 91, 222–23
inconsistency theme, feminine, 60
individualistic approaches in sex therapy, 53, 54
information processing model (IPM), 69n4
inhibited sexual desire (ISD), 15, 51, 52–53
intentionality, sexual, 199, 201, 203, 216–17
intercourse, penile-vaginal, social emphasis on, 131–33
interest: arousal and desire linked to, 118–24; in FSIAD, 84–87
International Society for the Study of Women's Sexual Health (ISSWSH), 66
International Wages for Housework Campaign (WfH), 153–54
intimate labor. *See* carework and embodied labor

Jagose, Annamarie, 3, 102, 172n3, 230
James, Selma, 154
Johnson, Lisa, 19, 144, 232–233
Johnson, Virginia, 38–45, 73, 96, 116

Kabat-Zinn, Jon, 95–96
Kaplan, Helen Singer, 44–52, 115, 210; Masters & Johnson and, 42
Kaye, Kerwin, 131
Kinsey, Alfred, 39
Klein, Melanie, 104
Kleinplatz, Peggy J., 16, 42, 49, 51n8, 89–90, 187
Kohut, Heinz, 194

Laan, Ellen, 69
labial thermistor clip method, 73
labor, embodied. *See* carework and embodied labor
Labuski, Christine, 10, 109, 131, 143, 150, 152, 164, 171, 178
Lalumière, Martin, 73n7, 143n10
Laplanche, Jean, 104
Lewontin, Richard, 53n10
liberal capitalist form of labor, 149–53, 178, 182–83
liberation, sexual, 41, 78
Loe, Meika, 93, 131, 132
Lo Piccolo, Joseph, 114

Lo Piccolo, Leslie, 114
Lorde, Audre, 111
love and sex, neurological linking of, 49–50
low female sexual desire: biopolitics and, 176–81; carework and, 152, 159; clinical category, women-with-low-desire as, 118; clinical history of, 14–17; coercion and, 175–76; desire-interest-arousal linkage, 118–24; "doing it anyway" and "going through the motions," 164–69; enhancing pleasure and, 206–17; faking it and affective performances of pleasure, 169–74; hermeneutics of, as frames of reference, 186; "men only want one thing" logic and, 161–64; nature/nurture binary and, 130–31; penetrative sex as the only "real" sex and, 131–33; phenomenological experience of gendered body and, 135–37. *See also* arousal; circular sexual response cycle; concordance and discordance; desire; FSIAD diagnosis; sex therapy models, history of
Lybrido and Lybridos, 93

Mac, Juno, 152
MacKinnon, Catherine, 110–11, 193n4
male hypoactive sexual desire disorder (MHSDD), 84, 87–89, 121
Mamo, Laura, 93, 132
Markowitz, Sally, 12–13
Marsden, Dennis, 151n1, 169
Marx, Karl, 153
masculinization of sex, 137–39, 162
masochistic desire, 34, 78, 125, 191–92. *See also* parasexuality, submission, and BDSM
Masters, William, 38–45, 73, 96, 116
masturbation, 127–29
McClelland, Sara, 108n1
McRuer, Robert, 19, 102, 144, 232–233
McWhorter, Ladelle, 12
medicalization: alternative wellness and neoliberal self-medicalization, 178–79; Big Pharma and anti-pharmaceuticalization, 66, 93–94, 116–17; feminists against, 52–53, 116; history of, 18–19; pathologizing-healing dialectic, 137–39. *See also* pharmaceuticals
men and women, construction of differences between. *See* sexual difference

Men Are from Mars, Women Are from Venus (Gray), 62n12
"men only want one thing" logic, 161–64
Meston, Cindy, 54–57, 83
"me" time, 127–29
#MeToo movement, 231–32
Miller, Jean Baker, 112, 115
mind/body disjuncture. *See* concordance and discordance; plethysmography and mind/body disjuncture
mindfulness: about, 6; BDSM and, 187, 207, 210–11, 219; Brotto's story of "Gianna," 230; bypassing and, 48–49; circular sexual response cycle and, 117; desensitization and, 43; new technologies, control, and, 231; sensate focus technique and, 44; therapeutic history of, 95–100
mindfulness-based sex therapy (MBST): about, 96–100; as bridge between traditional and alternative medicine, 209n8; carework and, 173; critiques of, 98–100, 104–5, 124; with men, 103n19; mind/body gap and, 81; trauma and, 122
mindfulness-based stress reduction (MBSR), 95–96
Moir, Jan, 192
Mollow, Anna, 19, 144, 233
Murphy, Michelle, 115
Murray, Sarah H., 87n14

National Health and Social Life Survey (NHSLS), 15
Natural History of Rape, A (Thornhill and Palmer), 58
nature/nurture binary, gendered, 130–31
neurocognitive emotion research, 70n4
neuro-drugs, 92–95
neurohormonal hypothesis, 77
neurological intimacies, 33
neuroscientific imaging techniques, 81–82
Newman, Andy, 74
new science of female sexuality, 1–5, 8, 76–77, 229–32
New Sex Therapy, The (Kaplan), 45–51
New View Campaign, 5n8, 67, 93, 116–17
nonbinary people, 8–9, 88, 123, 179, 185n1, 207, 229, 231–33
"non-sexual motivations interact with stimulus prepotency" hypothesis, 77

obviousness of body parts and functions, 135–37
Oedipus complex, 34–35, 48
Ogas, Ogi, 78, 190–91
Ogden, Gina, 51n8, 115
one-sex model, 33n2
orgasm: Basson on, 68; Brody on, 58; clitoral, 40, 41, 46, 58, 132; faking it and affective performances of pleasure, 169–74; Heiman, Lo Piccolo, and Lo Piccolo's *Becoming Orgasmic*, 114–15; in HSRC, 39–40; interview participants on, 124, 128–29, 132, 135, 145, 160, 169; Jagose on, 102, 172n3, 230; male, emphasis on, 91, 131; Masters & Johnson on, 39–41, 46; multiple, 41; "pre-orgasmic" women, 114–15; SSRIs and anorgasmia, 145; vaginal, 41, 46, 102
orgasmic reconditioning and conversion therapy, 3, 75, 102, 230
oxytocin, 37

painful sex: body shutting down, 145–46; carework and, 149–50, 170–71, 176–78; critiques of programs for, 124, 128; dyspareunia, 146, 150; genito-pelvic pain/penetration disorder (GPPPD), 43; low desire and, 146–47; penetrative norms and, 131; trauma and, 211, 226; treatments for, 22, 43, 95, 98; vulvodynia, 10, 43, 91, 143, 146, 150, 171
Palmer, Craig T., 58
parasexuality, submission, and BDSM: agency and, 187–88; catharsis, 203–4; definition of parasexuality, 187; discordance linked to submission, 190–91; feminism and, 192–95, 219; nonconsensual, 198; overview, 184–87; performing femininity, camp, and switching, 211–14; popular depictions, 188–93; queerness and rejection of heteronormative scripts, 214–17; reclaiming receptivity and subverting submission, 217–20; sexual power relations, social debates about, 193–95; taboo, trauma, and trust, 195–206; tempo, labor, and presence, 206–11
passivity: active, 125–26; Freud on, 29, 34–36; racialized sexual difference and, 11. *See also* receptivity; responsiveness
pathologizing-healing dialectic, 137–39
Patsavas, Alyson, 227n2
pelvic size in racist frameworks, 12–13
penetrative sex as only "real" sex, 131–33
penile plethysmography, 73
penile strain gauge, 75
penis envy, 35
performance of pleasure, affective, 169–74
performativity, 170, 174, 212
phallometry, 73, 75
pharmaceuticals: Big Pharma and anti-pharmaceuticalization, 66, 93–94, 116–17; neuro-drugs, 92–95
phenomenological experience: discordance and, 142; embodied experience of trauma, 144–47; of gendered body, 135–37
photoplethysmography, 73
physiological-psychological binary, 226
Pitts-Taylor, Victoria, 194–95
pleasure: affective performances of, 169–74; Kaplan on, 46, 47; performing femininity, camp, and switching, 211–14; queerness and rejection of heteronormative scripts, 214–17; tempo, labor, and presence, 206–11
plethysmography and mind/body disjuncture: about, 3–4, 73; assessment of sexual orientation with, 75; category-specificity and, 73–75; concerns and issues, 77–81; mind/body disjuncture and, 73–82; work of the gap, 3–4, 189–90. *See also* concordance and discordance
pornography, 79, 111, 172
post-traumatic stress disorder (PTSD), 99, 145
Preciado, Paul B., 10, 155
preference for responsive desire, 88, 120–21
preparation hypothesis, 31, 77, 143, 143n10, 189, 190n2
presence (being in the present), 209–11, 230
pronouns, 9
Przybylo, Ela, 89
psychoanalysis: affinities of later approaches with, 37–39; Freud's theory of female psychosexual development, 34–39; history of, 29–30; Kaplan and, 47–48; misogyny associated with, 31–32; post-Freud accounts of desire, dismissal of, 104; utility of, 32–33
psychological-physiological binary, 226

psychology of women subdiscipline, 110
psychosexual development, female (Freud), 34–37
psychosomatic approach, 43n6, 45, 50–52, 147
Puar, Jasbir, 20, 27, 102n18, 150, 179
push-pull framework, 70, 71

"quality over quantity," 30
queer excess, 229–30
queer failure, potential of, 183
queerness and rejection of heteronormative scripts, 214–17

race and racialization: carework and, 149, 152, 159, 163–64; expectation and silencing, 125; feminism and, 111; FSIAD and, 102–3; pelvic size and, 12–13; sexual difference and, 11–14; sexual violence and, 197; whiteness, 11–14, 19, 26–27, 109–10, 111
rape, 30, 58. *See also* trauma and gendered violence
rationalistic approach, 45–48, 52
receptivity: affective labor and, 175; as agentic, 187–88; boundaries of feminized body and, 227; evolutionary psychology and, 58–59; "expert" discourses, effects of, 10–11; feminism and, 117; FSIAD and, 86, 89–90; Kleinplatz on mediocre sex and, 89–90; men's lack of, 88; sexual optimization and, 182; sleeping beauty model of, 89; socialization and, 124–26; as submission, 103, 218. *See also* feminized responsive desire framework
regulatory control, 101–5
"remote" causes of sexual dysfunction, 45, 47–49
responsiveness: as agentic, 187–88; all human desire as responsive, 69; evolutionary psychology and, 58–59; feminism and, 117; FSIAD vs. MHSDD and, 87–88; history of sexology and, 5; Kaplan on, 46–47; MBST and, 98–99; in men, 87n14; normalization of, 72, 83, 89; socialization and, 125–26. *See also* specific models
Rich, Adrienne, 110–11
Rieger, Gerulf, 74
right to have sex, 52
Roiphe, Katie, 191–92

Rubin, Gayle, 110
Ruído, María, 157

Schuller, Kyla, 11
seduction theory of Freud, 34
selective serotonin reuptake inhibitors (SSRIs), 145
self-management, sexual, 100–106
self-optimization, 101–2, 150, 151, 182
Seltzer, Leon, 189–90
sensate focus technique, 43–44, 96–97
servicing, sexual, 90
Seto, Michael, 75
Sex, Explained (Netflix), 224n1
sex abuse. *See* trauma
Sex-Starved Marriage, The (Weiner-Davis), 177
sex therapy, field of, 41–42
sex therapy models, history of: continuity of, 31; evolutionary psychology, 30–31, 52–61; Freud and psychoanalysis, 29–30, 34–39; Kaplan and behaviorism, 45–52; Masters and Johnson, 39–45; naturalization of gendered conflict, 61–62; utility of psychoanalysis, 32–33
sexual aversion disorder (SAD), 15
sexual carework. *See* carework and embodied labor
sexual configurations theory (SCT), 113n5
sexual difference: Baumeister's erotic plasticity hypothesis, 59–61, 83; biological determinism, shift toward, 51–52; in evolutionary sexology and Meston & Buss, 52–61; Freud on, 29–30, 35–39; Gray's *Men Are from Mars, Women Are from Venus*, 62n12; incentive motivation model and, 70–71; Kaplan and, 46–47, 49–50; naturalization of, 61–62; neuroimaging and, 82; race, femininity, and whiteness of, 11–14
sexual difference socialization: about, 108–9; biology vs. socialization, 140–41; carework and, 156, 162–63, 174; as "certain kinds of sexual beings," 140; cultural feminism and, 110–18; emotionality and complexity, 133–34; gendered nature/nurture asymmetry and, 130–31; heterosexual intercourse as only "real" sex, 131–33; linkage of desire, interest, and arousal, 118–24; pathologizing-healing dialectic and masculinization of sex,

137–39; receptivity, 124–26; spontaneous desire, masturbation, and fantasy and, 127–30; visibility, "obviousness," and phenomenological experiences of gendered body, 135–37
sexual orientation: bisexuality, 29, 36, 74; "gynephilic," "androphilic," and "ambiphilic" women, 76–78; Kinsey on, 39; plethysmography, assessment with, 75; "reconditioning" of gay men, 3, 75, 102; women as not having, 58, 63–64
"sexual system," 50–51
sex workers, paid, 151n1, 152. *See also* carework and embodied labor
Silverman, Kaja, 225
Sims, J. Marion, 13
Skinner, B. F., 3
sleeping beauty model, 89
Smith, Molly, 152
Snorton, C. Riley, 11, 13
social constructionism: antimedicalization and, 19–20, 52–53; erotic plasticity hypothesis and, 59; evolutionary psychology and, 55; gender and, 27; looking beyond, 17; New View Campaign and, 116
socialization of carework. *See* carework and embodied labor
socialization of sex difference. *See* sexual difference socialization
social reproduction, 153–57, 175, 182
sociobiology, 38, 53–54
Somerville, Siobhan, 12
"sperm competition," 54
Spillers, Hortense, 11–12
spontaneous desire, 14–15, 65, 127–29
state theory of desire, 65n2, 70n4, 71n6, 76n11, 222
submission. *See* parasexuality, submission, and BDSM
Subramaniam, Banu, 113n5
Symons, Donald, 30

taboo, 197
target-specificity. *See* category-specificity
tempo and timing, 206–10
testosterone, 37
Thornhill, Randy, 58
Tiefer, Leonore, 40n4, 67, 116–17, 173

Toates, Frederick, 69
Tolman, Deborah L., 108n1
Tooby, John, 55
Toward a New Psychology of Women (Miller), 112
trans women, 8–9, 74, 122–23, 152, 228, 232–33
trauma and gendered violence: bodyminds and, 109; Brotto on, 122; bypassing, 48–49, 210; carework and, 164, 166; catharsis and, 203–4; desire-interest-arousal linkage and sexual abuse, 120–24; embodied experience of, 144–47; feminized violence, 196n5; fracturing and falling-apartness, 233–34; FSIAD and, 99; generational, 160–61; heteronormativity and, 199; Kaplan on, 50–51; Kleinplatz on, 51n8; ordinariness of, 122–23, 199–200, 226, 232, 234; "overcoming" and expectation of recovery, 228, 233–34; parasexuality and, 197–206; preparation hypothesis, 31, 77, 143, 143n10; PTSD, 99, 145, 227; racialization of, 197; rape, 30, 58; required and erased, 188; silencing and, 200–201; stress vs., 228n3; trans women and, 232–33; "valid," "authentic," and "exceptional" sexual abuse, 196–97; women of color and, 12
trust, 186, 201–6, 201n7
Tyler, Meagan, 89

unconscious, evolutionary, 55

vaginal pulse amplitude (VPA), 73
vaginal zone, Freud on shift to, 35–36
vaginismus, 42
van Anders, Sari, 113n5
Viagra, 92–94, 132, 135
violence, sexual. *See* trauma and gendered violence
visibility of body parts and functions, 136–38
visual stimuli and gender difference, 56
volumetric studies. *See* plethysmography
von Werlhof, Claudia, 154
vulvodynia, 10, 43, 91, 143, 146, 150, 171
Vyleesi (bremelanotide), 93

Weeks, Kathi, 149
Weiner, Linda, 43
Weiner-Davis, Michele, 177

whiteness, 11–14, 19, 26–27, 109–10, 111
"Why Humans Have Sex" (Buss and Meston), 54–55
"Why Sexuality Is Work" (Federici), 154–55
Why Women Have Sex (Buss and Meston), 55–56
Willey, Angie, 113n5
Wilson, Edward O., 53–54
Wilson, Elizabeth A., 33

women and men, construction of differences between. *See* sexual difference
"women" as term, use of, 9–10
work, liberal capitalist and neoliberal biopolitical forms of, 149–53, 178, 182–83. *See also* carework and embodied labor
"Working Women's Fantasies" (Roiphe), 191–92

Zola, Iriving K., 18

ABNORMATIVITIES: QUEER/GENDER/EMBODIMENT
SCOTT HERRING, SERIES EDITOR

This series explores the embodiment of gender identity and queerness within national and global frameworks of deviance that challenge hetero- and homonormative constructions of the body. The scope of the series is global and transnational, its time frame broad, and its focus interdisciplinary—from literary and cultural studies to history and anthropology and beyond.

Diagnosing Desire: Biopolitics and Femininity into the Twenty-First Century
  ALYSON K. SPURGAS

Asexual Erotics: Intimate Readings of Compulsory Sexuality
  ELA PRZYBYLO

Prevention: Gender, Sexuality, HIV, and the Media in Côte d'Ivoire
  CHRISTINE CYNN

www.ingramcontent.com/pod-product-compliance
Lightning Source LLC
Jackson TN
JSHW020314120426
100741JS00003B/19